INTERNATIONAL PERSPECTIVES IN PHYSICAL THERAPY 6

Ergonomics
The Physiotherapist in the Workplace

Edited by

Margaret I. Bullock BScApp PhD
Professor of Physiotherapy, University of Queensland,
Queensland, Australia

CHURCHILL LIVINGSTONE
EDINBURGH LONDON MELBOURNE AND NEW YORK 1990

CHURCHILL LIVINGSTONE
Medical Division of Longman Group UK Limited

Distributed in the United States of America by
Churchill Livingstone Inc., 650 Avenue of the Americas,
New York, N.Y. 10011, and by associated companies, branches
and representatives throughout the world.

First published 1990
  Reprinted 1992 (twice)

ISBN 0-443-03612-8

ISSN 0267-0380

British Library Cataloguing in Publication Data
Ergonomics: the physiotherapist in the workplace.
  1. Ergonomics. Role of Physiotherapists
  I. Bullock, Margaret I. II. Series
  620.8′2

Library of Congress Cataloging in Publication Data
Ergonomics: the physiotherapist in the workplace/edited by Margaret
  I. Bullock.
    p. cm. —(International perspectives in physical therapy,
ISSN 0267-0380; 6)
  Includes bibliographical references.
  ISBN 0–443–03612–8 (pbk.)
    1. Industrial hygiene. 2. Physical therapy. 3. Human engineering.
4. Occupational diseases—Prevention. I. Bullock, Margaret I. II. Series.
    [DNLM: 1. Accidents, Occupational — prevention & control. 2. Human
Engineering. 3. Physical Therapy. W1 IN827JM v. 6/WA 485 E67]
RC967.E68 1990
613.6′2–dc20
DNLM/DLC
for Library of Congress   89–24019

The
publisher's
policy is to use
**paper manufactured
from sustainable forests**

Produced by Longman Publishers Singapore (Pte) Ltd
Printed in Singapore

About the Series

The purpose of this series of books is to provide an international exchange of ideas and to explore different approaches in professional therapy practice. The books are written primarily for experienced clinicians. They are not intended as basic texts nor as reports on the most recent research, though elements of these aspects may be included.

Articles written by experts from a number of different countries form the core of each volume. These are supported by a commentary on the current 'state of the art' in the particular area of practice and an annotated bibliography of key references.

Each volume covers a topic which we believe to be of universal interest. Some are concerned with a troublesome symptom (for example Volume I on Pain edited by T. Hoskins Michel); others are related to problems and practice within a broad diagnostic category.

I. B.
N. T. W.

Preface

The value of applying ergonomic principles to work practices is well recognized and useful texts, offering a general overview of ergonomics or specific guidelines to the practitioner, are available. However, the science of ergonomics is so broad and the disciplines which contribute to its body of knowledge so varied, that books relating to ergonomics do not always meet the special interests of individual professionals.

Physiotherapists have been involved in the prevention of injury for many years, and in some countries their contribution to the implementation of ergonomic principles has been considerable. A need was perceived to publish a book which would outline principles of ergonomic practice in areas of special interest to physiotherapists as well as to illustrate the contribution which physiotherapists can make to the growth of knowledge in this field. This volume is intended to achieve that purpose.

The physiotherapist's role in the workplace is broad and includes such responsibilities as job analysis, work posture monitoring, measurement, design, education and rehabilitation. While focusing upon prevention of physical injury, the physiotherapist's concern extends to a consideration of psychological, social and environmental factors which may influence the quality of performance of an activity. The chapters of this book address these various aspects. In addition, the results of specific research studies provide guidance for design and practice.

Chapter 1 outlines the broad scope of the physiotherapist's contribution to ergonomics and lays the basis for the development of specific topics in succeeding chapters.

Chapter 2 dwells upon the development of optimum worker–task relationships and describes the types of measurements necessary for their definition. Illustrations within this chapter relate to research studies specifically concerned with measurements of body movements, body size, space requirements and force application, and they demonstrate the importance of gathering essential basic data for design.

Chapter 3 introduces the concept of postural work-load and describes the nature of various approaches to ergonomic job analysis. Methods of recording and analysing the work-site, work space, work methods, work postures and environmental load are outlined. The importance of facilitating the worker's self-analysis of workload and of monitoring the effects of load on the workers is emphasized.

The physiotherapist's role within industry has changed character over the years to take account of modified work practices and new technological demands. Chapter 4 illustrates this process of development through reference to the varied tasks carried out by physiotherapists in a large industry.

One of the major problems which has faced ergonomists in recent years has been the growing number of musculoskeletal complaints in workers engaged in repetitive work in fixed postures. Chapters 5, 6, and 7 address this issue. Chapter 5 offers an historic account of the development of the problem and describes different approaches for effecting a solution. The importance of epidemiological data in the development of a preventive approach is emphasized. The specific problem of pain emanating from neck and shoulder load is discussed in Chapter 6. Descriptions of factors influencing the loads and measures which might contribute to their reduction provide useful guidelines for the practitioner.

Workplace design is one of the most important methods of preventing the development of musculoskeletal disorders. In Chapter 7, the different approaches to ergonomic design are illustrated by reference to case studies carried out in a variety of occupational settings.

While the increase in the incidence of problems emanating from constrained postures during repetitive work has attracted the special attention of ergonomists, the continued incidence of back problems in many areas of work has maintained the need for research and development in methods of preventing back injury. Chapter 8 focuses upon one major cause of back pain—lifting—and offers a comprehensive overview of the nature, muscular activity and energy cost of lifting. The use of biomechanical, metabolic and psychophysical modelling to reduce hazards by predicting demands on the human body is also discussed.

While the importance of worker participation in the application of ergonomic principles to the workplace has been stressed by all authors, the particular challenge that this approach presents to professionals in ergonomics is addressed in Chapter 9.

The practice of ergonomics is meant to be applied to both the abled bodied and disabled. The latter group demands special attention from physiotherapists and two chapters focus on aspects of assessing a disabled worker's functional capacity and ensuring that work demands are matched to assessed abilities. Chapter 10 describes the development of the Activity Matching Ability System, which provides a means by which the appropriate level of demand in a job is matched to the specific limitations of the worker. Chapter 11 offers details of the philosophies and principles in assessment of the functional capacity of the worker and describes the ways by which the results of that assessment may be used for return-to-work statements, job or job-site modifications, the development of a work-hardening programme and resolution of a worker's compensation case.

While not intended to be a comprehensive text on ergonomics, this volume does provide background information, guidelines to practice and research results which should prove valuable to physiotherapists and others concerned for the welfare of people in the workplace.

I am grateful to Professor Nancy Watts and Miss Ida Bromley, the Churchill Livingstone Series Editors for International Perspective in Physical Therapy, for their constructive support during the preparation of this volume and to the authors for their cooperation and their contributions. I am also especially grateful to Miss Heather Buchanan for her patience, perserverance and perception during its production.

I hope that this book will not only provide some guidance to physiotherapists and others concerned with the prevention of injury in the workplace, but will also inspire some to undertake their own evaluative studies in the field of ergonomics.

Queensland, 1990   M. I. B.

Contributors

Marianne Gerner Björkstén MPT MMedSc

Marianne Gerner Björkstén qualified as a physiotherapist from Lund University, Sweden, and later completed a course in Industrial Health and Ergonomics for Physiotherapists. Her postgraduate studies included a Master's programme in Physiotherapy at the University of Minnesota, Minneapolis, USA, 1975–76 and a Master of Medical Science at the University of Uppsala, Sweden, 1987. The thesis for that degree was titled 'Ergonomic studies of Physical Workload' and comprised studies of muscular endurance and ergonomic and epidemiological investigations of railway engine drivers and medical secretaries.

Mrs Björkstén has worked within the Swedish National Board of Occupational Health and Safety as well as in two country Departments of Occupational Health and Safety. She is currently an ergonomist at the Department of Occupational Medicine, University Hospital, Uppsala, Sweden.

Margaret I. Bullock BScApp PhD

Professor Margaret Bullock graduated from the University of Queensland, Brisbane, Australia with a BScApp (Phty & Occ Thpy). She worked as a clinician in Australia and Boston, USA and as a university lecturer in physiotherapy for many years. Since 1967, Professor Bullock has been actively involved in pursuing or supervising ergonomics research and in teaching the subject to physiotherapy students at undergraduate and postgraduate levels. Her PhD, completed in 1973, focused upon an ergonomics topic, 'The determination of pedal alignments for the production of minimal spinal movements using a stereophotogrammetric method of measurement'. The Foundation Professor of Physiotherapy at the University of Queensland and the Head of the Department of Physiotherapy for 14 years (1974–1989), she has contributed significantly to both the physiotherapy profession and the discipline of ergonomics in Australia. Professor Bullock has published extensively on ergonomics and other professional topics and has delivered papers at many National and International conferences. She is currently the President of the Academic Board at the University of Queensland and the President of the Ergonomics Society of Australia.

Karin Harms-Ringdahl RPT DrMedSc

Dr Karin Harms-Ringdahl is an Associate Professor in Physiotherapy at the Department of Physical Medicine and Rehabilitation, Karolinska Hospital, Stockholm, Sweden. She is a senior lecturer in the postgraduate pre-research programme in physiotherapy and she is active in the kinesiology research group in the Karolinska Institute, focusing particularly upon research in occupational biomechanics, exercise biomechanics and assessments of load-elicited pain. Dr Harms-Ringdahl is the author of many scientific articles.

Susan J. Isernhagen BSc PT

Susan Isernhagen is a consultant and educator in functional capacities evaluation, work hardening and occupational medicine, and specializes in work injury management programmes.

Her past work includes development of the copyrighted Functional Capacity Assessment at Polinsky Medical Rehabilitation Center, Duluth, Minnesota and a multidisciplinary work injury programme at the same facility. Susan Isernhagen's professional experience includes work in private practice, hospitals, rehabilitation centres and nursing homes. She has also been a faculty member of a physical therapy school and a physical therapist assistant school.

Papers and seminars on functional capacity evaluation and work hardening have been given throughout the United States and in Australia, as well as at the World Confederation of Physical Therapy in 1987.

Mrs Isernhagen has edited a book *Work Injury—Management and Prevention* published by Aspen Publishers, Rockville Md in 1988 and other work includes a postgraduate lesson for physical therapists on 'Work Hardening and Ergonomics', published by Forum Medicum NY in 1988.

Lena Karlqvist BPT

Initially a physical education teacher at Stockholm University, Sweden, Lena Karlqvist qualified as a physical therapist from Lund University, Sweden. She has attended many courses relevant to ergonomics, including programmes in research and measurement in exercise physiology, Boston University, USA; occupational biomechanics; vision physiology; and industrial health and ergonomy for physical therapists.

After practising clinically, Lena Karlqvist worked at an Occupational Rehabilitation Centre which included ergonomics, and later was employed as an ergonomist in the Occupational Health Service in the Stockholm County Council. She then worked at the National Swedish Board of Industrial Safety until joining a small consulting firm—3 ERGONOMER—in 1980. Lena Karlqvist is currently working as an ergonomist in the Department of Occupational Medicine, Karolinska hospital, Stockholm, Sweden.

Shrawan Kumar BSc MSc PhD

Professor Shrawan Kumar gained his BSc in Biology and Chemistry and his MSc in Zoology in India, and his PhD in Human Biology (Ergonomics) from the University of Surrey, UK. After a series of science-orientated appointments, Professor Kumar was appointed in 1977 to the Department of Physical Therapy, Faculty of Rehabilitation Medicine, University of Alberta, Canada, where he became a full Professor in 1982. Professor Kumar has written over 60 scientific publications, including many chapters in several books, has been Conference Chairperson at Physiotherapy and Ergonomics Conferences and has contributed significantly to both the physiotherapy and the ergonomics fields in Canada.

Tuulikki Luopajärvi RSpPT BSc MSc

Tuulikki Luopajärvi qualified as a physiotherapist in Helsinki and later gained specialized qualifications in Public Health. She also holds a BSc and an MSc in

Health Care Administration. Following a period of clinical practice, Mrs Luopajärvi was appointed Chief Occupational Physiotherapist at the Institute of Occupational Health in Helsinki in 1976 and Associate Professor of Physiotherapy at the University of Jyvaskyla 1985–1987. Mrs Luopajärvi is a council member of the Nordic Ergonomics Society and the International Ergonomics Society and has served on important committees concerned with ergonomics and prevention. Mrs Luopajarvi has published widely, her earlier works focusing on physiotherapy treatments for patients with back disorders, but later works focusing on the prevention and causes of work-related musculoskeletal disorders.

Ian L. McClelland CDipTech MSc

Ian McClelland graduated from Middlesex Polytechnic with a CDipTech in Mechanical Engineering and later gained an MSc in Ergonomics from Loughborough University. While working as a Project Officer and Project Manager with the Institute for Consumer Ergonomics, Loughborough University, he undertook research and consultancy work for a wide range of clients within industry, commerce and government. In 1986, Mr McClelland joined the Philips Company in the Netherlands as the Manager of the Applied Ergonomics Group at Corporate Industrial Design. His special interests are the integration of usability principles into the user interface for end-user products, user instructions and product evaluation methods.

Barbara McPhee DipPhty MPH(Syd) MAPA MCPA

Barbara McPhee was educated as a physiotherapist in Sydney, Australia, graduating in 1969. After working in Sydney, England and Canada she entered the fields of ergonomics and occupational health in 1975 when she joined the Occupational Health Section of the School of Public Health and Tropical Medicine at the University of Sydney. During the 10 years until 1985 she undertook a wide range of teaching and consultancy work, mostly in the field of occupational ergonomics.

In 1977, she was granted an NH&MRC Travelling Fellowship to study the scope, teaching, organization and practice of occupational physiotherapy and its role in occupational health research in North America and Europe.

In 1983, she commenced a research project on work-related symptoms in keyboard and clerical workers, in which work and personal factors were examined in relation to musculoskeletal and other complaints. In 1989, she was awarded the Master of Public Health (Occupational Health) degree from a thesis based on this research.

Barbara McPhee has been involved in a number of professional activities in Australia and internationally. In 1988, she was Scientific Convener of the International Ergonomics Association Congress held in Sydney, and she is currently National Chairman of the Special Interest Group in Ergonomics and Occupational Health of the Australian Physiotherapy Association and Chairman of the NSW Branch of the Ergonomics Society of Australia.

Elizabeth Melin PT PGDipOH

After her graduation as a physiotherapist, Elizabeth Melin worked as a clinical physiotherapist in the orthopaedic field. This encouraged her to further development resulting in a work tour in France and the United States with rehabilitation as the point of focus.

In 1965, Mrs Melin commenced work in the Physiotherapy Department of the Ericsson Company. It was at this time that a patient work-station related activity developed. Initially, working alone and almost entirely with patient treatment, this unit has developed the physiotherapy contribution within the company so that today there are physiotherapists in 30 different Ericsson locations in the world, whose main task is to develop ergonomics. These colleagues meet once a year to develop a consistent medical policy as well as an ergonomic approach. Elizabeth Melin assumes the responsibility for all ergonomic decisions taken within the Ericsson Company.

Mrs Melin lectures to the graduating physiotherapists at the Karolinska Institute in Stockholm. In addition, she shares responsibility for the further education of physiotherapists in the occupational health course offered by the Swedish Employers Association. Mrs Melin has been involved in various research projects where the overall aim has been to seek answers to the relationship between work and injuries in the musculoskeletal system. Some of these projects have been published or reported at conferences.

Robert Rustad MNFF MPH

Mr Robert Rustad gained his physiotherapy qualifications from Statens Fysioterapihogskole in Oslo, Norway and a Masters degree in Public Health at the Nordic School of Public Health in Gothenburg, Sweden in 1988. Mr Rustad initially practised as a physiotherapist at Sunnaas Hospital, Oslo in the field of rehabilitation, later practising as an industrial physiotherapist in Oslo. Subsequently, he worked as a physiotherapist and ergonomics advisor to the Norwegian Labour Inspections Department in Oslo.

Besides being a physiotherapist, Robert Rustad is also educated in pedagogics and preventive health care, environmental health work and ergonomics. He has written several articles on the organization and work of the occupational health services in Norway. Robert Rustad was elected as vice-president of the Norwegian Physical Therapy Association in November, 1987.

Kristina Schüldt MD PhD

Dr Kristina Schüldt is a physician at the Department of Physical Medicine and Rehabilitation, Karolinska Hospital, Stockholm, Sweden and she has specialized in rehabilitation medicine and rheumatology. Active in the Kinesiology Research Group, Karolinska Institute, her research work has concentrated upon areas concerned with occupational biomechanics, exercise biomechanics and technical aids. Dr Schüldt is a lecturer in the Karolinska Physical Therapy programs—both at an undergraduate level and in the postgraduate physiotherapeutic programme in vocational rehabilitation.

Hilary J. Watson BSc PhD

Dr Hilary Watson qualified as a physiotherapist following education at St Mary's Hospital in London. She worked in the National Health Service in the UK and private practice in France before studying for a BSc (Combined Honours) in Ergonomics and Sociology at the University of Aston in Birmingham, UK. Dr Watson joined the Institute for Consumer Ergonomics, University of Loughborough in 1982 as a Research Associate with a special interest in functional assessment, and was appointed to work on projects funded by a number of sponsors including the European Coal and Steel Community in conjunction with the British Steel Corporation. In 1984, she joined the

Rehabilitation Studies Unit at the University of Edinburgh as a Research Officer where she incorporated the functional assessment techniques described in this chapter in the study of lower limb fracture. This research, funded by the Association of British Insurers, formed the basis of her thesis for a PhD which was awarded in July, 1988.

Susan Whalley BSc PhD

Dr Susan Whalley graduated from Aston University with a BSc in Combined Honours in Ergonomics and Education. She joined the Institute for Consumer Ergonomics specifically to work on the ECSC project at British Steel, that work leading to the development of AMAS. This was followed by a short period working with ICE's accident research unit prior to undertaking a PhD. The thesis topic was 'Factors affecting human reliability within the chemical process industries'. From this research a computerized technique for identifying the causes of human error has been produced: PHECA, the Potential Human Error Cause Analysis technique. Since 1986, Dr Whalley has been working within the Loss Prevention industry as a consultant providing human factors and reliability advice to the chemical and nuclear industries. She is currently employed by RM Consultants Ltd to set up and manage a human factors and reliability unit to provide advice and undertake research for the process industries.

Contents

SECTION ONE

1. Introduction. Ergonomics—a broad challenge for the physiotherapist

M. I. Bullock

Designers of equipment, of products which people use and of environments within which people work have responsibilities which have a direct bearing on work performance and human welfare. These responsibilities, emphasized by McCormick as early as 1957, are embodied in the study and application of Ergonomics. LeGros Clark (1954), in his discussion on the 'Anatomy of Work', pointed out that if a man is to operate a machine with maximum efficiency and minimum fatigue, it is important to ensure that the design and location of instruments, apparatus, hand and foot controls and seating take into account the natural positions and movements of the human body. At a later date, Hodsdon (1967) asserted that while the improvements which must be introduced in order to fit the machine to the worker are reasonably easily ascertained, the changes which must be made 'on the human side' are much less obvious, although they may be more important.

During the last few decades, major changes have taken place in industry. Mechanization, automation and the introduction of intensive safety campaigns have produced a safer working environment. Nevertheless, although the likelihood of a major accident is low, the chances of occurrence of other 'minor' injuries are high. Work procedures have been designed to increase productivity through streamlining the process and economizing on effort, but in many instances, the constant use of the same muscle groups through repetitive performance of one task, or the demands for constant attention and perception while a worker receives and processes information continuously, have been increased. The need for a reduction in these physical and psychological stresses has been recognized and the techniques for combating them are found in the science of ergonomics.

The scope of ergonomics is broad and its practice embraces several major topics. For example, it is concerned with the particular characteristics of the person, both physical (including body size, physical ability, working posture) and psychological (e.g. learning ability, reacting to directions and decision-making). Ergonomics relates to a person's relationship to the workplace and his effectiveness while working within it, his reaction to work-load and stress, his level of endurance and the rate at which he becomes fatigued. Safety factors and the likely incidence of accidents are also points of concern. Man–machine–task relationships are an important consideration within ergonomics and encompass reference to physical use of controls or equipment within the work arrangement or visibility and interpretation of displays. Since all activity takes place within an environment, ergonomics is concerned also with environmental conditions including lighting, noise, temperature control and ventilation.

In analysing the physical aspects of a work situation, it is interesting to note the extent to which the performance of activity is dictated by the limitations and design of tools and equipment and by the nature of the workplace. A poorly designed workplace and clumsy tools could lead to and perpetuate inadequate work methods and prevent their improvement. On the other hand, properly designed workplaces and tools not only allow the worker the opportunity of applying the principles of good working techniques if he so wishes. but they also prevent that misuse of the body which is a direct result of poor design.

Of the many factors which contribute individually or collectively to the production of detrimental effects on the human body, those which are particularly relevant to the physical aspects of work include the use of space and spatial relationships, the demands of static posture, the neglect of the principles of good dynamic posture and the physical demands placed on the operator by required movements.

Ergonomics is often called a multidisciplinary activity, because many branches of learning, co-operatively and separately, contribute to the body of knowledge of this discipline. Engineers, psychologists, medical practitioners, physiotherapists, architects and others contribute their individual knowledge of anatomy, biomechanics, physiology, psychology, engineering principles, anthropometry and kinesiology to solve work-stress problems whether at home, school or place of employment. Physiotherapists fit into this study of the man–machine–task relationship because of their special ability to analyse body movements in detail and evaluate postural abuse during dynamic situations. Thus the physiotherapist can help to eliminate misuse of the body and assist in the design of equipment and work areas so that the situations so arranged are better suited to the physical well-being of the person using them.

It is many years since it was realized that physiotherapists had more to contribute to total health care than the rehabilitation of the disabled. The concept that physiotherapists could also play a significant part in a programme of prevention was acknowledged in some countries as early as the 1920s. But it was the Second World War and the subsequent changes in industry and technology which provided the impetus for the growth of ergonomics as a science and the greater use of physiotherapists in prevention programmes.

The physiotherapist has a large part to play in the modern industrial scene and contributes to the control of injury and production loss in many ways. The physiotherapist's role falls broadly into the three categories of injury prevention, therapeutic activities and rehabilitation, and research. The balance between these major roles for the physiotherapist varies between countries and companies (Bullock 1986). For example, physiotherapists in industry in Scandinavia can spend 50% of their time in the preventative role. In contrast to this many of the physiotherapists working in industry in other countries offer therapeutic and fitness programmes and fewer have the opportunity to offer 'advice on the floor'.

There are many facets to the preventative role of the physiotherapist. They include such responsibilities as job analysis, work posture monitoring, task design, personnel selection and placement, education, supervision of work methods, the influencing of motivation and attitudes, and the provision of activity breaks and physical fitness programmes.

The thorough analysis of the physical aspects of a job is a task of considerable magnitude. It includes surveys of the nature of the task, the work layout and the work environment. But it also involves a comprehensive evaluation of the worker's method of performing the task. Job analysis should be approached from two angles. The first is the analysis of the work-site and the second is the analysis of the physical and mental demands on the worker. In considering physical aspects, job analysis involves a detailed quantitative study of work postures and this can be done in several ways. This volume provides a background to job analysis and work task monitoring and provides some interesting examples of studies carried out within industry where different systems have been used.

Both simple and more complex methods of job analysis are available and some physiotherapists prefer the simpler and quicker methods. However, all physiotherapists acknowledge that where industrial managers need to be convinced that a problem exists and that a solution needs to be implemented, objective facts and figures such as those produced by more complex methods of job analysis are essential.

Ergonomists are involved in assessing the workplace for many reasons. For example, the workplace itself, the work process undertaken within it, the equipment used in the process or the surrounding environment which influences task performance may each need assessment to determine those features which need modification to ensure the safety and comfort of the worker (Murrell 1965, Singleton et al 1967, Kvålseth 1983, Corlett 1988). Redesign for the purpose of injury prevention is an important purpose of work-site assessment. On the other hand, if a worker has already sustained an injury, workplace assessment can reveal the cause of the problem. Not only might this provide the evidence for compensation payments, but it can also establish the basis for modifications necessary to allow re-placement of the handicapped worker. The design or redesign of a workplace can properly proceed once the deficiencies of the job have been highlighted by survey and analysis. But the introduction of new designs or modifications needs acceptance by those who are to work with them.

Indeed, as a multidisciplinary science, the development of ergonomic solutions demands co-operative consideration by an appropriate team. In addition, communication with those who are to adopt the new proposals is fundamental to the application of ergonomic solutions to the workplace. Such communication recognizes that the worker has a first-hand knowledge of the task and the workplace. In Sweden and Finland, where the team approach is well exemplified, it is necessary to have 'labour safety and environment committees', where employee representatives and union delegates meet with the professionals. This arrangement acknowledges that without the worker's co-operation, few changes could be implemented successfully. Unless the worker perceives the appropriateness of a possible solution during discussion, its incorporation into the workplace is likely to be ignored subsequently. One chapter in this volume focuses specifically on this fact. Some of the work studies included in this volume demonstrate and emphasize the collaboration of physiotherapy ergonomists with those involved in the work process.

Because the effectiveness of any man–machine–system depends upon the integration of the biological characteristics of the operator with the mechanical design of the equipment and working areas, there are some who believe that the routine examination of new personnel can provide useful information for their placement. It has been suggested that an evaluation of the physical, psychological and functional capacities of the employee ensures his proper placement in the work situation based on job analysis. During the past few years, the concept of pre-employment screening has attracted interest. In some countries a form of screening is undertaken, particularly with the identification of factors of skin, respiratory or back problems which would preclude the placement of the employee in certain occupations. However, in other countries, the workers' unions do not permit either pre-employment screening or a probationary period for the employee.

One of the most important roles of the physiotherapist in industry is in the education of various categories of people (Bullock 1988). Ergonomic education programmes aim to provide sufficient relevant information to help in the implementation of measures to prevent physical, psychological or emotional injury or stress. When first introduced, the emphasis of educational programmes tended to be upon the teaching of lifting and handling techniques to workers, reflecting the high proportion of injuries which originated from this type of work. However, appreciation of the many causes of musculoskeletal injuries associated with repetitive tasks has emphasized the need to offer educational programmes more broadly (for example to managers, supervisors and workers), so that each group can appreciate their own role in the prevention of injury or stress. Courses can be offered to the new employee, the worker in general, workers in specific areas, workers suffering chronic back pain, employees in special circumstances (e.g. the ageing, disabled), safety officers, foremen and managers. The physiotherapist involved must direct the course work according to the special needs of each group. Reference to educational programmes used within industry by physiotherapists is made within this volume.

Supervision of work practices and consultation with employees is an important role for the physiotherapist in industry. The physiotherapist's regular assessment of the capacities of all employees and the inspection and supervision of working methods allows opportunity for correction of operating difficulties or undesirable postures and for reinforcement of good work methods. It also allows investigation of possible causes of frequently occurring injuries and these could reveal the need to re-design either the task itself or the relationship of the worker to it. The presence of the physiotherapist on the job site encourages consultation by employees uncertain of their posture or work methods, so allowing correction before the development of a soft tissue lesion or injury. Descriptions of the physiotherapist's activity within industry in this volume highlight the importance of this aspect of the physiotherapist's role.

The increase in the number of repetitive tasks requiring a static posture during their performance and the effect of industrial noise or tension have led to the physiotherapist's promotion of brief exercise periods during the working day. These take various forms, including 'pause gymnastics', 'mini pauses' or job rotation. The brief exercise periods are designed by the physiotherapist to provide physical activity not included in the working process, to encourage relaxation either generally or of specific muscle groups and to promote health and physical fitness.

The two areas of the body reported as having the highest incidence of complaint in industry are the back and the neck (Ferguson & Duncan 1976, Hagberg 1984, Itani et al 1983, Kilbom et al 1986, Rowe 1969, Ryan et al 1987, Wallace & Buckle 1987). The challenge to the physiotherapist of assessing work areas producing these injuries is described within this volume. Reference is also made to use of different approaches to back care in industry and their evaluation.

The second major area for the physiotherapist in industry is in therapeutic activities. It has been shown that intensive physiotherapy applied in the acute phases of occupational illness or injuries is desirable for rehabilitation and limits the total period of treatment. The adequate provision of physiotherapy within industry means that the treatment is available immediately, can be given as frequently as necessary and may be scheduled at times most convenient to the employee work programme.

For the physiotherapist in industry, physical rehabilitation is not limited to the acute condition. Not only should physiotherapists continue treatment until patents are restored to the highest functional level, but they should reassess their changed capacities and abilities to cope with job demands. With experience in handling handicapped workers, the physiotherapist is well aware that capacities and skills may be re-established through rehabilitation and that, in fact, some permanent disabilities are no handicaps to employment

(Isernhagen 1988). The physiotherapist's consideration of the abilities of the seriously disabled worker and of the demands of the various jobs in the factory could suggest modification of a job to fit the employee's changed capacity or guidance into alternative employment. Two chapters within this volume are devoted to this area and are concerned with the assessment of the functional capacities of the worker and with developing and testing assessment techniques to identify jobs suited to the varying abilities of differently disabled workers.

Research is one of the important roles of the physiotherapist in industry and there are several areas for fruitful involvement. Carefully designed surveys of the incidence of fatigue, pain or injury provide evidence for further study. Experimental projects at the work-site allow redesign of problem areas, while laboratory studies provide more extensive data for use in a general population. Each of these approaches to research is essential for the collection of data relevant to ergonomic design. It is gratifying to know that major research projects are being mounted throughout the world which provide data basic to ergonomic design. Reference to some of these are included in this volume.

Whereas the economic advantages which flow from research in ergonomic areas are welcome, such investigations should be undertaken primarily from the point of view of considering workers as human beings and particularly with the aim of preventing injury, discomfort or disability during the performance of activity. Recognition has been given to the fact that ergonomic problems can exist in the work, home, play or school environment and that there is a need to investigate design features in a variety of settings if particular problems have been suspected or identified for men, women or children. In this volume, reference to 'task' and 'work' can be taken to apply generally to performance of activity in any environment.

The preparation of the physiotherapist for work in industry has been approached in varying degrees in different countries throughout the world. In some countries, education in ergonomics is provided at undergraduate level and the contribution of physiotherapists to the ergonomic field is so important that attitudes to prevention and approaches to ergonomic management should surely be encouraged from an early level of physiotherapy education. In a number of countries, such study is also offered for postgraduates, either as part of a formal higher degree or in short specialized courses. For example, in Australia postgraduate qualifications in areas concerned with ergonomics are offered by Schools of Physiotherapy. Also in that country, the skills pertaining to the practice of ergonomics are included in such courses as the Master of Health Administration, the Master of Public Health the Master of Safety Science. The physiotherapist's broad knowledge of anatomy, physiology, biomechanics, psychology and clinical implications of poor working postures, which are the foundations of physiotherapy practice, provide a strong base for such postgraduate study.

In other countries, too, physiotherapists may develop the specialized skills necessary to practise as an ergonomist. For example, the Department of Ergonomics and Cybernetics at the Loughborough University of Technology in the United Kingdom offers both undergraduate and postgraduate programmes in this field, while the University of London is well known for its Master of Science (Ergonomics) course. Many physiotherapists have already taken advantage of furthering their education in one of these institutions.

In Scandinavian countries, specific concentrated short postgraduate courses are offered to physiotherapists planning to work in the ergonomics field, while higher degrees are available to physiotherapists in a number of institutions, including the Karolinska Institute and the Nordic School of Public Health in Gothenberg.

The professional 'continuing education' courses offered by Physiotherapy Associations are also an important avenue for physiotherapists seeking to learn the skills relevant to ergonomics practice. In a number of countries, e.g. Scandinavia, the United Kingdom and Australia, Special Interest Groups for physiotherapists in ergonomics have been developed. These provide a focus for continuing education activities and also serve to promote the contribution of physiotherapists in the ergonomics field.

Many physiotherapists have become active members of Ergonomics Societies (or similar bodies, such as the Human Factors Society). Through such involvement, physiotherapists are exposed to the multidisciplinary nature of ergonomics and can share new ideas and developments with professionals with differing basic backgrounds. Such contact, through scientific meetings and conferences, can only enhance the knowledge of physiotherapists interested in the preventative approach, while introducing other professionals to the particular contribution of the physiotherapist. Collaborative programmes organized jointly by Ergonomics Societies and Physiotherapy Special Interest Groups are also considered to be of great value to participants. Physiotherapists contemplating entering this field would benefit from initial involvement in local Ergonomics Societies and their conferences and in their professional Special Interest Groups, where they exist. Communication with others working in the field is an important aspect of any education process. Lists of National Societies affiliated with the International Ergonomics Association and some of the primary journals in ergonomics are provided in Appendix 1.

In line with developing technology and changing community needs, physiotherapists must explore new possibilities, develop new interests, apply their knowledge and their expertise in broader ways and they must accept the challenge of working in fields other than the traditionally 'clinical'. Prevention is not a new concept in the health field and there are some who have applied the principles of prevention as carefully as they have administered treatment. But this is not a universal approach and there is considerable scope for advancement of the physiotherapist's knowledge in ergonomics, so that more effective use of broad-ranging skills may be applied to problems within the working situation. In presenting descriptions of work and study undertaken by physiotherapists in a variety of settings, to fulfil varied objectives and in countries around the world, this volume demonstrates the capacity of physiotherapists to contribute to this important field in a most significant way.

REFERENCES

Bullock M I 1986 Overseas observations of the physiotherapist in the workplace. Australian Journal of Physiotherapy 32:3: 151–156
Bullock M I 1988 Health education in the workplace. In: Isernhagen S (ed) Work injury—management and prevention. Aspen, Rockville 9–18
Corlett E N 1988 The investigation and evaluation of work and workplaces. Ergonomics 31(5): 727–734
Ferguson D, Duncan J 1976 A trial of physiotherapy for symptoms in keyboard operating. The Australian Journal of Physiotherapy 22: 61–72
Hagberg M 1984 Occupational musculoskeletal stress and disorders of the neck and shoulder: a review of possible pathophysiology. International Archives of Occupational and Environmental Health 53: 269–278
Hodsdon D F 1967 Remarks from a representation of farm workers. Ergonomics problems in agriculture. Meeting at Nottingham University School of Agriculture April 1967
Isernhagen S 1988 (ed) Work injury—management and prevention. Aspen, Rockville
Itani T, Kondo T, Matsubayashi S, Ose Y, Watanabe A, Ohara H Aoyama H 1983 Occupational cervicobrachial disorder and the effect of improved work conditions on prevention. Journal of the Science of Stress and Rest 2: 15–23
Kilbom Å, Persson J, Jonsson B 1986 Disorders of the cervicobrachial region

among female workers in the electronics industry. International Journal of Industrial Ergonomics 1: 37–47

Kvålseth T O 1983 Ergonomics of work-station design. Butterworth, London

LeGros Clark W E 1954 The anatomy of work. In: Floyd W F, Welford A T (eds) Symposium on human factors in equipment design. Lewis, London

McCormick E J 1964 Human factors engineering, 2nd edn. McGraw-Hill, New York

Murrel K F H 1965 Ergonomics. Chapman & Hall, London

Rowe M L 1969 Low back pain in industry. A position paper. Journal of Occupational Medicine 11: 161

Ryan G A, Hage B, Bampton M 1987 Postural factors, work organization and musculo-skeletal symptoms. In : Buckle P (ed) Musculo-skeletal disorders at work. Taylor & Francis, London, pp 251–253

Singleton W T, Easterby R S, Whitfield D 1967 The human operator in complex systems. Chapman & Hall, London

Wallace M, Buckle P 1987 Ergonomic aspects of neck and upper limb disorders. International Reviews of Ergonomics 1: 173–200

2. The development of optimum worker–task relationships

M. I. Bullock

INTRODUCTION

One of the principal contributions which the physiotherapist can make to ergonomics is as a researcher, where major problems affecting the physical well-being of people may be studied and recommendations made as a basis for design or redesign. Physiotherapists' understanding of body motion, their skill in movement analysis and their understanding of the implications for injury provide them with an appropriate background to contribute significantly to research in the physical aspect of ergonomic design.

Research projects which aim to improve the relationship between the person and the machine or the task can include studies which assess and define the problem, which collect basic data or which involve experimentation to find a solution.

Assessment of the nature and magnitude of an ergonomic problem may be achieved in several ways. These might include examination of industrial records or insurance and compensation claims to reveal the incidence of injury or disease, or surveys of people by interview or questionnaires to gauge their opinions of the conditions of work and its effect on their physical well-being. Historical case studies, in which details of factors in the environment or the background contributing to the incidence of a specific injury are ascertained through interview, provide alternate means of assessing the nature of a problem.

Observational studies, including task analysis, in which the researcher analyses the job demands, observes the operator's performance and notes movements and actions which are not consistent with the principles of good working techniques, are important components of some investigations (Corlett & Bishop 1976, Karhu 1977, Corlett et al 1979, Aaras et al 1988). Longitudinal studies, which monitor changes in procedure or developments of specific problems, may also be pursued.

13

More extensive studies may apply techniques for the detailed analysis of movements involved during performance of a task. These usually include some form of photography.

Recommendations for a solution to the identified problem rely on the application of ergonomic principles for design and the use of data which are relevant to the particular task or work area. Physiotherapists may be involved at different stages in the development of suitable recommendations. Through suitable research, they may collect the basic data relating to the physical activity of the work process and provide advice to the designers of equipment for future incorporation into design specifications. For this purpose, they may be closely involved in the development of appropriate experimental techniques. Alternatively, they may construct 'mock ups' based upon known ergonomic design principles in which various designs may be evaluated at the work-site. This approach is particularly relevant where the problem relates to a specific work area, but can be applied with caution to other similar situations. Frequently, important new designs emanate from such studies. The former type of contribution, involving basic data collection for a defined group of the population, can be applied more frequently to design which will be used generally in the activity in question.

Physiotherapists working as ergonomics consultants usually collect data at the work-site as it relates to a particular group of employees, because concern is usually focused upon a problem within a specific company. Occasionally, however, experimental studies must be undertaken in the laboratory because of the sophistication of measuring techniques required or where data involves sampling subjects from a variety of locations.

The projects described within this chapter illustrate some of the research approaches used within the Ergonomics Research Unit in the Department of Physiotherapy, University of Queensland, Australia, in collecting data of importance to ergonomic design.

In undertaking research projects concerned with the establishment of optimum worker–task relationships, various parameters have been used. These include measurements of body movements, body sizes, spatial requirements, forces applied and physiological processes. This chapter outlines the details of projects which were concerned with the first four of these parameters.

BODY MOVEMENTS AND WORK POSTURE

Pedal operation

It was brought to the attention of the Research Unit that owing to prolonged use of heavy and often awkwardly placed controls and foot pedals, pedal operators in industry and agriculture were complaining of physical fatigue and pain by the end of their working day. It was considered that since both of these conditions could influence the performance of the operator, they might be included as essential factors in the sequence of events leading to an accident. At the time, the Department of Physiotherapy was developing a method of analysing body movements in detail and it was decided to explore the problem of pedal operation as part of a large scale experimental programme.

Preliminary surveys

In order to assess the frequency of occurrence of backache and of similar physical problems in workers whose employment required repeated pedal operation and to collect information regarding pedal orientations and specifications, surveys were undertaken amongst pedal operators both in agriculture and in industry.

Tractor drivers. Questionnaires were distributed at random to approximately 700 tractor drivers concerned with agriculture, road works or garden maintenance and a return of almost 60% was received. Relevant data were collected from the drivers in relation to the availability and use of seat adjustments and to the different methods of pedal operation on the 54 different models of vehicle reported. Through inspection of the equipment currently in use the tractor pedal–seat relationships were assessed in terms of the physical demands placed on the driver during operation of the vehicle, the availability of adjustments to suit individual needs as well as pedal design and orientation.

Many makes and models of tractor were found to exist, each having its own unique features. For example, the pedals on the tractors were reported as being between 7 and 30 cm above the platform, 38% being depressed along an almost vertical path, 51% moving forwards and downwards and the remainder moving over an almost horizontal path during pedal depression. A little over half of the tractor operators reported having to depress the pedal fully to engage a power-take-off for use of extra equipment, and of these,

60% considered that this manoeuvre was difficult, as was maintenance of the pedal depression.

Some tractor drivers reported awkwardness in depressing the pedal, 25% describing the need to grasp the steering wheel firmly for stability and 24% reporting that during the movement they relied on the back rest for firm stabilizing support. During pedal depression, 25% of the operators found that they had to extend their leg to its fullest extent and 16% reported that they had to rotate or flex their trunk to complete the action.

Considering the awkwardness of postures reported, the frequency of operation (ranging between 3–300 times per hour) and the resistance to pedal depression (19% considering it to be heavy, 59% medium and 20% light), it was not surprising that 88% of tractor drivers found that they were tired or aching while working. 50% of operators reported problems in the neck and lower back. As many as 21% of the drivers had sought medical attention for ailments which had developed through working their vehicle, and the majority of these conditions had been concerned with back problems. It was obvious that considerable work needed to be done to improve the tractor operator's working environment and the man–machine–task relationship.

Pedal operators in industry. Visits to seven industrial plants using foot-operated presses in their manufacturing process provided the opportunity of objectively examining the man–machine–task relationship and collecting information through the distribution of questionnaires to operators. Analyses of responses revealed that the size and alignment of the pedals used in industry differed markedly between machines and that they were located at heights ranging between 3 and 33 cm above floor level. Of the pedals measured, 75% travelled over a horizontal path, the remaining travel paths being at angles of 30–45° with the horizontal. 31% of the pedal operators found that they needed to extend their hip and knee fully during pedal use.

Pedal operation in industry is a highly repetitive task.. While the frequency of pedal depression reported by the subjects in different factories varied between 500 and 15 000 times, the average frequency of the task was close to 8000 times per day. The high repetition of the industrial process allowed little chance for muscle relaxation, and the development of a mild degree of muscular fatigue would not have been surprising. 90% of the operators admitted to the presence of such problems. Undoubtedly, the 40% of operators who suffered low back pain did so, at least partly, because of the repetitive task required of the lower limb, whose actions were noticeably associated with pelvic and trunk movements. These 'associated movements' varied in their range and this fact could have been due to the pedal's relationship to the operator, its resistance or the manner in which it was depressed.

Experimental study

The statistics collated from the studies of both tractor operators and industrial press operators demonstrated the inadequacy of the pedal–operator relationship and indicated the need for research in this field. The frequency of back problems in pedal operators emphasized the importance of focusing on a study of pedal design which might help to prevent their production. It was considered that the minimal detrimental effects on the operator's spine and its supporting structures would be produced by use of a pedal which, during its depression, required the least amount of spinal joint movement in any direction. Observations of the body movements occurring during pedal depression showed that a three-dimensional analysis was necessary. It was therefore planned to study the effects on the spine of depressing a pedal through varied pedal paths, altered according to their proximity to the operator's foot on the platform, as well as to their angles with both the horizontal and sagittal planes. The pedal orientation defined as being optimal would be that with which minimal spinal movements were associated. By using spherical co-ordinates to locate the pedal in space, the optimal pedal–operator relationship with regard to minimal spinal movements could be defined in terms of the range of hip flexion and abduction and of leg extension required to place the foot on the pedal.

Development of a method of measuring three-dimensional body movements. As the patterns of motion in the pedal activity involved movement in three dimensions, systems of two-dimensional motion analysis were inadequate. The systems of recording body movements in three dimensions available at that time were considered unacceptable in terms of data recording and reduction, as well as accuracy. The feasibility of adapting the stereophotogrammetric procedure used by surveyors for topographical mapping was assessed and, subsequently, an experimental procedure was developed which allowed data to be collected relatively simply and reduced quickly. An evaluation of the accuracy demonstrated that, with a mean error of 2 mm in a measurement

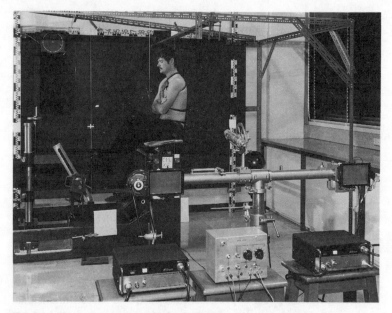

Fig. 2.1 Stereophotogrammetric set-up for three-dimensional movement analysis. The subject is seated on the experimental seat and pedal assembly for the study of spinal movements during pedal operation.

of 2–3 m, this method of measuring three-dimensional body movements was acceptable for this study (Bullock & Harley 1972).

Two photo-theodolite survey cameras supported on a stable base bar provided the stereophotography. To provide suitable images during photography, small pieces of reflective transfer film were applied directly or on pointers at appropriate points on the subject (see Fig. 2.1).

Electronically-synchronized repeating flash units were fired when the camera shutters were opened and the pedal operator was asked to raise his foot and depress the pedal. The pair of negatives so produced contained multiple images of each of the reflective tape spots, representing the trajectories of the marked body points. Each set of negatives was placed in a Galileo Santoni Stereosimplex IIC plotting instrument in order to read the XYZ co-ordinates of all points. By using computational procedures, joint movements in the horizontal, sagittal and frontal planes could then be determined by reference to the same sets of three co-ordinate values.

The determination of the optimal pedal–operator relationships.
An experimental seat and pedal assembly was built so that a desired
pedal–operator relationship could be easily obtained (Fig. 2.1). The
pedal position could be altered anteriorly, laterally and vertically in
relation to the operator, while its travel path was set at 15°, 45° or
75° to the horizontal and either parallel to the saggital plane or in a
line continuous with the line of force from the hip to the foot on
the pedal. The pedal could be depressed over 135 different travel
paths, each related in a specific way to the starting position and,
by using spherical co-ordinates for the pedal orientations, altera-
tions in position could be effected by making specific changes to
the angulations of the hip joint or to the extent of the operator's
leg reach.

Measurement of both spinal and leg movements was necessary to
determine the effects of repeated pedal depression on the operator.
Accordingly, three pointers were fixed to the articulating surfaces
between C7 and T1, T12 and L1 and L5 and S1 so that they
pointed in the direction of the articulating surfaces of the respective
vertebrae, while a fourth pointer was fixed at a lower point on the
sacrum. Small pieces of reflective tape were glued in position over
darkened areas of skin on the iliac crest, at the estimated joint
centres of the hip, knee, ankle and fifth metatarsophalangeal joint
and on the centre of the lateral surface of the pedal.

The stereo-photogrammetric method of monitoring body motion
was applied during pedal depression from each of the 135 pedal
positions. Interpretation of the analyses carried out revealed that the
optimum relationship of pedal to operator was where the pedal path
was at a 45° angle, continuous with the 'hip to foot' line and when
the pedal was positioned within a minimal forward leg reach of the
operator, requiring very little hip flexion or hip abduction to place
the foot upon it. On the other hand, pedal positions demanding
quite a lot of hip movement upwards or outward to reach were
considered to be disadvantageous regardless of the pedal angle, as
they produced three to four times as much spinal movement as occurred at the optimal locations. In addition, where the pedal
travelled at a specific angle, certain pedal locations were found to
be inadvisable: for example, the 'almost horizontal' 15° pedal
should not be located in a low, medial position, where it produced
five times as much spinal movement as in the optimal location. The
'almost vertical' 75° pedal should not be located in high medial
positions, for in these locations, up to 6.5 times as much spinal
movement is involved as in the optimum pedal–operator relation-

ship (Bullock 1974a,b). This information was provided to engineers concerned with tractor design.

It might appear that an obvious solution to this problem of reduction of driver stress would have been the use of power-operated pedals in all work situations. However, regardless of the mechanism by which the pedal is activated, certain pelvic and spinal movements are associated with the lower extremity movement involved in raising the foot from the platform to the pedal tread. Their magnitude would vary with the pedal location and also with the pedal orientation during its depression. In addition, prolonged intermittent repetitive work, even if performed against light resistance, has been shown to impose definite physical stresses on the operator. These would undoubtedly be increased if because of poor work-layout design, the performance of pedal depression involved the holding of awkward postures or the use of other than functional patterns of motion. While many new tractors are fitted with power-operated pedals, many older tractors do not have this facility. The recommendations provided as a result of the study described here allow relatively simple modifications to be made to seat–platform–pedal dimensions to ensure a more satisfactory pedal arrangement for the individual operator.

The effect of vibration of pedal operation

The ergonomist researcher is interested not only in the measurement of body movements but also in assessing the influence of other physical demands on the ability of the worker to control movement, position or balance. Other studies within the Department of Physiotherapy have reflected that interest. For example, the magnitude and nature of vibration associated with tractor driving could have a serious effect on the operator's performance. The high incidence of changes seen on x-ray, particularly in the thoracic and lumbar spine, and of low back complaints among drivers of trucks and heavy work machines (Rosseger & Rosseger 1960) focused interest on a possible relationship between low back pain and vibration. Other effects of vibration on the human body have also been reported (Grether 1971, Mishoe & Suggs 1977, Griffin & Lewis 1978, Lewis & Griffin 1978, Moseley & Griffin 1987), and the need for designs which will restrict vibration to acceptable limits has been recognized. As part of a large study concerned with the ergonomic design features of load-haul-dump vehicles (commonly called LHDs) used for rock and earth moving, it was observed that vibration produced from travelling over uneven ground appeared to prevent the driver from maintaining the accelerator pedal in the required semi-depressed position. Apparently for stability, the drivers were apt to fully depress the accelerator and then control the vehicle's speed through manipulation of the gear selector. Accordingly, a study was made within the Department of Physiotherapy of the ability of the seated operator to retain the pedal at specified points through its path of depression while being subjected to vibrations of varying frequency and amplitude (Boyling 1979).

For this laboratory-based experiment, the support frame of an experimental seat-pedal-steering wheel apparatus which simulated the known relationships in a load-haul-dump vehicle was attached to a hydraulic ram. A hydraulic system connected to the ram supplied sinusoidal vertical vibration to the seat-pedal arrangement to simulate the vibration conditions found to exist during field testing.

Each of the 20 subjects was exposed to 10 conditions of vibration combining four low frequencies and four high amplitude vibration displacements while seated on the apparatus and grasping the steering wheel with both hands. In each case, the subject attempted to maintain his foot in a constant, partially-depressed position, monitoring this by watching the needle of a display device set to indicate the mid point at the designated pedal position. Measurements of vibration displacements and frequencies, the root mean square (RMS) error and the magnitude of pedal movements were recorded. Recordings of the RMS error of pedal movement for the vibration periods were examined against the non-vibration control periods of each subject.

Analysis revealed a definite deterioration in the ability of subjects to control an accelerator foot pedal while exposed to vibration, and indicated the need for a careful review of the design of this particular work layout. Accordingly, the engineers involved in this major project incorporated this information into their considerations of the design needs of LHD vehicles.

Roof tiling

All movement consists of postural adjustment to a situation. The extent to which movements can be performed effectively and tasks completed with safety may be influenced by many factors, the importance of each being dependent upon the activity involved. Frequently, a small change in one feature of a work design can increase the difficulties of a task to such a degree that the efficiency, comfort and postural safety of a worker are significantly reduced.

This appeared to be the case in the job of roof tiling, where an alteration in roofing specifications led to an increase in the distance between rafters from 610 mm to 915 mm. Because of the difficulties experienced by the workers while stepping on these widely separated rafters, the Department of Physiotherapy was commissioned by the Building Workers' Industrial Union to analyse the activity and to determine whether the job performance under the newly imposed constraints followed principles governing safe, effective movement.

Observation of the work process revealed that during roof tiling, a conveyor belt carried the tiles to the roof to a workman, standing in a stride position on the sloping roof, used one of two methods to unload the tiles. In some instances he took a pair of tiles, weighing approximately 9 kg, and threw them onwards to the next workman. In other cases he unloaded five tiles together (a weight of 23 kg) and carried them across the sloping roof.

When the workman stood on 610 mm centred rafters facing upwards, his weight was evenly distributed between the two feet and he had a firm base for catching and throwing tiles or later for positioning them on the battens. However, when facing down the roof slope the weight was borne mostly through the heels and therefore the feet were not in a position of readiness for walking. Also, the width of the stride was greater when facing down the slope than when facing up the slope because of the tiler's need to place the feet across both the rafter and the batten for stability (see Fig. 2.2). An increase in the separation between rafters as was proposed, could have led only to an uncomfortably wide stride standing position, with a possible increase in the strain on the hip joints and on the medial ligaments of the knees and ankles. It also demanded a greater range of ankle eversion and made it difficult for the tiler to move rapidly or to alter position for catching and throwing tiles.

This project involved a photographic analysis of lifting, lowering and carrying tiles and of walking patterns, as well as consideration of the influence of such factors as body weight, age, step length, speed of walking, energy expenditure, load carrying and restriction of balancing arm movements, the process of skill learning and the implications of accident proneness.

The ability to remain stable is extremely important for the safety of a workman in a situation such as this. It is essential that he be able to balance while standing on one leg, while shifting his body weight or when maintaining a wide stride position, and that he can

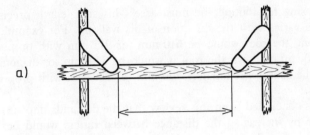

a)

b)

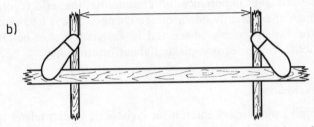

Fig. 2.2 Comparison of stride widths when the roofer faced up or down the roof slope.

continue to do so while carrying out the vigorous activities entailed in tiling. Studies relating to equilibrium in various stances suggested that the increase of base from 610 to 915 mm would result in greater subject instability and an increased sway in the forward direction. Because of the need to change positions rapidly, the tiler is often not in the correct position for catching and he could easily overbalance if tiles were thrown short or too hard. The tiler's method and speed of walking is regulated by the positioning and spacing of the rafters, the angle of slope on the roof and the danger of falling from a height. When carrying his 23 kg load of tiles along the roof, the tiler has to make frequent postural adjustments so as to maintain the centre of gravity of his body plus load over his base. Naturally, any constraint on walking while carrying this heavy load would increase his difficulty.

Normally, when walking with a load, step length is decreased and the period of support, especially that of double support, is prolonged. Step length is also normally reduced when walking up or down an incline. But it is not possible for the tiler to reduce his step length to suit the physical demands. Neither is it possible for him to walk using a consistent natural rhythm because in order to avoid losing his footing, he must assess his step length precisely and this varies with the direction of his walking. For example, a step along the roof would be 610 mm (or 915 mm with proposed changes), up or down the roof it would be 340 mm, or diagonally across the roof approximately 700 mm (or 980 mm with proposed changes).

It was concluded from this review that the demands imposed on the tiler by increasing the distance between rafters would be too great and that the continued implementation of such a proposal would be unwise. The Building Workers' Industrial Union was advised accordingly (Unkles & Bullock 1976). This particular study emphasized the importance of considering the effects on the workman of apparently minor design changes. It was heartening to find the Union seeking advice and it was gratifying to be able to contribute to the decision-making about future policy.

BODY SIZES

A second major area of interest for ergonomic studies relates to the measurement of body sizes. A knowledge of the variability of body size and proportions is vital to the solution of equipment and work-space design problems if safe, comfortable and posturally correct accommodation is to be offered to all users. If design specifications are to be applied to particular types of working areas in any location anthropometric measurements must be taken on a sample of subjects who represent the parent population in terms of relevant criteria, so that the dimensions of the full size range of the population may be estimated. Two types of anthropometric mesurements are commonly used. For example, static or structural measurements are taken in standardized positions, while dynamic or functional measurements are taken in the postures assumed during the activity relevant to the work situation being investigated.

Anthropometric data may be used for many purposes, including the design of clothing and personal articles and the planning of equipment or work spaces which will allow safe use by a specified percentage of the population. Such data should be applied not only to industrial situations but also to the planning of other work areas such as the school, the home, the office and various forms of transportation. Ideally, the anthropometric dimensions of the proposed user population should be considered early in the design sequence. Where they are not, modifications to the work layout may be necessary to satisfy individual demands.

Measurements of specified anthropometric dimensions are usually taken by ergonomists at the work-site when establishing or correcting a worker–task relationship. However, where design specifications are required for application to a particular type of workplace, then a broader collection of data is necessary. The following sections describe anthropometric studies carried out to satisfy a need for data which would describe the space requirements of a specified group of the population in the performance of a particular task.

Cockpit accommodation

A work area where safe accommodation is important is in the cockpit of light aircrafts. The Department of Civil Aviation in Australia (now renamed the Department of Transport) held concerns about the adequacy of cockpit accommodation for pilots in light aircraft, particularly since they were eager to investigate the relative appropriateness of various types of seat restraint. The Ergonomic Research Unit was requested to carry out investigations relevant to this area.

Preliminary survey

It was realized that any planned improvements to cockpit design must take account of pilots' safe, secure and adequate restraint, their comfortable accommodation and accessibility to hand and foot controls. To determine the pilots' perception of their accommodation, questionnaires were sent to 407 commercial and private pilots chosen at random (340 male and 67 female pilots). A 48% return was achieved, providing a total of 194 replies.

At the time, the installation of upper torso restraint in light aircraft was not mandatory. Indeed, the absence of a shoulder harness in some light aircraft and the potential for injury which that presented was one of the reasons prompting the initiation of the study. Analysis of responses revealed that twice as many pilots flew with lap belts only as with a shoulder strap. Although the pilots using lap belts reported that they wore them all the time during flight, up to 20 of these found that they had to stretch unduly to reach certain cockpit installations, including the cowl flap control, the stowed microphone, the rudder trim and the fuel tank selector. Some (8%) pilots complained of knocking other controls and more than half reported loss of vision through the windscreen during this reaching. Of the pilots whose aircrafts were fitted with an upper torso restraint without inertia reel, 25% stated that they did not wear it all of the time, frequently because of their inability to reach to various low controls when wearing their restraint. It was found that 90% of pilots always adjusted the seating arrangement to suit their own space requirement, half to accommodate leg length and the remainder to allow use of both hand and foot controls.

Quite a large proportion of pilots experienced some discomfort in their cockpits, and 20% reported knocking their knees on the instrument panel, 16% had difficulty fitting their thighs under the control yoke and 33% stated that they had inadvertently operated controls while entering or leaving the seat. Comparison of the frequency of occurrence of these accommodation problems between men and women revealed a larger proportion of male pilots reporting cockpit accommodation problems. Analysis of their stature showed them to be in the upper level of the height range.

The statistics and comments showed that the problem of control accessibility was sufficiently significant to warrant a re-examination of cockpit design.

As a result of this survey, suggestions for improvements in light aircraft cockpit design based on consideration of ergonomic design principles were made (Bullock 1973a). These included the following:

— Standardization of instrument panel layouts is needed
— Increased adjustability is required (particularly in seat height) to cater for a wide range of pilot size
— The layout of controls and gauges should be improved (in terms of grouping, spacing and positioning) to ensure the pilot's manipulation of the correct instrument and to eliminate unnecessary movements from one area to another
— The identification of control knobs by touch alone would be desirable
— Pilot error in selection of controls might be reduced if shape and colour coding were used
— The on–off switch on controls, such as the fuel control, should be more definite in its action
— The instrument panel should be faced with non-reflective glass
— Instruments should be angled to face the pilot, rather than being positioned in one plane
— The entry door should be on the left of the cockpit to allow the pilot to check its security when he/she is seated

— Map storage on the left wall of the cockpit would be an advantage for easier accessibility
— A wider field of view is required
— Attention should be given to the installation of safety features, such as providing a padded instrument panel, the illumination of protruding knobs and fittings to ensure the easy extraction of the fire extinguisher.

Collection of structural anthropometric data

Although there is growing recognition of the need for anthropometric data, comprehensive information is still urgently required for most adult civilian populations. As little information was available concerning the Australian adult civilian population, it was decided to collect anthropometric data which would specifically represent the dimensions of male and female light aircraft pilots, so that the information so gained could be applied in the design of the the light aircraft cockpit.

Stratified samples of 75 male and 35 female civilian pilots of light aircraft were randomly selected to represent exactly the height distributions of the Australian light aircraft pilot population. The mean weights of the male and female subjects (76.2 kg and 58 kg respectively) were very close to those of the parent populations (74.1 kg and 58.1 kg respectively).

The dimensions selected for measurement were included either because of their apparent relationship to functional arm reach or because of their relevance to the problems of cockpit design (Fig. 2.3). Stature provided data which could influence the ease of entry to and exit from a cockpit. Eye height was considered to be important as a basis for the number and magnitude of vertical seat adjustments necessary to provide all pilots with a satisfactory, wide visual field. Measurements of biacromial breadths gave an indication of required back rest widths as well as the minimum lateral distance of the upper harness anchorage from the seat reference point (SRP, the centre of the line joining the seat and the back rest). The maximum 'shoulder height sitting' dimension provided valuable information on the optimum vertical location of this anchorage. The range in measurements of popliteal height sitting, knee height sitting and sitting height provided the minimum and maximum vertical dimensions necessary for seat height in relation to the floor, instrument panel, control wheel and cockpit ceiling, to allow comfortable accommodation for the pilots. Abdominal and

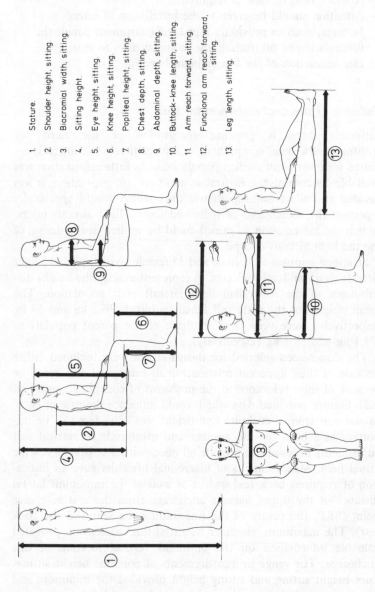

1. Stature.
2. Shoulder height, sitting.
3. Biacromial width, sitting.
4. Sitting height.
5. Eye height, sitting.
6. Knee height, sitting.
7. Popliteal height, sitting.
8. Chest depth, sitting.
9. Abdominal depth, sitting.
10. Buttock-knee length, sitting.
11. Arm reach forward, sitting.
12. Functional arm reach forward, sitting.
13. Leg length, sitting.

Fig. 2.3 Structural anthropometric dimensions applicable to aircraft cockpit design.

chest depths and buttock-to-knee lengths were included for the specification of adjustments for fore-aft seat positions to allow proper use of the control wheel during take-off and landing and to prevent knee contact with the instrument panel. The relationship of the seated operator to hand controls and foot pedals is important in the provision of fore-aft seating adjustability, and measurements of arm and leg reach are an important part of this design calculation.

Various methods have been used for taking anthropometric measurements. Early investigators such as Randall et al (1946), Hrdlicka (1947) and Montagu (1951) referred to basic equipment such as an anthropometer, a sliding caliper, a spreading caliper and several types of anthropometric tapes. The anthropometer used for measuring large dimensions, such as stature and sitting height, consists of a long graduated rod with fixed and sliding horizontal branches. The sliding caliper enables measurements of smaller body dimensions to be made by approximating to the body surfaces the edges of its two horizontal, flat and parallel branches. For measurements of body parts not accessible to the flat arms of the sliding caliper, a spreading caliper with two bowed arms is used. In addition to these simple methods, more sophisticated means of collecting anthropometric data have been applied for many years. For example, anthropologists have been using photography for the collection of structural anthropometric data since such a method was described by Sheldon in 1940. Tanner & Weiner (1949) took body measurements directly from enlargements of three photos of each subject, but later Gavan et al (1952) pointed out the need for standard scaled pictures to minimize some of the inherent errors in photography. Such errors could be eliminated by the use of stereophotography and this approach was introduced as early as 1957 by Hertzberg et al. At a later stage, Chaffin et al (1972) provided a means of collecting anthropometric data by the use of four orthogonal cameras triggered simultaneously by an electronic shutter release to provide frontal, side, rear and overhead views of the subject, while at much the same time, Owings et al (1974) described a computer-controlled system for collecting anthropometric measures. Automated systems were also described by Garn (1962), Garn & Helmrich (1968) and Prahl-Andersen (1972). The stereophotogrammetric method developed by Bullock for measuring three-dimensional body motions (Bullock & Harley 1972) was also applicable to the collection of anthropometric data. The Metrecom, produced by Faro Medical Technologies Inc.,

Canada, utilizes an electrogoniometer for digitization of body points. Its skeletal analysis software package provides both graphical and tabular data relating to a wide variety of three-dimensional skeletal measurements. The vector stereograph, which is a microcomputer-based system and which uses three potentiometers as a basic space-positioning transducer, has also been designed to obtain spatial information (Pynsent et al 1983). The CODA-3, manufactured by Charnwood Dynamics Ltd in the UK, uses light scanning instruments in which rotating planar mirrors are used to produce beams of white light sweeping across the field of view, reflecting back pulses of light from markers on the subject. The system then calculates the true three-dimensional XYZ co-ordinates of each marker and displays the output numerically and graphically in real time, concurrently with the subject's movement (Mitchelson 1977, 1988). While such sophisticated methods are costly, they offer exciting opportunities for laboratory studies.

For the study of light aircraft pilots, a three-sided anthropometric cubicle was used in which three movable vertical rods, with attached metric scales, rolled in front of horizontal metric scales fixed on the cubicle walls. Small projecting horizontal rods could be moved freely up and down the vertical bars and, by moving the vertical bars laterally and the horizontal rods vertically, the rods could be approximated to any desired point on the body and both horizontal and vertical measurements read quickly from the relevant scales. Basic positions and measurement definitions described by Garrett and Kennedy (1971) as being most frequently used in the major studies of structural anthropometry were selected for use.

In applying anthropometric data to design specifications, consideration is given to the use of 'maximum' or 'minimum' dimensions or to the allowance for adjustability. Application of maximum dimensions ensures that the smaller members of the community are catered for in such design features as seat height, bench height and eye height. The measurement used must not exceed the stipulated maximum if the smaller person is to be able to sit, see and work comfortably. Similarly, application of 'minimum' dimensions protects the larger members of the population. Certain design features must not be reduced below the specified minimum (e.g. head height in sitting or standing) if the taller persons are to be given sufficient space. Where the range of the dimension is considerable, adjustability must be provided to satisfy both the spatial and operational needs of the large and the small persons.

Anthropometric dimensions are expressed in terms of percentiles which indicate the proportion of the population who will be accommodated by a design whose specification uses that particular value. For example, to accommodate the pilots with the greatest sitting height dimension, the 97.5th percentile measurement would be likely to be used for specifying ceiling height. On the other hand, to ensure that pilots with the shortest leg length can reach the pedals, the 2.5th percentile measurement would most probably be used when specifying the minimum distance from the seat reference point to the heel point.

With regard to the ascending array of values for each structural anthropometric dimension, the 5th percentile measurement is that value which is exceeded by the values of 95% of the pilot population, while the 90th percentile measurement is that value which is exceeded by only 10% of the pilot population. To provide information for all design specifications, 2.5th, 5th, 10th, 20th, 50th, 80th, 90th, 95th, 97.5th percentiles as well as the means and standard deviations of each structural anthropometric measurement for the male and the female samples were presented. Comparisons were also made of these data with similar dimensions of overseas personnel, for reference by the Department of Civil Aviation in their consideration of design specifications (Bullock 1973b).

Measurements of spatial requirements

Not only are the static dimensions of the working population required for the design of adequate man–machine relationships, but also information is needed in regard to the operator's spatial requirements in particular working environments. As the maintenance of good dynamic posture during activity demands both adequate space for positioning the feet and placement of controls within comfortable arm or leg reach, the definition of the reach capabilities of the relevant working population is essential. Functional anthropometric measurements are required for these specifications.

Part of the concern of the Department of Civil Aviation regarding the accommodation for light aircraft pilots related to its recognition of the value of a shoulder strap as well as a lap belt in the restraint of vehicle occupants. At the time, Australian light aircraft were being required to have their front seats fitted with upper body restraint. Cockpits had been designed when pilots were restrained by lap belt only and, as the survey described above revealed, the placement of certain manual controls would not allow their manipulation by all pilots when they were confined by a shoulder strap also. It was therefore important at the time of compulsory lap and sash harness introduction, to have access to data which could illustrate the reach capabilities of all Australian male and female light aircraft pilots while so restrained. As a result of analysing such data, modifications could be made to the aircraft or to its installations which would ensure the provision of safe restraint for pilots while allowing them to reach all controls.

To provide a design suitable for a specified group of the population, measurements of a representative sample are needed. By selecting subjects representative of the total parent population, the results can have wider use than a study of selected subjects from a particular work-site where the results would apply to people in that work-site only. The criteria used for stating that a subject sample represents a parent population depends on the data required and, frequently, several criteria are considered. For example, because age, gender, race and occupation have a bearing on an individual's body dimensions, they should be considered in the sample selection for anthropometric studies. Also, in projects concerned with the determination of a functional measurement, dimensions which are relevant to the attainment of good dynamic posture should be taken into account. These usually include height and weight, as they are known to be correlated with body lengths and breadths respectively. For these reasons in this project, stratified samples of 75 male and 35 female pilots who represented the Australian pilot population in terms of height were selected.

This project is an illustration of a study which must be undertaken in the laboratory where equipment may be constructed to simulate working conditions. The functional arm reach measuring device consisted of a rigid, vertical rod suspended from a horizontal rail, so that it could be moved along the mid-sagittal plane of the chair in its 0° degree position through the seat reference vertical (SRV, the vertical line through the SRP). Thirteen coloured, numbered flat buttons were fixed to the rod from 30 cm below to 126 cm above the SRP at intervals of 13 cm. A thumb tip arm reach was measured for both right and left arms at angles of $-15°$, $0°$, $15°$, $30°$, $60°$, $90°$, and $110°$ to the mid-line at 13 horizontal

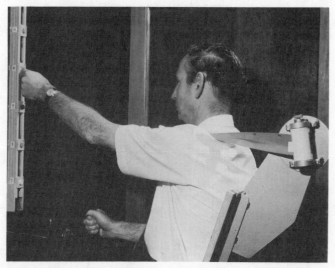

Fig. 2.4 The pilot reaching maximally within shoulder restraint, to the measuring device.

levels. The pilots were instructed to push the buttons whose colours and numbers were displayed in turn in front of them and their maximum reach for each position was recorded electronically (Fig. 2.4). The measurements for all pilots were processed so that the boundaries which could be reached by certain percentages of the pilot population could be defined (Bullock 1973b, 1974c). The diagram of the boundaries reached by a small female and a tall male pilot level gives an indication of the type of difference in space envelopes which was produced by the full size range in the sample (Fig. 2.5). The lines showing the various locations of instrument panel and cockpit floor (of seven light aircraft in current use at the time) in relation to the seat in its forward, high position and to a right arm reach at 15° to the mid-line indicated that for those aircraft in which the instrument panel was more than about 650 mm anterior to the SRP, the small pilot would have considerable difficulty in reaching high- or low-placed controls, while the tall pilot might also have reaching difficulties in the low forward area.

Subsidiary measurements to determine the effect of changing backrest angles or restraint conditions on the space envelopes were also taken. With the backrest angled at 13°, 18°, 23°, and 28°, func-

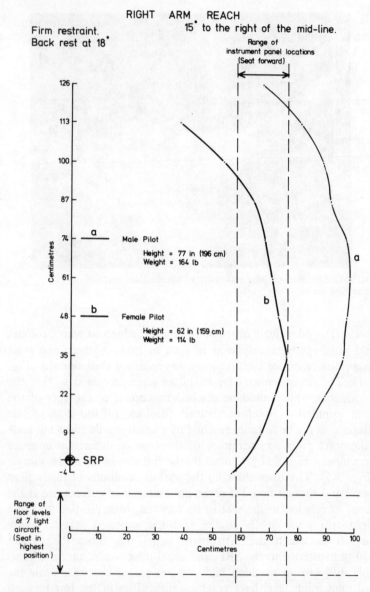

Fig. 2.5 Arm reach boundaries attained by a tall male pilot and a small female pilot at 15° to the right of the sagittal plane. The range of instrument panel locations, indicated by dotted lines, illustrate the potential difficulties of small pilots in reaching some high or low placed controls.

tional arm reach decreased progressively and instrument panel controls placed to the side of the mid-line became increasingly difficult to reach.

The effect of allowing the shoulder strap to unwind from the inertia reel as the pilot pushed the button away from him was also studied. Results showed that with a reduction of the firm restraint, significant increases to the reach boundaries appeared to occur where they were most needed: that is, to the front and up to 60° to the right and left of the mid-line and in the areas corresponding to the lowest sections of the central control panel.

On completion of this project, the Department of Civil Aviation required the installation of inertia reels as part of the restraint system in all light aircraft cockpits.

Seating problems in a secondary school

School students vary greatly in their physical characteristics, principally because of their varying age, but partly because of genetic, racial and environmental factors. However, the provision of furniture within schools often does not reflect this fact. The implications of providing children with desks and chairs which do not match their own dimensions, include poor posture, fatigue, inattention and even pain. Unfortunately, in the educational setting there are some who regard chairs and tables only as equipment to be provided, without appreciating the importance of matching the furniture to the needs of the children (Bullock 1987). Concern expressed about such problems in one secondary school for girls led to the involvement of the Ergonomics Research Unit in a study of that school environment.

Initially, observations were made of the 'working' situations and working postures of students in selected classrooms requiring sitting and/or standing. A general observation of the girls' posture was that it was consistently poor. Taller students stooped over their work, assuming either a thoracic kyphosis or a postural scoliosis. Indeed, the latter was the most common posture observed. Inadequate space for knees under the desks meant that the girls' feet were often twined around the legs of their chairs or stools or that their legs were often stretched out awkwardly. Some smaller girls had to sit on the front edge of their seats to reach the desk and consequently made little use of their backrests. Students described pain in the thoracic or lumbar regions, knees and legs, particularly in classrooms furnished with benches and stools only. Some smaller girls complained of muscular soreness in the mid-scapular and shoulder regions by the end of the day. Soreness in the posterior cervical region after classes using audio-visual aids was particularly prevalent. The major complaint described after art classes related to fatigue in the upper arm, shoulder and scapular region. Surprisingly, it was found that the students had given little thought to the reasons for muscle fatigue or soreness which they experienced.

The 30 staff members interviewed appeared not to have thought deeply about the design of furniture or of its effect on the girls' posture. Their concern was to achieve certain educational aims within the class periods and they noted that consideration of furniture and posture was peripheral to their interests. It appeared that during their own education, teachers had not been made sufficiently aware of the importance of furniture to students' posture, nor of its influence on the receptivity of students during class.

As a basis for comparison with student sizes, the dimensions of the furniture in each type of classroom were recorded. It was found that all chairs, stools and desks were of standard heights.

In this school, each grade or level consisted of five classes. To provide a representative sample of the parent population for measurement purposes, girls in one class of each level were measured, providing a total sample of 107. Structural anthropometric measurements were taken of stature, elbow height sitting and popliteal height using a portable anthropometer. Percentiles for each dimension were computed (see Table 2.1). The students ranged in stature between 146 and 187 cm, and the distribution of percentiles for

Table 2.1 Structural anthropometric measurements of female students at secondary school level (n = 107)

Antropometric measurements	Percentiles				
	5th (cm)	20th (cm)	50th (cm)	80th (cm)	95th (cm)
Elbow height standing	52.5	92.3	95.8	102.5	105.8
Elbow height sitting	19.7	23.2	25.4	28.0	30.3
Popliteal height sitting	37.5	38.6	40.0	42.0	44.1
Knee height sitting	46.5	48.2	50.5	53.0	55.0
Buttock to popliteal	41.1	43.1	45.5	47.3	49.2
Hip width	28.8	31.6	34.2	37.0	38.7
Height lumbar curve, sitting	15.4	16.6	19.1	21.3	24.0
Scapula height, sitting	34.4	37.9	40.6	42.9	45.7
Arm reach forward	46.5	51.4	54.2	57.7	58.8
Height upward reach	150.0	160.9	170.7	180.4	193.8
Height downward reach	79.3	82.3	88.3	93.4	100.1
Stature	149.9	155.9	163.0	168.0	173.4

stature revealed a marked difference between the students aged between 12 and 18 years. Such differences have also been reported in the literature (Meredith & Knott 1962, Rauh et al 1967).

To be effective, a seat must support the person to ensure not only the maintenance of stable, upright, but adaptable postures during the seated activity, but also the relaxation of muscles not required for that activity. Its dimensions in relation to the person and to the desk must be such that these characteristics for effectiveness are protected. Ideally, a seat matches the anatomical dimensions of the person using it, according to recommendations outlined clearly in the literature (for example, by Åkerblom 1948, Floyd & Roberts 1958, Barkla 1964, Damon et al 1966, Oxford 1969, Grandjean 1969). Where matching occurs, the feet can rest either on the floor or on a suitable footrest and the desk is at approximately elbow height. In some work situations, matching can be achieved through use of adjustable chairs and tables. However, this would be impossible economically and practically in situations such as schools, where there are multiple users.

Because the period of secondary education coincides fairly closely with the rapid growth spurts characterizing puberty, postural habits formed during this period are likely to have a strong influence on the skeletal and muscular system, thereby setting a pattern which is likely to persist throughout the remainder of life. It is all the more important, therefore, that during this period appropriate education should be provided about the need to maintain correct posture and that such education should be carried out in a physical environment which is inducive to success. To this end, the installation of ergonomically designed furniture in secondary schools is essential.

As a result of this study, recommendations for modification or replacement of existing furniture were made. To reduce the range of sizes of students using each room, it was suggested that timetables be organized so that each room was not used by all class levels. To take account of the differing sizes of students in each individual class, it was recommended that chairs and desks be supplied in two sizes, distinguishable by differing colours. Two sizes of footrest were also recommended, to cater for the shorter girls in the class for whom the recommended seat heights might be too great. Sizes advocated were:

chairs   — 40 and 44 cm
tables   — 66 and 72 cm
footrests   — 4 and 8 cm

Table 2.2 Recommended stool heights for use at a fixed 90 cm high bench by secondary school girls

Size of student	Stool height (cm)	Footrest height (cm)
Small	72	35
Average	67	27
Tall	62	20

The benches installed in the classrooms were fixed at a standard height of 90 cm. To cater for the range of sizes in the students, stools for use at these benches were recommended to be at three heights with footrests set at specified levels, as shown in Table 2.2. It can be seen that for effective use of a bench of fixed height, the smallest students needed the highest stool, with the footrest positioned within their leg reach in the sitting position. In laboratories where computers were in use, adjustable seats and tables were recommended.

Teachers were introduced to the ergonomic principles of seating and advised to assist students in determining their own combination of seat and desk. Students were also educated in the basic principles of ergonomic seating and encouraged to ascertain the heights of seats and desks most appropriate to them at the commencement of each year.

A further survey undertaken in the school 2 years after the introduction of the new furniture revealed that in many instances, students had selected furniture more appropriate to their needs. Although the adoption of inadequate postures occurred less frequently, they did still exist. It was obvious that the education of teachers and students needed to be prolonged and that as new students and teachers entered the school, further advice would need to be given to ensure consistent use of guidelines. Such a continuing programme was instituted within the school.

Wheelchair dimensions and patient needs

It has been observed clinically that wheelchairs sometimes fail to provide the mobility and support required by patients with neuromuscular disability. For many disabled persons, the wheelchair has offered the difference between a life of loneliness and confinement and a freer, more active and comprehensive life-style.

For some, it is an essential aid in compensating for loss of muscle power, mobility, balance or co-ordination. While the provision of carefully designed seats is important for all people, the availability of wheelchairs which match the specific requirements of the individual user is essential. Observations that for some, the wheelchair does not provide the source of support, control or mobility anticipated by the patient, led to a study aimed at comparing the needs of certain patients with the specifications of available wheelchairs (Nitz & Bullock 1983).

In each of three categories studied, the subjects selected were representative in terms of age, gender and degree of disability of a larger group surveyed in a number of Rehabilitation Centres. Those studied included seven persons (4 women and 3 men) with multiple sclerosis aged between 34 and 67 years; five spinal injured patients (3 women and 2 men) aged between 19 and 65; and three subjects (2 women and 1 man) aged between 25 and 64 years suffering from muscular dystrophy. In each group, patients with varying degrees of disabilities or differing levels of spinal injury were included.

Initially, observations of the subjects within their wheelchairs were made. Attention was focused upon the areas of support, ability to apply the brakes and methods of propulsion and transfer. Of the 15 subjects, not one displayed a good, erect, well-supported posture in the wheelchair, although all might have obtained a better posture with some alteration to wheelchair design. An increase in thoracic kyphosis appeared to have been induced in two subjects by a too high backrest, while a change in the degree of lumbar curvature appeared to have occurred in nine subjects due to inadequate lumbar support. A scoliotic curve had developed in four of the subjects, apparently due to lack of vertical and/or horizontal support from the backrest to counteract the effect of gravity on the patient's trunk.

Although propulsion of a rear wheel drive chair requires arm extension, four of the subjects found that the backrest interfered with that movement. Further, eight found that wheel access was difficult because of armrest placement, and the efficiency of one subject was limited because of inappropriate seat width. Only nine of the 15 subjects could reach and handle their brakes effectively, three being unable to reach them and the remainder too weak to apply the brake correctly. Methods of transfer from the chair varied between subjects.

The nature and magnitude of the problems revealed in this study suggested that either the patients had been supplied with an inappropriate wheelchair for their disability, or that wheelchairs in general did not satisfy the requirements of patients with neuromuscular disabilities. This emphasized the need to review the specifications of wheelchairs in common use and to match them against the anthropometric dimensions of the subject sample.

Sixteen different models produced by seven manufacturers were studied and dimensions of seat height, width and depth, backrest and armrest heights and footrest length adjustability were noted. Anthropometric measurements were taken of the patients. Using the basic position of sitting with the thighs horizontal, knees at right angles and shoulders at 25° flexion and abduction, the anthropometric dimensions of shoulder height, olecranon height, two-thirds buttock–knee length, biacromial width, popliteal height, buttock width, height of lumbar curve and height of thoracic curve were measured.

A comparison of the anthropometric dimensions with the mean measurements of the wheelchairs revealed a number of inconsistencies. For example, while the mean olecranon (elbow) height of the subjects was 148 mm, the height of the wheelchair armrest varied between 188 and 238 mm. For many occupants, this additional height demanded that the arms be lifted over the armrests to reach the drive wheels, an awkward position for applying a propulsive force. This armrest level was also uncomfortable when being used as an arm support. Even with the use of a 100 mm foam seat cushion, which compresses by approximately 70 mm during seating, the user was placed at a disadvantage. Subjects also complained of a 'shut in' feeling when using wheelchairs with armrests so much higher than their own elbows. It was recommended that the possibility of reducing armrest heights or of providing a choice of two levels of armrest might be considered. Further, it was recommended that in prescribing wheelchairs, health personnel should ensure that the armrest height was suitable for the needs of the particular person concerned.

Deficiencies in wheelchair backrests were also obvious. Many wheelchairs have a straight backrest mounted at varying angles to the seat, supposedly supporting the normal anatomical curves of the trunk. In some chairs, the lowest part of the backrest was vertical to the level of the forward lumbar curve and then sloped backwards at 15–20° to the vertical to allow for the convexity of the thoracic curve. Unfortunately, in many instances this design appeared to exaggerate the lumbar lordosis. The survey demonstrated that while the height of the maximum thoracic curve in the subjects was fairly constant for all users (390–405 mm), the level above the seat of the maximum forward curve in the lumbar region was more variable, ranging between 140 and 200 mm. To provide for individual support on standard wheelchairs, it was recommended that some adjustability of lumbar contouring was necessary and that this might be achieved by designing the backrest in two parts. For example, a sacral segment could be mounted vertically to extend upwards for 120 mm and a lumbar support could be attached to this by means of clips. Use of such telescoping uprights could provide the necessary height variation for lumbar support. A forward curve in this section of the chair flowing to a backwards and upwards projection to accommodate the thoracic curvature could offer better support and ensure good trunk posture and prevention of deformity. It was suggested that for those patients with weak trunk extensors, rather than inclining the backrest posteriorly to ensure trunk stability, the chair itself could be tilted backwards by a few degrees on the rear wheel axles. This would also control increased extensor tone in the trunk and lower limbs. The inclusion of padding and contouring could control pressure on the sacrum.

Comparison of the dimension 'two-thirds buttock to knee length' with wheelchair dimensions revealed that many chairs were too deep. This can force a patient to move forward so as to maintain a right angle at the knees and the feet on the footrests. This change in position tends to encourage the development of a kyphotic posture and this was observed in a number of the patients. It was recommended that seat depths be made available in two sizes for each type of chair. As different wheelchair manufacturers provide varying seat depths, the most suitable design for the individual patient would need to be ascertained.

A study of the effective use of brakes on commonly-used wheelchairs demonstrated that a brake based on a lever mechanism was the most effective and easily applied. Weaker patients could be provided with a longer lever arm attached to the brake handle and, by angling this extension, it could also be made accessible to those patients with limited upper limb movement.

Comfort, safety, durability, manoeuvrability and low propulsion effort have been defined as the most desirable features required in a wheelchair. As a result of this study, it was found that these features are not always satisfied by the wheelchairs prescribed to patients with neuromuscular disorders. While recommendations to manufacturers can lead to improved design, the importance of physiotherapists selecting a wheelchair from the available models which provide design specifications matching the patient's individual needs must be emphasized (Nitz & Bullock 1983).

FORCE MEASUREMENT

Because of its importance to the long-term well-being of the worker, the force that may be applied by an operator has been a subject of considerable study by researchers. In most cases, studies have been made to determine the relationship of hand or foot controls to the operator which would allow maximum application of force. Related to these tests are experiments designed to estimate the operator's strength during pushing and pulling activities in various working postures and the use of force platforms on which the subject stands so that the forces transmitted through the feet while handling objects at various heights may be monitored.

Strength tests have been made on subjects of all ages for most of the voluntary muscle groups of the human body. Consideration has also been given to the relationship of anthropometric measures to arm strength, particularly in view of the demand for pushing activities in work situations. Although static strength is not dependent on gross body size, a combination of size and body build provides a fairly adequate representation of the factors determining strength.

One ergonomic study undertaken at the University of Queensland was concerned with application of force during a sporting activity. Besides providing an example of force measurements, this project illustrates the importance of considering ergonomic factors in the design of equipment for sport and leisure.

Pull force capability for parachute ripcord release

Comparisons of arm strength in men and women have revealed the superior strength of males over females (Laubach 1976, Hoffman et al 1979, Hosler & Morrow 1982, Bishop et al 1987). This fact was of concern to the Department of Civil Aviation which had noted that the ratio of fatalities involving female and male sporting parachutists (1:3) in relation to the ratio between the number of women and men participating in this sport in Australia (1:10), indicated that women were over-represented in fatal parachute accidents while sky diving.

The sport of parachuting, which began seriously in France in the late 1940s, has grown in popularity throughout the world. It has developed to the point where the experienced jumper can perform a series of manoeuvres in a given time and manipulate a parachute canopy so as to land accurately on a specified target and can also move in space as part of a jumping team, forming predetermined patterns. Safety in sport jumping depends on many factors, including the parachutist's ability to control both his emotions and his body in unusual circumstances, the accuracy of his instruments, the proper function of his parachutes and his ability to take effective corrective action in emergencies. Rigorous training is given to all parachutists, and followers of the sport maintain its safety as long as careful rules and guidelines are followed. However, the chances of survival if neither of the parachute canopies inflates are minimal. As half of the total deaths of parachutists in Australia at the time had been associated with failure to deploy the main or reserve parachute and as a disproportionate number of women were involved in fatal parachute accidents, the Department of Civil Aviation commissioned a study of maximum pull forces relating to ripcord release in Australian female parachutists. It was considered that specification of maximum pull capabilities for the 97.5th percentile of female parachutists would easily meet the requirements of male parachutists.

For this study, a laboratory project was necessary as data needed to be collected using equipment simulating parachute use. Subjects needed to be representative of the entire Australian female sporting parachutist population, so that the data collected could be applicable to the design of equipment used by all parachutists. At the time, there were 62 registered female parachutists in Australia and information was available on their individual heights, weights, builds and ages. It was therefore possible to specify the way in which the subject sample should be stratified so that it was fully representative of the parent group under study. Thirty-seven subjects (60% of the parent group) were included.

It was important for this experiment to simulate the conditions in which the parachutist releases the ripcord. The most important of these was the fact that in free fall the parachutist receives no external counterbalancing support for the effort applied in releasing the ripcord. For the experiment to be valid, any apparatus designed had to be independent of external support, that is, totally confined to the subject herself. Forces applied by the subject in pulling the ripcord had to be counterbalanced by apparatus on the subject, but not by the subject. A light-weight frame was built to satisfy these

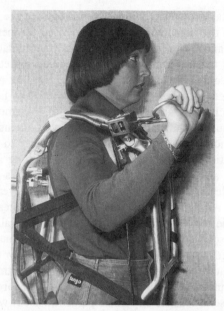

Fig. 2.6 The light weight frame and force transducer fitted to the parachutist to provide a means of recording forces applied from various positions relevant to ripcord release.

constraints. Its design allowed for body contact through foam-contoured pads at bony points of the body (Fig. 2.6). Fittings on the experimental frame allowed force measurements for handle extraction from pockets on the right and left shoulder straps, and for ripcord release of both the main and the reserve parachute in their various positions. While under normal circumstances, a ripcord will release instantaneously, in cases of 'hard-pull', force may have to be exerted for a longer period. For this reason, measurements of both the effort applied in one forceful pull and force as a function of time were taken using an electric resistance strain gauge. Data were collected on an x–y recorder while the subject applied and maintained her maximum effort of pulling on the parachute handle. Repeatability tests were carried out to determine a subject's consistency of performance.

The traces produced by the x–y plotter provided a ready means of extracting relevant data: the peak force exerted by the subject during the 5-second period, the duration of application of the peak force, the time taken for the subject to reach peak force, the maximum forces which could be maintained continuously for any single period of 1, 1.5, 2 and 2.5 s during the 5-second pull, and the maximum force which could be maintained continuously for a 1-second period during the first 2 seconds of the pull.

Percentiles were calculated to indicate the physical ability of various proportions of the population to apply a certain force. In applying data from a study of this nature, interest must be focused on the capabilities of the weakest group of the subject population. For any handle location, the fifth percentile pull force measurement could be achieved by 95% of the parachutists, while a decreasing percentage of parachutists could apply greater forces. That is, the fifth percentile force measurement represented the 95th percentile of pull capability of the subjects. Examination of the results revealed that the maximum forces were not large, the 95th percentile pull force capabilities ranging from 3.5 kg for a 2.5 s pull to 7.1 kg for a 0.25 s pull (Bullock 1978).

At the time, most sporting parachutes used in Australia were manufactured in the USA, where they were required to meet the Federal Aviation Agency Technical Standard Order (TSO) C23B. This specification demanded that the 'pack opening device shall be tested by use of an accurate spring balance to indicate its positive and quick functioning with no more than 22 pounds (10 kg) pull'. In practice, the forces required to extract the handle from its pocket and to release the ripcord pins can be influenced by many factors. These include the size, design and tightness of the handle pocket, the type of canopy, the method of packing (which in turn could be dependent on the interval of repacks), the tension of pack-opening bands, the size of the container, the extent of insertion of the pins and general maintenance. Where one or more of these factors acts to increase the force required to release the pins, the parachutist is likely to experience a 'hard-pull' if he or she cannot supply sufficient force to overcome the resistance offered. The results of the study showed that only 72% of the female subjects could exert the 10 kg pull force when releasing a ripcord over the right shoulder and only 5% could do so when over the left shoulder.

Subsidiary tests were made to determine the effect of varying some of the factors involved in ripcord release. For example, parachutists grasp the clover-leaf type handle in two ways: either with all of the fingers or with the base of the handle passing across the base of the thumb. Measurements of forces applied in each of these grasps revealed that less force could be applied using the 'thumb grasp' than the 'hand' grasp. An alternative handle shape, the 'blast', is not housed in a pocket so that the parachutist does not have to struggle with handle extraction before releasing the rip-cord. It was found that less force could be applied by using a blast handle than a clover leaf handle. When experiencing a 'hard pull' during jumping, a parachutist may apply a double-handed pull to the rip cord. Measurements revealed that an increase of force of 69% could be achieved by using two hands.

During this experiment, the subjects had maintained an erect standing position, chosen for reasons of comfort and convenience. However, in free fall, the parachutists are in a forwardly inclined position. To determine whether a change in body posture would affect the force which could be applied to the ripcord, pull forces applied in the erect position were compared with those applied during the forward leaning position for a small subgroup of the subjects. All subjects were able to apply a slightly greater force while leaning forward than when standing erect. However, con-sideration of the increases produced by a combination of leaning forward and using two hands did not raise the level of the pull capabilities of the weakest group of the parachuting population (as presented in the 97.5th percentile pull force capability figures) to the 10 kg specified by the Parachute testing standard.

Results from this test were supplied to the Department of Civil Aviation for use in consideration of specifications for design and for standards applied in parachute testing (Bullock 1977).

CONCLUDING REMARKS

Physiotherapists involved in ergonomics research can contribute in many ways. The examples offered in this chapter provide illustra-tions of a number of approaches. In particular they emphasize the importance of the laboratory-based study which provides the fun-damental data for design purposes.

REFERENCES

Aarås A, Westgaard R H, Stranden E 1988 Postural angles as an indicator of postural load and muscular injury. Ergonomics 31(6): 915–934
Åkerbolm B 1948 Standing and sitting posture. Stockholm A B Nordiska Bokhandeln
Barkla D M 1964 Chair angles, duration of sitting and comfort ratings. Ergonomics 7(3): 297–304
Bishop P, Cureton K, Collins M 1987 Sex differences in muscular strength in equally trained men and women. Ergonomics 30(4): 675–688

Boyling J D 1979 The effect of vibration on foot pedal control. Proceedings, 16th Annual Conference, Ergonomics Society of Australia & New Zealand 91–96

Bullock M I 1973a Cockpit design—pilot accommodation and accessibility to controls. Aerospace Medicine, November 1295–1299

Bullock M I 1973b Arm reach boundaries for cockpit control operation. Aviation Medicine Memorandum No 31, Department of Transport, Melbourne

Bullock M I 1974a The determination of an optimal pedal-operator relationship by the use of photo-grammetry. Biostereometrics 290–317. Proceedings of the Symposium of Commission and International Society for Photogrammetry, Washington, USA

Bullock M I 1974b The determination of pedal alignments for the production of minimal spinal movements using a stereo-photogrammetric method of measurement. PhD thesis, Department of Physiotherapy, University of Queensland, Australia

Bullock M I 1974c The determination of functional arm reach boundaries for operation of manual controls. Ergonomics 17(3): 375–388

Bullock M I 1977 Pull force capabilities for parachute ripcord release. Aviation Medicine Memorandum No 33, Department of Transport, Melbourne

Bullock M I 1978 Ripcord release capability of female parachutists. Aviation Space and Environmental Medicine 49: 117–118

Bullock M I 1987 Posture in the School Room, Australian Educational Computing. Journal of the Australian Council for Computers in Education 2(1): 22–25

Bullock M I, Harley I A 1972 The measurement of three-dimensional body movement by the use of photogrammetry, Ergonomics 15(3): 309–322

Chaffin D B, Schutz R K, Snyder R G 1972 A prediction model of human volitional mobility S A E 720002

Corlett E N, Bishop R P 1976 A technique for assessing postural discomfort. Ergonomics 19: 175–182

Corlett E N, Madeley S J, Manenica I 1979 Posture targetting: a technique for recording working postures. Ergonomics 22(3): 357–366

Damon A, Stoudt H W, McFarland R A 1966 The human body in equipment design. Harvard University Press, Cambridge, Mass

Floyd W F, Roberts D F 1958 Anatomical and physiological principles in chair and table design. Ergonomics 2: 1–16

Garn S M 1962 Automation in anthropometry. American Journal of Physical Anthroplogy 20: 387–388

Garn S M, Helmrich R H 1968 Next step in automated anthropometry. American Journal of Physical Anthropology 1(26): 97–99

Garrett J W, Kennedy K W 1971 A collation of Anthropometry, AMRL TR 68, 1, Wright-Patterson Air Force Base, Ohio

Gavan J A, Washburn S L, Lewis P H 1952 Photography: An anthropometric tool. American Journal of Physical Anthropology 10: 331–353

Grandjean E (ed) 1969 Sitting posture. Proceedings of a Symposium. Taylor & Francis, London

Grether W F 1971 Vibration and human performance. Human Factors 13(3): 203–216

Griffin M J, Lewis C H 1978 A review of the effects of vibration on visual acuity and continuous manual control. Part I: Visual acuity. Journal of Sound and Vibration 56(3): 383–413

Hertzberg H T E, Dupertius C W, Emanuel I 1957 Stereophotogrammetry as an anthropometric tool. Photogrammetric Engineering 23

Hoffman T, Staufter R W, Jackson A S 1979 Sex differences in strength. American Journal of Sports Medicine 265–267

Hosler N W, Morrow J R 1982 Arm and leg strength compared between young women and men after allowing for difference in body size and composition. Ergonomics 25: 309–313

Hrdlicka A 1947 Hrdlicka's Practical Anthropometry (3rd edn). In: Stewart T D (ed) The Wistar Institute of Anatomy and Biology, Philadelphia

Itani T, Kondo T, Matsubayashi S, Ose Y, Watanabe A, Ohara H, Aoyama H 1983 Occupational cervicobrachial disorder and the effect of improved work conditions on prevention. Journal of the Science of Stress and Rest 2: 15–23

Karhu O et al 1977 Correcting working postures in industry, a practical method for analysis. Applied Ergonomics 8: 199–201

Kilbom Å, Persson J, Jonsson B 1986 Disorders of the cervicobrachial region among female workers in the electronics industry. International Journal of Industrial Ergonomics 1: 37–47

Laubach L L 1976 Comparative muscular strength of men and women: a review of the literature. Aviation, Space and Environmental Medicine 47: 534–542

Lewis C H, Griffin M J 1978 A review of the effects of vibration on visual acuity and continuous manual control. Part I: Continuous manual control. Journal of Sound and Vibration 56(3): 415–457

Meredith H V, Knott V B 1962 Descriptive and comparative study of body size of United States schoolgirls. Growth 25: 283–295

Mishoe J W Suggs C W 1977 Hand arm vibration. Part II: Vibrational responses of the human hand. Journal of Sound and Vibration 53(4): 545–558

Mitchelson D 1977 CODA: A new instrument for three-dimensional recording of human movement and body contour. Proceedings of Orthopaedic Engineering Conference, Oxford, pp 128–131

Mitchelson D L 1988 Automated three dimensional movement analysis using the CODA-3 system. Biomedizinische Technik 33: 179–182

Montagu M F A 1951 An introduction to physical anthropology (2nd edn). Thomas, Springfield

Moseley M J Griffin M J 1987 Whole body vibration and visual performance: an examination of spatial filtering and time-dependency. Ergonomics 30(4): 613–626

Nitz J C, Bullock M I 1983 Wheelchair design for people with neuromuscular disability. Australian Journal of Physiotherapy 29(2): 43–47

Owings C L, Snyder R G, Spencer J L, Schneider L W 1974 New techniques for infant and child anthropometry: mini-computer controlled anthropometry and center of gravity measurement. Proceedings. Conference on Engineering, Medicine and Biology, p 375

Oxford H W 1969 Anthropometric data for educational chairs. Ergonomics 12(2): 140–161

Prahl-Andersen B A, Pollman J, Roaben D J, Peters K A 1972 Automated anthropometry. American Journal of Physical Anthropology 37: 151–154

Pynsent P B, Fairbank J C T, Clark F J, Phillips H 1983 Computer recording of anatomical points in three dimensional space. Journal of Biomedical Engineering 5: 137–140

Randall F E, Damon A, Benton R S, Patt D I 1946 Human body size in military aircraft and personal equipment. U.S. Army Air Forces Technical Report No. 5501 Wright Filla, Dayton, Ohio

Rauh J L, Schumsky D A, Witt M T 1967 Height, weights and obesity in urban school children. Child Development 38: 151–530

Rosseger R, Rosseger S 1960 Health effects of tractor driving. Journal of Agricultural Engineering Research 5(3): 241–275

Sheldon W H 1940 The varieties of human physique. Harper and Row, New York

Tanner J M, Weiner J S 1949 The reliability of the photogrammetric method of anthropometry, with a description of a miniature camera technique. American Journal of Anthropology 7: 145–186
Unkles E L, Bullock M I 1976 Analysis of the physical activities involved in roof tiling. Report to Building Worker's Union, 39 pp

3. Ergonomic analysis of workplace and postural load

T. Luopajärvi

INTRODUCTION

Although physically heavy jobs have decreased in number, work-related musculoskeletal disorders and symptoms have increased continuously during the last decades in most industrialized countries. These disorders cause considerable human suffering and are also economically very costly because of reduced working capacity and lessened production. Promotion of the health of musculoskeletal organs and prevention of their disorders are therefore becoming increasingly important tasks for occupational health care services, and especially so for the occupational physiotherapist.

The relationship between some musculoskeletal disorders and work-load is known. Indeed, a fair amount of evidence already exists on the injurious effects of some work-load factors, and knowledge about health-maintaining factors has grown.

Improvements in working conditions have been achieved by detecting existing health hazards and designing the workplace and activities in accordance with the workers' physical and psychosocial abilities and requirements. A central tool here is the application of ergonomics. This involves the application of knowledge about the physiology and functioning of human beings in technical solutions to working methods, work organizations and work-sites. To achieve this, good co-operation is necessary between the technical and health care professionals at the workplace.

Ergonomic analysis is a mechanism which may be used to facilitate the identification of particular problems in the workplace. Through a process of systematic recording of specified aspects of the work done or of the effects on the person of that work, ergonomic defects and possible health hazards may be defined and subsequently eliminated. Such ergonomic analyses can also provide a tool for better mutual understanding of the existing and future problems between the different occupational groups.

51

As physiotherapists have a great deal of knowledge about the musculoskeletal system and its disorders, their main task in the application of ergonomics is usually to analyze and prescribe corrective measures for musculoskeletal and postural load. The methods of analysis presented in this chapter therefore concentrate on the factors and problems related to the well-being, loading and functions of musculoskeletal organs. Experience has also demonstrated their suitability for use by physiotherapists in field studies and at workplaces. Methods requiring special instruments or laboratory conditions are only briefly discussed.

The recommendations and advice offered about ergonomic analysis in this chapter stem from the research undertaken and experience gained in this field by physiotherapists working in occupational health care in Finland or within the Institute of Occupational Health, Helsinki, Finland.

POSTURAL WORK-LOAD

The term 'postural work-load' implies both work postures, i.e. the positions of the different parts of the body during work, and work movements, i.e. the movements of the body and extremities required to perform the work.

Postures and movements are necessary during all kinds of physical work. The work-load is affected by the necessary exertion of muscle forces, the configuration and maintenance of the work postures, as well as the form and speed of work movements.

During the last decades, the physical load pattern has changed dramatically with mechanization of work. The need for heavy dynamic work involving the whole body has diminished greatly. The developmental trend has been towards minimized physical work-load and rationalized movements, resulting in an increase in sedentary work, general physical inactivity, constrained work postures and repetitive, stereotyped work movements with high speed and pace. However, this development has caused many problems already. In particular, the incidence of so-called cumulative trauma disorders has increased rapidly among many worker groups. It is obvious that dynamic muscle work with suitable load provides the basis for more natural and healthy functioning for the human being.

The major postural health hazard today is static muscle work. It can be caused by improper design of the work-site, poor organization of work or working methods, and poor individual working techniques. Static contraction of the muscle compresses blood vessels and thus reduces blood irrigation of the muscles. The supply of oxygen and energy decreases while the waste products caused by muscle work accumulate in the muscles. These wastes hasten muscle fatigue and can eventually cause pain, hardenings and cramps. The holding time of a muscle contraction is related logarithmically to the proportion of the maximum force required, so that the maintenance of a posture depends on the most highly loaded muscle group. Corlett (1983a,b) and Björkstén & Jonsson (1977) have shown that the muscle work in static contraction should not require more than 5–6% of the maximal voluntary contraction (MVC) of a muscle in conditions which last over one hour. Very rapid repetitive movements and a high demand for accuracy may also cause static contraction in the muscle or overuse of tendons, ligaments and muscles. In addition, some work environmental factors, such as cold and noise, and some mental work-load factors, may increase the static muscle load and its effects.

Other known musculoskeletal hazards include too heavy continuous loading (over 50% of MVC), high peak loads (over 70% of MVC), extreme working positions and sudden, jerky loadings.

Some examples are given below of the most common and well-known load factors on the different parts of the body, as described in the pertinent research literature. A knowledge of the influence of such factors is important to those considering ergonomic analyses. In the neck, most of the work-related disorders and pains seem to be associated with exposure to:

— static muscle work which exceeds the 5–6% of MVC
— sustained positions with a bend or twist of over 20 degrees
— sudden jerky movements which may cause microtraumas,
  that is, minor injuries, even unnoticeable at the time
— mental stress
— local chilling or draft
  In the shoulders, the disorders are often related to:
— repeated elevation of the arms to more than 30 degrees from
  the body
— forceful, jerky movements.

In the elbows and hands, the reported causes of disorders and occupational diseases are:

— unaccustomed movements
— forceful, jerky movements

— repetitive movements executed with high speed
— extreme positions of wrists and fingers
— direct local trauma
— cold environment.

In the low back, the commonly known and generally agreed risk factors are:

— lifting of heavy objects, especially below knee level and above shoulder level
— prolonged sitting, especially in a poorly fitting chair without proper back support
— sustained twisted and/or stooped postures
— jerky movements by which microtraumas may be induced
— whole body vibration
— mental stress.

Although work-load in the legs has not been studied as much as the other parts of the body mentioned, some risk factors have been nominated, such as:

— prolonged sitting or standing
— one-sided loading
— deep squatting.

CRITERIA FOR SELECTION OF AN ERGONOMIC ANALYSIS METHOD

The number of work analysis methods available today is enormous. However, it is typical for the practice of ergonomics that the screening must occur in a multidisciplinary and extensive way, even though the actual problems concern the musculoskeletal organs. In selecting an appropriate method, several factors must be taken into account. In the first instance, the purpose of the analysis must be defined. This may be:

— designing or re-designing a working environment, worksite, work process or equipment
— preventing work injuries or work-related health disorders and disabilities
— replacing or maintaining of the work ability of a handicapped or aged worker
— finding grounds for compensation of an occupational disease or injury

— planning a health care or research programme where measures must be based on the assessment of work and its characteristics.

The level of accuracy and the degree of specification of information to be gathered are related to the purpose of the analysis. For research and legal purposes they must be as high as possible, but for the solution of practical problems a less exact record of the work may be sufficient.

The quality of the end-product and the nature of the work done in the enterprise or workplace must also be taken into account. For example, the methods of analysis used for manual handling would include different components from those used in the analysis of work with a VDU.

In many cases, the practical possibilities and available time are so limited that the method chosen cannot be complex, and cannot require any special equipment or a long education. In most cases a simple method is sufficient for determining a solution to the problem. Not only does this minimize misinterpretation and mistakes, but it also keep costs to a low level.

The reliability and validity of the chosen method should always be as good as possible. If the analysis is for research purposes it is obvious that reliability must always be assessed by every analyst and, if necessary, improved to an acceptable level. But even in more practical circumstances, these matters must be addressed. Both 'retest-reliability' (that is repeatability of results for repeated analyses at different times), as well as inter-observer reliability must be checked.

The use of any measuring equipment or special test batteries for the ergonomic analysis should be considered carefully. Even if they are readily available, their use can often create problems and absorb time for relatively little return. If such special methods or instruments are applied during the ergonomic analysis, they should be calibrated and serviced carefully and their method of use properly taught.

The interpretation and evaluation of the results and information gathered should also be considered in the selection of the method. Musculoskeletal health risks and problems are more difficult to define than some other risks (for example chemical hazards), as there are few norms or standard values for reference. Nevertheless, research on the functions and health of musculoskeletal organs during the last 15–20 years has increased the knowledge of both harmful and beneficial factors. Information acquired through such research should be so clear and comprehensive that practical conclusions can be drawn and decisions reached about feasible measures at the workplace. In many countries some ergonomic recommendations, based on research, have been established (e.g. lifting guidelines by NIOSH 1981) . They can serve as background data when individual loads or ergonomic defects are evaluated.

ERGONOMIC WORK ANALYSIS METHODS

Ergonomic work analysis methods can be divided into two main categories according to the object of the study:

1. Methods which are focused on the recording and analysis of the work which causes the load in question.
2. Methods which are aimed at assessment of the effects of the work-load on the person working.

In practice, the methods in these two categories often overlap and each may be used to confirm the findings of the other.

The usual pattern of a work analysis is shown in Figure 3.1. Each

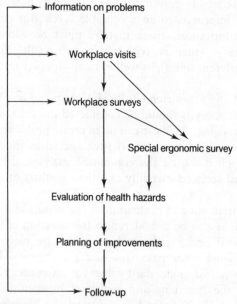

Fig. 3.1 Workplace analysis—a continuous process.

phase must be considered separately for each individual situation, but in an ergonomic survey the working conditions should be evaluated from both the technical and the human angles so that all pertinent factors are included.

Examples of methods of ergonomic analyses within these two categories, which have been used successfully in research studies at the Institute of Occupational Health, Helsinki, are worthy of mention. These methods may be used as a form of memorandum or as an aid in the planning of a new modified method.

Methods of recording and analysing work

a. Checklists

The general ergonomic checklist is based on a comprehensive checklist prepared by the International Ergonomics Association. It is intended as an indicator of the type of questions which should be asked in connection with an ergonomic analysis.

General

1. What is the operator expected to do? What data are required?
2. Is there an important physical or mental load?
3. What environmental effects on the worker are likely?
4. What is the work organization method? Is shift work or overtime involved?
5. Can the operator be replaced entirely or partly by a machine?
6. What training is required, and over what period?
7. Is the task insignificant, disagreeable, or otherwise dissatisfying?
8. What are the characteristics of the available labour force?
9. What physical, mental, emotional qualifications are required?
10. Is the task suitable for males or females or both? Is age an important factor?

Work-space—physical demands

1. Is the work-space adequate?
2. Does the work layout permit satisfactory posture and control?
3. Can the worker be seated during all or part of the working time?
4. Is the working level satisfactory for good vision?
5. Is the working surface suitable as to hardness, smoothness and colour?

6. Are the pedals suitable in size and in a suitable position? Can they be operated from a seated position only?
7. Are hand controls suited to the operating forces? Are the forces acceptable?
8. Is seating provided, and is it satisfactory in design?
9. Are foot-, arm-, hand-, back-, or headrests needed?
10. Are hand tools used? Are they satisfactory?
11. Are containers used? Is their position, size and weight satisfactory?
12. Can machine speed be adjusted to the operator's skills?
13 Are design and layout satisfactory for maintenance and repairing?
14. Are some parts of the body subjected to undue mechanical pressure?
15. Are personal protective devices required?
16. Is vibration present to an adverse degree?

Work-space—mental demands

1. Do the tasks impose high visual demands?
2. Is more general or local light needed?
3. What is the degree of contrast between working surface and surroundings?
4. Is there glare? What is the source?
5. Is colour or very fine visual discrimination required in the tasks?
6. Are tasks within a comfortable visual range?
7. Are warning lights needed and if used are they centrally placed?
8. What auditory signals are used?
9. Is verbal communication needed? Does noise permit it?
10. Can auditory signals be easily detected and distinguished?
11. Can controls be recognized by touch or position?
13. Do tasks require good balance or kinaesthetic sense?
14. Do tasks require discrimination of smells or tastes?

Work method—physical demands

1. Is the muscular load heavy?
2. Are the muscle groups involved large or small?
3. Is work done in sitting, standing, walking position, or in combination?
4. What is the amplitude, frequency and duration of peak loads?

5. Are heavy weights carried? How? When? Why? Where? By whom?
6. Is the muscle load mainly static or dynamic?
7. Is alternation possible?
8. Are the movement patterns optimal?
9. Are unstable or twisted body postures required?

Work method—mental demands

1. Are the directions of the control movements and their effects compatible?
2. Is great accuracy of movement required?
3. Have many data to be processed or compared before action?
4. Are data estimated? Are there standards or comparison values available?
5. Are the data required obvious, unequivocal, relevant?
6. Are unnecessary data excluded?
7. Does information overload or underload mental capacity?
8. Is one sensory channel overloaded? Can the load be distributed evenly?
9. Is much short-term memory retention required?
10. Can signals from different sources occur simultaneously?
11. Can preferred signals be easily distinguished?
12. Is there rapid feedback of the results of control actions?
13. Are factors for decision-making presented in the right sequence and in adequate time?
14. Can controls be recognized easily by shape, size, colour, position labelling? Even in emergency?
15. Are controls near to corresponding information sources?
16. Are workers informed enough about process flow and output?

Environmental load

1. Are conditions within thermal comfort limits?
2. Is there discomfort from air temperature and movement, humidity, radiation? What is the range of these conditions?
3. Is climatic control needed? Does the control method impede performance?
4. What is the noise level? Does it interfere with communication, distract, irritate, reduce performance, deafen? Can it be eliminated?
5. Do atmospheric contaminants constitute a hazard, or hinder performance?

Checklist for investigating handling tasks. A checklist based on the expert work done by NIOSH was prepared in Helsinki for the investigation of handling tasks. It is included here as an example of a checklist focused on a specific problem area.

General

1. What is the purpose of handling? Consider infrequent and common tasks.
2. Are restrictions of cost and time impediments to possible improvements?
3. Will improvements be in conflict with handling within a larger system?

Handling task

1. What accidents or injuries have arisen or may arise from any action?
2. List size, shape, weight and packaging materials to be handled.
3. List actions required.
4. Note rate, accuracy, regularity and rhythm of handling required.
5. Are simultaneous actions needed? Do major static components exist?
6. Do any actions require more than one person for safe handling?

Operators

1. Do the physical dimensions of the operators need consideration?
2. Have the actions been planned for persons of average capabilities?
3. Are many actions incompatible with human limitations of strength, speed, accuracy, reach?
4. If the loads have been designed for males, do females have to cope with them?
5. Are the capacities of the operator being overloaded or not fully utilized?

Equipment, work-space and environment

1. Are passages, seats, work-spaces adequate for the dimensions of the operators?
2. Is protective clothing available, if necessary?

3. Are suitable, easy-to-use mechanical aids provided and used?
4. Is allowance made for maintenance and housekeeping? Are they done?
5. Are work-places adequately lit?
6. Does the thermal environment affect well-being or performance?
7. Does noise hamper communication? Is vibration a problem?

Selection and training

1. Are operators of suitable intellectual and physical capacity selected?
2. What training is needed and given?
3. Have written instructions been supplied and understood?
4. Do operators understand the purpose of handling and the methods used?
5. Is testing of operators carried out, or necessary?

Supervision and work organization

1. Do operators get adequate feedback on results of the performance?
2. Is appreciation of good work shown?
3. Have the opinions of foremen and experienced operators been sought?
4. Has allowance been made for the relief and rest of operators, or the rotation of duties, if the work cycle does not allow adequate impromptu pauses and variation of activities?
5. Is there dynamic or static overload of any one muscle group, and if so can it be engineered out, or reduced by variation and alternation?
6. Are all actions necessary, or can some of them be eliminated or modified so as to be more effective, or combined or co-ordinated with further stages?
7. Can all or some actions be better done by a machine?
8. If isolation, boredom, fatigue and environmental or emotional stress is likely, could a person be replaced by a machine?
9. Are handling injuries adequately investigated? Is correction applied?
10. Are planning and supervision of handling activities planned?

These two checklists presented demonstrate the variety of items covered by ergonomics and which should be addressed in connection with the ergonomic analysis of postural load. The use of such checklists relies upon a basic knowledge and understanding of ergonomics and its application.

b. Work-site analysis

Ergonomic work analysis method. At the Institute of Occupational Health in Helsinki, a more detailed, systematic method of recording called the Ergonomic Work Analysis (1987) has been developed for ergonomic surveys.

The method consists of a formula for recording the data at the workplace and a guidebook with ergonomic criteria and recommendations based on pertinent literature and on experience gained through research at the Institute.

The principal survey methods consist of observations at the workplace and interviews of workers, supervisors and labour safety representatives. Prior to commencing the surveys, the analyst should collect background information from the company records concerning absences, accidents, occupational diseases and employee characteristics such as age, sex, education requirements etc.

The analyst should also have fundamental knowledge of ergonomics, some training in the use of the method, and know the work tasks and workplace as well as possible.

The Ergonomic Work Analysis method developed at the Institute of Occupational Health at Helsinki comprises 14 entities of workplace characteristics. These are: work-site, general physical activity, lifting, work postures and movements, accident risk, job content, job restrictiveness, worker communication/personal contacts, difficulty in decision-making, repetitiveness of the work, attentiveness, air temperature and noise.

The ergonomic conditions are judged on a five level rating scale, where level three (3) is considered acceptable and fairly normal. Ratings one (1) and two (2) are 'above average' and 'satisfactory' respectively. The most loaded areas and urgent improvement requirements in the profile are designated by levels four (4) and five (5) which imply the presence of serious ergonomic defects and health risks, and indicate that there is a problem that should be handled immediately or as soon as possible. In the report of the analysis the results can be summarized as a simple profile of the whole task (Fig. 3.2).

The method is practical and fairly simple and it provides an informative tool for the occupational physiotherapist.

ERGONOMIC JOB ANALYSIS

Evaluation form _____ date _____ no. _____

_____ analyst _____

Firm/workplace Steampan factory   department Pipehall

Job Welding   work-site Welding of pipes

Work object _____

Equipment, machines _____

Job description, work phases (1, 2, 3...) _____

_____

_____

_____

Drawing of the work-site and photograph

Levels

Level 1. Meets high quality recommendations
Level 2. Is a satisfactory level
Level 3. Is acceptable, some improvements possible
Level 4. Is difficult or there are some ergonomic problems, situation should be improved in connection with annual planning
Level 5. Is very difficult or dangerous, immediate corrective measures are necessary

Load factor	Estimation					Corrections required
	Level 1.	2.	3.	4.	5.	Remarks
1. Work-site			X			
2. General physical activity			X			Pulling of ø mm pipes
3. Lifting				X		
4. Work postures/movements					X	
5. Accident risk			X			
6. Job content			X			
7. Job restrictiveness		X				
8. Worker communication Personal contacts		X				
9. Difficulty of decision making		X				
10. Repetitiveness of the work						
11. Attentiveness			X			
12. Lighting				X		
13. Air temperature			X			
14. Noise				X		Hand tools

Special: Item 4. A more accurate postural analysis is required

Remarks/improvement suggestions:
A new machine coming, in the planning the problems of
the existing machine will be taken into consideration

Fig. 3.2 An example of recording of an ergonomic job analysis.

An English translation of the original Finnish description of this method is available from the Institute of Occupational Health, Helsinki.

AET, ergonomic job analysis procedure. The AET (Arbeitswissenschaftliches Erhebungsverfahren zur Tätigkeitsanalyse; Ergonomic Job Analysis Procedure) is an example of a more sophisticated method of job analysis (Rohmert & Landau 1983). It was developed in Germany by Rohmert and Landau and since 1976 has been applied to the analysis of over 4000 different industrial situations from shop-floor to management jobs.

According to Rohmert and Landau, the AET has been developed for the universal analysis of work systems, the content of work ranging from production of forces to production of information. The procedures can be used for selection, placement and training of employees as well as for job classification, rehabilitation, job design, occupational medicine, work safety etc.

The AET method comprises three entities as illustrated in Figure 3.3:

Part A. Work system analysis, which deals with the types and properties of work objects, the equipment used in work and the physical, organizational and social working environment.

Part B. Task analysis, which covers the behavioural requirements of the work.

Part C. Job demand analysis, which describes the resulting demands upon the working person.

The analysis is based on the analyst's observations of the work and on interviews of the worker, his/her superior and union representatives. The general course of any AET analysis is shown in Figure 3.4. The complete analysis programme includes 216 characteristics of the task, from which a profile of the task and its contents can be drawn.

By application of the cluster-analytic method, the collected data can be reduced to a more practical quantity. The results can also be statistically interpreted and evaluated, which improves the reliability of the conclusions made.

This method of ergonomic analysis was used in a study of work, health and retirement age in municipal occupations conducted at the Institute of Occupational Health, Helsinki (Nygård et al 1988). The work contents and demands of 88 municipal occupations, deduced from the jobs of 62 women and 71 men, were analysed by researchers.

PART A — Work System Analysis

1. Work objects
    1.1 material work objects (physical condition, special properties of the material, quality of surfaces, manipulation delicacy, form, size, weight, dangerousness)
    1.2 energy as work object
    1.3 information as work object
    1.4 man, animals, plants as work objects

2. Equipment
    2.1 working equipment
        2.1.1 equipment, tools, machinery to change the properties of work objects
        2.1.2 means of transport
        2.1.3 controls
    2.2 other equipment
        2.2.1 displays, measuring instruments
        2.2.2 technical aids to support human sense organs
        2.2.3 work chair, table, room

3. Work environment
    3.1 physical environment
        3.1.1 environmental influences
        3.1.2 dangerousness of work and risk of occupational diseases
    3.2 organizational and social environment
        3.2.1 temporal organization of work
        3.2.2 position in the organization of work sequence
        3.2.3 hierarchical position in the organization
        3.2.4 position in the communication system
    3.3 principles and methods of remuneration
        3.3.1 principles of remuneration
        3.3.2 methods of remuneration

PART B — Task Analysis

1 tasks relating to material work objects
2 tasks relating to abstract work objects
3 man-related tasks
4 number and repetitiveness of tasks

PART C — Job Demand Analysis

1. Demands on perception
    1.1 mode of perception
        1.1.1 visual
        1.1.2 auditory
        1.1.3 tactile
        1.1.4 olfactory
        1.1.5 proprioceptive
    1.2 absolute/relative evaluation of perceived information
    1.3 accuracy of perception

2. Demands for decision
    2.1 complexity of decision
    2.2 pressure of time
    2.3 required knowledge

3. Demands for response/activity
    3.1 body postures
    3.2 static work
    3.3 heavy muscular work
    3.4 light muscular work, active light work
    3.5 strenuousness and frequency of movements

Fig. 3.3 The contents of the AET analysis method (from Rohmert and Landau, 1983).

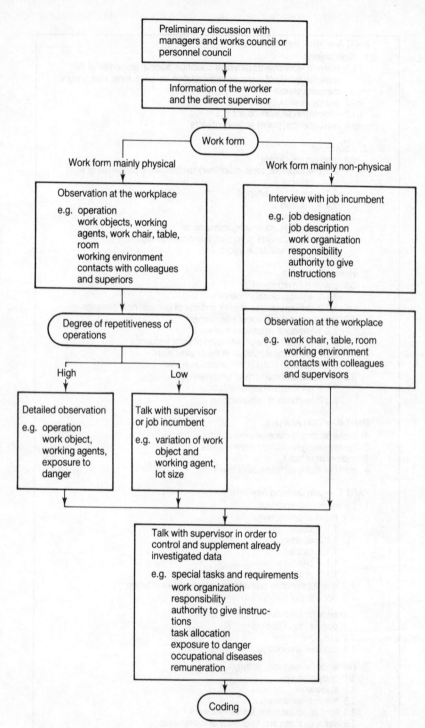

Fig. 3.4 The course of an AET analysis (from Rohmert and Landau, 1983).

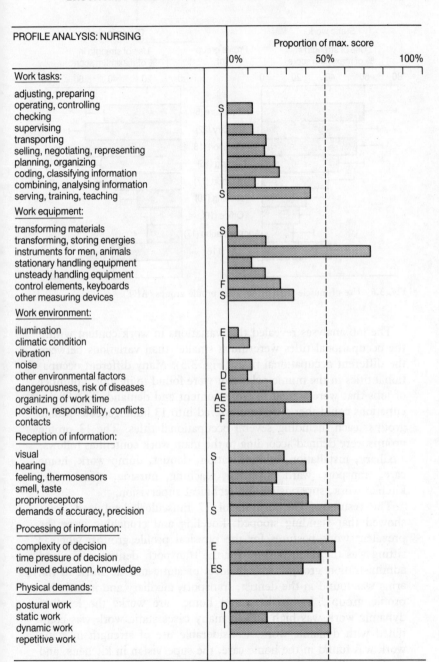

Fig. 3.5   An example of the profile analysis of AET.

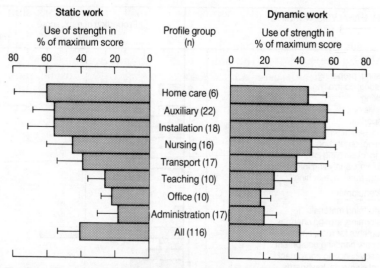

Fig. 3.6 Use of muscle strength in some profile groups (AET).

The job analyses revealed that variations in work content within the occupational titles were much smaller than variations between the different occupational titles (Fig. 3.5). Many different occupational titles in the municipal sector were found to include a number of jobs that were similar in work content and demand. The 88 occupations could therefore be clustered into 13 homogeneous profile groups, each including several occupational titles. The 13 profile groups were defined according to the main work content as follows: auxiliary, installation, administration, dentist, dump work, home care, transport, ward physician, teaching, nursing, office work, kitchen work, supervision and technical supervision.

The results of the analysis of 17 musculoskeletal load items showed that standing stooped, kneeling and crouching were the prevalent work postures for the physical profile groups, whereas sitting was the main posture for the transport, dentist, office and administration groups. A high level of static muscle work in the arms was found in the dentist, transport, auxiliary and installation profile groups. In auxiliary and home care work, the level of dynamic work was high and in many cases static work was combined with dynamic work. Considerable use of strength in static work was found in the home care, the supervision in kitchens, and in the auxiliary and installation work groups, where the extensive use of strength was also needed over a long period of work shift (Fig. 3.6).

AET method has been applied and its results compared to perceived work-load in the study of 981 women working in eight different health care occupations (Luopajärvi 1989). The most noticeable differences were found in the analyses of the work-load of bath attendants and orderlies. In AET, the physically heavy work-load was seen as the main hazard, but the workers themselves reported that the feeling of responsibility for the patients and lack of knowledge of their condition were the most important overloading factors. Altogether the information of the perceived work-load completed nicely the picture obtained by AET and, thus, the simultaneous use of an objective and subjective analysis method can be recommended.

The AET method was shown to be a satisfactory means of classifying the occupations into different characteristic groups and of evaluating the quantity of static work. The method proved to be very suitable for use by a physiotherapist.

c. Observations of working postures and movements

In the methods described above, the analysis of postural load has been part of a comprehensive work-load and workplace analysis. Quite often, however, occupational physiotherapists are requested to do more precise analyses of work-load and of problems caused by work postures and movements.

Observation and recording of working postures and movements is one of the primary ways of carrying out a work analysis. According to Corlett et al (1979), posture observation has been known for at least two or three thousand years, as posture symbols have been found in ancient Tibetan, Egyptian and Chinese writings. Today, numerous observation methods are available. Some methods are 'pencil and paper' techniques based on direct visual observations, but advanced and scientifically orientated methods with computerized data recording and processing have also been developed. The usual aids are photography and videotaping, the latter permitting more accurate observation of posture sequences and measurement of their holding times.

Several instruments have been developed to facilitate collection of data relating to measurement of exerted force. Such instruments include the Flexion Analyser developed in Gothenburg, Sweden;

strain gauge electrodes placed in hand tools for measurement of exerted forces; telemetric EMG units, biomechanical models and catalogues; and rating scales such as the Rating of Perceived Exertion (RPE) and the Analog-Visual Scale (AVS) by Borg & Noble (in Nordin 1982).

OWAS. One example of a method of observing postural load is the Ovako Working Posture Analysis System (OWAS), which was developed in a Finnish steel company for use by work-study engineers in their daily work (Karhu et al 1977). The method has been successfully implemented also by occupational physiotherapists.

The OWAS method aims at recording and identifying poor working postures and at setting criteria for the redesign of working methods and places. In this system, postures are grouped according to the general features of the tasks (e.g. standing, sitting and to the position of the back, arms and legs (Fig. 3.7). Based on the ergonomic improvements required, these postures were divided into four operative classes. These particular criteria were developed through the combined judgements of 32 experienced steel workers and a small group of internationally recognized ergonomists.

1. A normal posture which, except in special cases, needs no attention
2. A posture which should receive attention at the next regular check-up of the working method
3. A posture which must be attended to in the near future
4. A posture which requires immediate attention.

The observation is based on work sampling (either variable or instant interval sampling), which gives the frequency and duration of each posture. The number of observations needed for a reliable analysis depends on the variety of the work postures involved in the task and must be estimated beforehand. The more complex and varied a task is, the longer must be the observation time and the greater the number of observations. The instant observations at the work-site are recorded on a special form. In the assessment of overloading and uncomfortable postures, a decoding transparency is used where the four operative classes are marked with different colours.

In addition to being used originally in the steel industry, the method has been applied widely in a number of branches of industry (Oja & Kuorinka 1981). The method has also facilitated the charting and improvement of ergonomic problems. Some studies

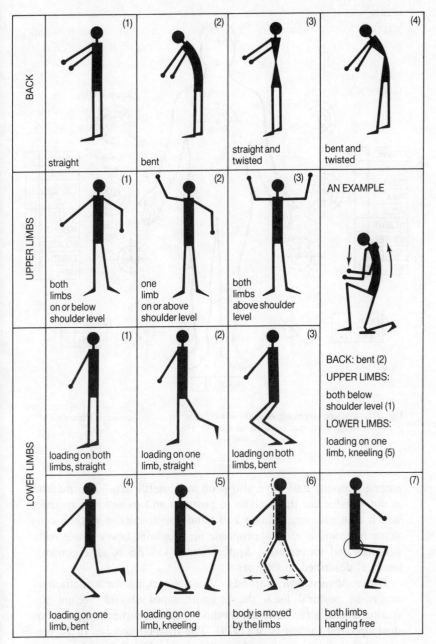

Fig. 3.7 List of items classified by OWAS. Each posture is given a three-digit code. The example in the right, thus, gets the code 215.

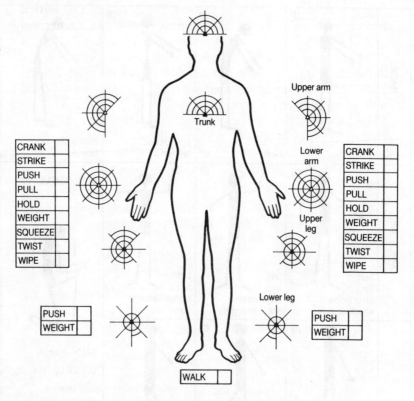

Fig. 3.8 Posture targetting diagram showing the 'standard' position from which postural changes are estimated (from Corlett 1983).

among hospital staff have also produced useful data. The method is not suitable for the analysis of postures and movements in tasks which comprise small finger and hand movements, e.g. on a conveyor belt, and is most appropriate for jobs with heavy whole body postures and movements. Application of OWAS to an ergonomic study is described in Chapter 4.

Other observation methods. When searching for a method of analysing postural load, the physiotherapist should become acquainted with a fundamental method such as Posture targetting, as developed by Corlett et al (1979). The method consists of 10 prearranged targets on a ready made form (Fig. 3.8) referring to different parts of the body in the standing position. The vertical displacements are recorded by concentric circles with a numerical scale of 45, 90, 135 from the target centre. For instance, a vertical displacement of 90 from the standard position is marked on the second circle. An attempt is also made to evaluate the exerted forces involved, so that any forces exerted by a limb should be indicated with a certain sign in the pertinent area.

Several video-computer based methods have also been developed. The work of Chaffin from the University of Michigan in this regard is known world-wide. In Sweden, a well-known method is ARBAN—which was developed by Holzman.

These methods usually consist of four phases:

1. recording the workplace situation on videotape or film
2. coding the posture and load situation in a series of closely-spaced 'frozen' situations
3. computerization
4. evaluation of the results.

Methods require preferably two videocameras and are fairly complex and arbitrary. The results are calculated by a computer in terms of the total ergonomic stress on the whole body, as well as on different parts of the body. They are presented as ergonomic stress/time curves with the heavy load situations showing as peaks on the curve. These are not 'everyman's' methods, but may be recommended if especially accurate information is needed.

A new approach, which could also be useful to physiotherapists, is the 'ergoshape' system developed at the Institute of Occupational Health in Finland. The system is constructed inside a micro-CAD programme called AutoCAD, which is the most used CAD programme in the world.

The 'ergoshape' system consists of three parts:

— anthropometric man models, with the help of which working space can be assessed and fitted to human dimensions and requirements of movement
— biomechanical calculations, which enable the evaluation of postural stress in the designing or analysis of working conditions that require manual material handling or static postures
— recommendation charts, which give direct design guidelines to particular work situations and workplaces.

d. Worker's self-analysis checklists

A problem connected with the application of ergonomics often lies in the fact that only a few ergonomic experts or enthusiasts in the enterprise participate, whereas the majority of the employees remain as uninterested outsiders. This is why many good ideas either remain undiscovered, or the implementation of a planned improvement programme does not succeed, or succeeds only partially. This problem is explored in greater detail in Chapter 9. One way of encouraging worker participation and involvement is the development of self-analysis checklists.

In Finland, such checklists are available for typists, data operators and cashiers in shops. The methods have been developed by occupational health experts together with representatives of the workers in question, so that the nature of the work and its demands are taken into account. The method includes a small booklet which describes in relevant and meaningful terms the main physical and psychosocial characteristics of the tasks, the usual work-sites, existing ergonomics recommendations and criteria for detecting the defects, plus some simple advice on how to improve the situation. The purpose is to encourage the worker, together with his/her closest superior, to undertake as many corrections and improvements as possible. Outside help is sought only if they cannot solve the problems together.

Before such checklists are forwarded to the target group, they must be evaluated to make sure they will be understood and considered relevant. The support of the employer must also be ensured, because the general atmosphere at the workplace has a marked influence on the extent to which the self-help guidelines may be used to solve practical problems.

The typist's guidebook and the cashier's guidebook have been checked as to functioning and reliability. Observations made by groups of typists and cashiers compared favourably with those of occupational physiotherapists and ergonomists in 15–20 workplaces. The lists of improvements perceived to be necessary were almost identical in each case.

There is evidence to suggest that information directed to the workers themselves enables them to make relevant suggestions as far as far as their own work and workplace are concerned. Participation motivates people to acquire new behaviour more effectively than a visit by an outside expert. Moreover, this approach is economical. Occupational physiotherapists could apply this experience and consider the development of similar methods as a means of affecting the working environment, with perhaps even longer-lasting results.

The benefits of these methods are that the workers learn the ergonomic guidelines thoroughly and through personal involvement, become more motivated to rectify the situation. The corrections and improvements are carried out on-the-spot by the persons concerned.

Measurement of musculoskeletal load

Laboratory methods for the measurement of postural load have been actively developed during the past few years. The application of occupational biomechanics has been useful for this purpose. Several static and dynamic biomechanical models based on automated data processing have been developed (Chaffin 1984). Other important measuring methods are electromyography in its different forms, measurements of intra-discal pressure of the spine, and intra-abdominal pressure using a radiotransmitter pill.

Analysis of the effects of load

Analysis of effects means the analysis of the body's response to a load. The analysis of work-load effects on the musculoskeletal organs still presents many difficulties as it is often difficult or almost impossible to distinguish between the pathological findings caused by work and those caused by ageing.

The effects of work-load may be both positive and negative. rapid or slow. The body needs a certain amount of exercise and physical activity to maintain or improve its functional capacity. Thus, if the work-load, postures and movements are optimal or within the performance capacity of the individual, the work-load is acceptable. If the work is so overloading that it leads to immediate symptoms of overstrain or even to a disease, the deficient relationship is easy to identify. Such work injuries are caused for instance by sudden, external overload ('an accident') or by an occupational disease compensated by the insurance company, and which can be related directly to a work-load factor.

The most common and difficult form of harmful work-load is continuous, slightly overloading work. The short-term effects are usually temporary fatigue, experienced as unpleasant feelings or discomfort by the worker. However, the permanent changes, im-

The date of inquiry	___/___/___ year month day	☐☐☐☐☐☐
Sex	1 ☐ Female 2 ☐ Male	☐
What year were you born?	______	☐☐
How many years and months have you been doing your present type of work?	______ years + ______ months	☐☐☐☐
On average, how many hours a week do you work?	______ hours a week	☐☐
How much do you weigh?	______ kg	☐☐☐
How tall are you?	______ cm	☐☐☐
Are you right-handed or left-handed?	1 ☐ right-handed 2 ☐ left-handed	☐

NORDIC COUNCIL OF MINISTERS.
PROJECT 170.21—330

Fig. 3.9 The Nordic questionnaire (from Kuorinka et al 1987).

pairments and disabilities are so similar to the changes caused by physiological ageing that in most cases they are impossible to distinguish from each other.

An ergonomic workplace analysis may be confirmed by an investigation of effects and this is often a duty of the occupational physiotherapist. Most commonly, it is achieved through an analysis of the company's disease records, if available and sufficiently reliable, by inquiry or interview of the workers' complaints and symptoms and/or by clinical examination of the workers.

As the implications of the results depend on the knowledge of the incidence of such disorders in the general population, it is beneficial to compare the results to other respective or national epidemiological data.

For this reason, there has been an increasing interest in the development of standardized methods. In the Nordic countries a questionnaire has been developed for this purpose (Fig. 3.9). It includes two entities: a general questionnaire and two specific questionnaires focusing on the low back and neck/shoulder region (Standardized questionnaire for musculoskeletal disorders, Project of Nordic Council of Ministers 1984 (Kuorinka et al 1987)).

Experiments have also been conducted to develop functional test batteries which could be used both locally for the neck and upper extremities and generally for the whole body, but the need for valid and reliable methods is still urgent.

Reporting of the ergonomic analysis

The results of an ergonomic work analysis should always be summarized so clearly that both technical personnel and laymen are able to understand the message.

A ready-made system for reporting, as in the AET, OWAS, ensures easy and rapid reporting. If recommendations are included, it is usually advisable to discuss the problems and plans with the decision makers and to set a schedule for implementation.

SUMMARY

Any one method of work analysis is rarely suitable for all circumstances, because there are as many different working situations as there are workers. The occupational physiotherapist should become acquainted with existing models, choose the most suitable and try to modify the method according to the acute and local needs. It is also important that in the analysis of musculoskeletal load, attention is focused not only on the physical factors, but on the whole working environment, including mental and social factors.

By learning and adapting the principles of ergonomic work analysis methods, occupational physiotherapists may improve the quality of work and achieve more economical and successful ways of preventing musculoskeletal disorders.

REFERENCES

Björkstén M, Jonsson B 1977 Endurance limit of force in long-term intermittent static contraction. Scandinavian Journal of Work Environment and Health 3: 23–27

Chaffin D B 1984 Biomechanical models for evaluation and design of manual materials handling. In: Prevention of occupational low back pain international Course, Espoo, March 1984, pp 19–23

Corlett E N 1983a Analysis and evaluation of working posture. Ergonomics of work-station design. Butterworths, London

Corlett E N 1983b In: Kvalseth T O (ed) 1983 Ergonomics of work-station design. Butterworths, London

Corlett E N, Madeley S J, Manenica I 1979 Posture targetting. A technique for recording working posture. Ergonomics 22: 3

Ergonomic Work-site Analysis 1987 Section of: Ergonomics and occupational physiotherapy, Institute of Occupational Health, Helsinki

Karhu O, Kansi P, Kuorinka I 1977 Correcting working posture in industry: a practical method for analysis. Applied Ergonomics 8: 4

Kuorinka I, Jonsson B, Kilbom Å, Vinterberg H, Biering-Sorensen, Andersson G, Jørgensen K 1987 Standardized Nordic questionnaires for the analysis of musculoskeletal symptoms. Applied Ergonomics 18(3): 233–237

Luopajärvi T 1989 Perceived work-load and musculoskeletal strain among middle-aged women working in eight health care occupations; a four-year follow-up.

National Institute for Occupational Safety and Health NIOSH 1981 Work practices guide for manual lifting. DHHS, NIOSH Publication No 81: 122

Nordin M 1982 Methods for studying work-load with special reference to the lumbar spine. Thesis. University of Gothenburg, Sweden

Nygärd C-H, Suurnäkki T, Landau K, Ilmarinen J 1988 Musculoskeletal load of municipal employees aged 44 to 58 years in different occupational groups. International Archives of Environmental Health

Oja P, Kuorinka I 1981 A method for assessing postural stress in industry. In: Corlett E N, Richardson J (eds) Stress, work design and productivity. Wiley, New York

Rohmert W, Landau K 1983 A new technique for job analysis. Taylor & Francis, London

4. Occupational physiotherapy in a large industry

E. Melin

INTRODUCTION

The position of occupational physiotherapist at the Ericsson Head-quarters has a long-standing tradition, having been established as early as 1927. Since that time, the occupational role has changed a great deal as a result of the development of the Swedish Occupational Health System and due to technical changes in the production system. Until the mid-60s, the major work task consisted of treating patients. At that time, the physiotherapist's introduction to work environment studies took the form of patient work-station visits. By this means, the physiotherapist was able to obtain information about disorders in the musculoskeletal system which were closely related to work.

As ergonomic problems have changed character over the years, the work of the physiotherapists has altered accordingly. Today, the ergonomic problems associated with lifting heavy objects and other physically 'heavy' work have almost been eliminated. Instead, there has been an increasing emphasis on eyesight, precision work and perseverance, which follows naturally from demands created by new electronic technology. In such situations, not only the physical design of the work stations, but also the actual organization of the work must be considered. Early training in a correct working position is of utmost importance. Thus the fields where the occupational physiotherapists must gain more knowledge and place more emphasis are several. They include production technique and work organization, the influence of pauses on work-load and the optimum design and method of utilization of those pauses, the determination of a correct working technique and how it should be taught and learnt.

To be able to solve the problems created by injurious work-loads, the whole company must be involved and motivated to participate.

Early efforts at Ericsson's consisted of collecting information about the effect of different types of work-load and of making ad hoc contributions as possible solutions. Some examples of such early work accomplished by the physiotherapists are given within this chapter. At a later stage, the physiotherapist's work focused upon the control and management of musculoskeletal injuries in the company. Today, the efforts of the physiotherapists are also concentrated on spreading acquired knowledge to operators, foremen and production technicians, so that the application of ergonomic principles can set appropriate standards for design during the planning phase. In other words, more educational tasks are needed from the physiotherapist.

Today, occupational physiotherapists are involved in projects in which the basic idea of implementing ergonomic principles in a company is to share the responsibility with employees through increased knowledge, by which they might develop their own proposals for ergonomic improvements. Good educational assistance in these programmes may be rendered by using the videocamera and biofeedback equipment.

Production technicians and foremen are also important personnel categories with regard to further education in ergonomics. The responsibility of and knowledge in good ergonomics and design should be solidly anchored among such staff. Indeed, today that is an absolute prerequisite for obtaining an optimum work environment. At present in the Ericsson group, occupational physiotherapists are engaged in and co-operate with the safety engineers in offering such educational programmes, as the experts in ergonomics.

During the 80s, the Ericsson group has established itself as a world-wide organization in telecommunications, employing approximately 70 000 people in most countries of the world. The provision of occupational health is compulsory to all employees of Ericsson in Sweden (approximately 30 000). Most of these have the services of occupational physiotherapists. The headquarter's occupational physiotherapist staff today number six professionals. Examples of their work and investigations over the years are included in this chapter. This provides a summary sketch of the evolutionary work of the occupational physiotherapist in a large company.

PREVENTION

Connection work—complaints

It was through the patients that the occupational physiotherapist was first introduced to the preventative programme. The physiotherapist started to visit the patients' workplaces as soon as she suspected any causal relationship between the patients, their symptoms and their work situation, often doing this visit with the safety engineer. After some years, special routines were developed to make more systematic analyses. During 1972–73 (a one year period), four physiotherapists and two safety engineers undertook a study to estimate to what extent a relationship existed between symptoms in the musculoskeletal system and the work situation, and what possible interventions could be introduced to prevent medical relapses as well as to improve the patient's work situation (Johansson & Melin 1973). This study was the first real attempt to collect information about the ergonomic needs in the Ericsson company. In retrospect, this study stands out as a breakthrough in establishing the connection between complaints and the workplace design.

Material and methods

A total of 555 consecutive patients who visited the physiotherapy department during one year were included in the study. Of these, 320 were men and 225 women, while 264 worked 'on the workshop floor' and 291 worked in offices.

At each workplace visit, two different forms were completed (Fig. 4.1 and Fig. 4.2). The first form was designed to detect a possible connection between the complaints and the workplace. Furthermore, it contained a section where suggestions for interventions could be included. On the other form, an attempt was made to identify various symptoms for different anatomical regions. Examples would be the cervical region or the lumbar region.

Results

The following results were considered to be most interesting in that study:

— One third of the patients had a rather unsatisfactory working situation, bearing in mind the pattern of symptoms.

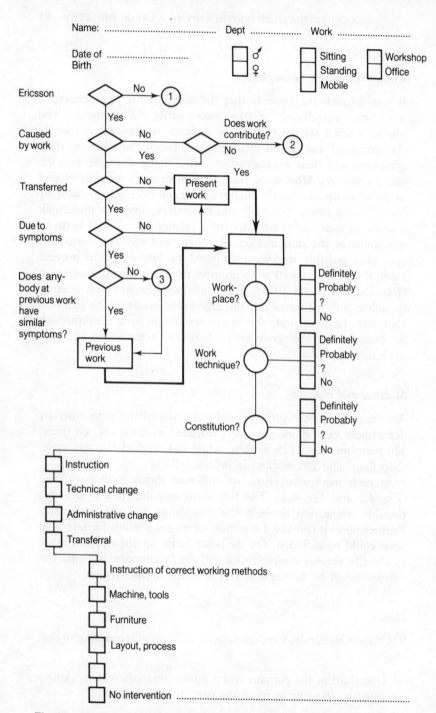

Fig. 4.1 The basic schedule followed when assessing possible relationships between workplace and complaints among patients, including suggestions for intervention.

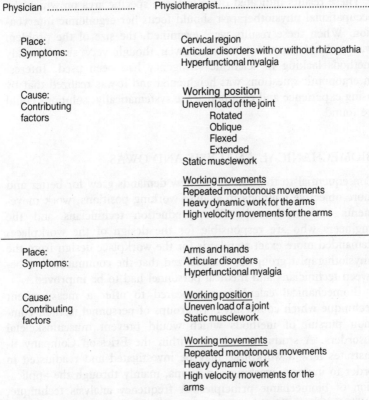

Physician	Physiotherapist...
Place:	Cervical region
Symptoms:	Articular disorders with or without rhizopathia
	Hyperfunctional myalgia
Cause:	**Working position**
Contributing	Uneven load of the joint
factors	Rotated
	Oblique
	Flexed
	Extended
	Static musclework
	Working movements
	Repeated monotonous movements
	Heavy dynamic work for the arms
	High velocity movements for the arms
Place:	Arms and hands
Symptoms:	Articular disorders
	Hyperfunctional myalgia
Cause:	**Working position**
Contributing	Uneven load of a joint
factors	Static musclework
	Working movements
	Repeated monotonous movements
	Heavy dynamic work
	High velocity movements for the arms

Fig. 4.2 The form used to identify symptoms in the cervical region and upper extremities. Other forms focused upon the thoracic and lumbar regions and the lower extremities.

— Factory workers were over-represented compared to the office staff.
— Women were over-represented compared to men.
— Disorders from the neck and shoulders were the most common as far as work-related problems were concerned.
— A short distance between the worker's eye and the object could often produce a flexed neck and a static load for arms and shoulders, with complaints developing as a consequence.
— Repeated movements and static muscle load associated with monotonous work caused disorders in arms and shoulders. (One patient a week on average reported these complaints.)
— Individual instruction with regard to correct working technique was necessary to improve the work situation.

These results indicated quite well the specific area on which the occupational physiotherapist should focus her ergonomic intervention. When these results were examined, the size of the problem was realized for the first time, even though very simple study methods lacking in scientific stringency had been used. Interest in ergonomic questions was heightened and it was realized that by using experience and common sense systematically, solutions could be found.

BIOMECHANICAL ANALYSIS AND OWAS

Consequential to these findings, new demands grew for better and more objective methods to analyse working positions, work movements and work-loads. The production technicians and the engineers who are responsible for the design of the workplace, demanded more exact standards for the workplace design from the physiotherapist group. It was realized that the communication between technicians and medical personnel had to be improved.

Biomechanical calculations appeared to offer a measurement technique which could suit both groups of personnel in their common pursuit of methods which would prevent musculoskeletal disorders. A study carried out within the Ericsson Company illustrates how a workplace may be investigated and readjusted in order to improve working conditions, mainly through the application of biomechanic principles. A frequency analysis technique, OWAS (Ovaco Working Posture Analysing System), was also used for the first time in this project (Reisig & Seijmer-Andersson 1981).

Annealing work station

The working place which was analysed in that study was an annealing work station (Fig. 4.3). Disorders from the lumbar region had been reported from the staff, so that, subsequently, the recruitment to the department was difficult.

The work consisted mainly of moving items from boxes into pans, which would be heated to approximately 800°C, and subsequently putting the details back in the boxes, once they had cooled down. Throughout this task, the pans and boxes were stacked in two piles and one pile would increase in height while the other decreased. The weight of each pan was 30 kg and the boxes would be filled with goods up to 28 kg. Finally, the boxes were piled onto a stool (32 boxes).

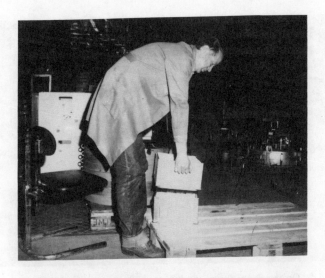

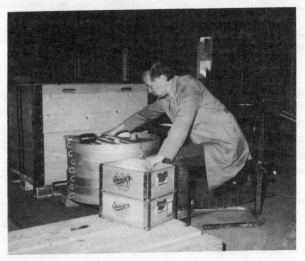

Fig. 4.3   An annealing work station.

Material and methods

Photographs were taken of the workers throughout the activity.

The flexing external torque on L5 (lumbar disc 5) was estimated according to the formula:

$$Torque = force \times moment\ arm$$

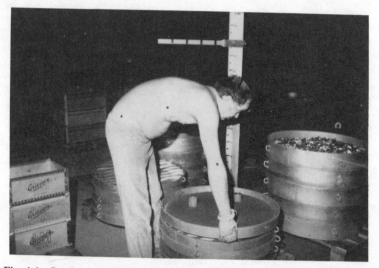

Fig. 4.4 On the photo above, the flexing external torque on L5 was estimated to be 359 Nm. Compared to the bodyweight, that load is more than 10 times greater. As a comparison it can be said that in an optimal lifting situation (i.e. with the box close to the body in the upright position), the flexing external load on L5 is 180 Nm.

As almost all lifts were symmetrical, a 2-dimensional analysis was considered to be sufficient and the lifts were analysed from side projection (see Fig. 4.4). On the photo, the centre of gravity was indicated by a black dot for the head, the trunk, the arms and the full mass of the whole body. The distance between each dot and L5 was measured (the moment arms) and the external torque on L5 was estimated.

In this study, the basic OWAS system was used as a complement to the biomechanical analysis. Basic OWAS, outlined in Chapter 3, is suitable when the task involves the whole body. The method can only be recommended when the work involves large dynamic movements, since it provides information as to how many times during the working day an individual assumes a certain position. It does not take into consideration whether the load is static or dynamic. The OWAS method thereby is a type of frequency analysis technique, and the observer only needs paper, pen and a watch. The working position assumed by the subject is observed every 30 seconds and is then registered using 3 or 4 digit codes, which are recorded in a co-ordinate system. A number of basic postures of the back, arms and legs are represented in those codes, so that different positions of the back, arms and legs can be recorded. Even the weight of the material being lifted can be registered according to three different classifications. Altogether, there are 84 types of possible working positions and these are divided into three weight classes. Each type of working position (registration) is classified according to four different 'intervention' categories, depending upon how quickly the intervention should be made, for the sake of the person's safety.

Conclusion

The biomechanical analysis and the OWAS study were complementary to each other and, together, they revealed that instruction in lifting techniques to the personnel concerned was insufficient. It was also obvious that useful tools which would facilitate the handling of goods and prevent injuries at the workplace needed to be developed (Fig. 4.5). Recommendations to change the design of the workplace and to introduce lifting aids were made, as shown in Figure 4.6.

Once the adjustments had been implemented, further biomechanical and OWAS analyses were carried out. These re-evaluations indicated that the maximum load on the lumbar spine had been halved from 10 to 5 times the body weight and the load-

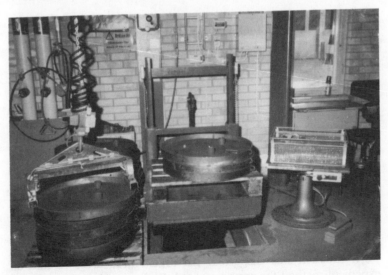

Fig. 4.5 Lifting aids.

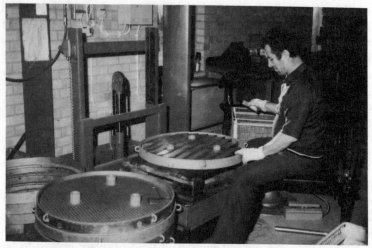

Fig. 4.6   Height adjustable workplace.

creating movements were not repeated by the operators as frequently as they had been previously.

Through this particular study, more objective methods had been introduced into the company by the physiotherapist and new forms of communication and understanding had started to develop between the health department and staff responsible for production.

VIDEO REGISTRATION AND QUESTIONNAIRE

As the production system in the main factory of Ericsson changed from one of electromechanics to one of electronics, the ergonomic problems also changed in character and so did the nature of the complaints from some personnel. The demands for precision increased dramatically and the movements of the arm became more and more restricted. This new work situation resulted in the operators assuming a considerably more static work position. The major area of strain ascended from the lumbar spine to the cervical region. This 'elevation' of pain centralization in the labour force occurred in less than half a decade.

An increasing number of patients with soft tissue disorders in neck and shoulders visited the physiotherapy department, and frequently a relationship between the patient's complaint and his/her work situation was suspected. An urgent need arose to find an expedient method for recording work-load on neck and shoulders.

In co-operation with the National Swedish Board of Occupational Safety and Health, two physiotherapists and a safety engineer developed a method to register work positions and movements reliably. Simultaneously, attempts were made to examine other factors, such as life-style habits, psychological balance and other features which could influence human well-being (Cardell & Melin 1981). In developing this method, specific requirements were imposed by the occupational physiotherapists and the safety engineers. For example, it was considered that it should show a measurable difference between various work situations, it should be useful when planning working methods and it should be a help when evaluating ergonomic measures. For the purpose of testing the use of the method and at the same time increasing knowledge about the relationship between work-load and neck–shoulder pain, it was decided to carry out a controlled case study where a questionnaire could also be included.

A study of work-load on the neck

Is was hypothesized that patients seeking help from the Occupational Health Department at Ericsson for soft tissue disorders in the neck and shoulder region had a heavier work-load on the neck and shoulders than a control group without complaints. It was also hypothesized that the method of recording the work-load would show a difference in the degree of strain on neck and shoulders between the group of patients and the control group.

It was also considered that apart from work, there could be other factors such as physical condition, mental condition and leisure time activities which could affect the muscle tension of the patient, thereby preconditioning soft tissue disorders. The incidence of such factors could also be investigated. The study was carried out by physiotherapists at four of the Ericsson Group's factories where, for several months, patients with neck and shoulder disorders were requested to participate in the project. Twenty-eight such patients agreed to be involved. Forty-five control subjects matched for age, sex and jobs were included in the study. The study methods included examination and questionnaire, photography and videofilming.

Methods

Both the patients and the control subjects were examined in

accordance with a special standardized protocol established by the occupational physiotherapists and used in each of the different occupational health departments. Structured interviews according to a questionnaire dealt with the development of the complaints in the patient group and the nature of work in both groups. Attempts were made via the questionnaire to assess the incidence of 'other factors' such as previous infections, nervous disorders and leisure time activities in both groups.

In order to estimate the load on the neck in its most flexed position during work, the persons were photographed in profile in this position. The necessary measurements were performed on the photograph, and biomechanical calculations were made.

The movements of arms and head were recorded by means of videofilming. A representative part of the work (usually an entire work cycle) was filmed in two projections; from the rear to record the abduction of the arms and from the side to record forward–backward flexion of the arms and head movements. Different coloured tape was applied on the medial and lateral sides of the arms and on the side of the trunk, to indicate their relative positions (see Fig. 4.7). The videofilm was then shown on a monitor. A keypad with three functions was connected to a printer. Each key represented a certain angle area and the chain of movements was transferred to the printer by pressing the keys manually.

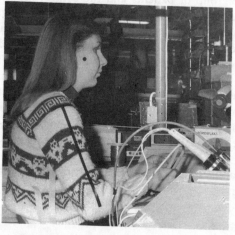

Fig. 4.7 Photograph of subject during activity.

Results

Results of the questionnaire showed:

— that patients had been subjected to a situation in their work for which they were not trained, more frequently than the control subjects
— that increased muscular strain on the shoulder–neck was more common among the patients, either because of an increased level of stress or as a result of leisure time activities which involved movements analogous to the work movements
— that patients more often than controls were absent from work for periods longer than 2 months prior to the onset of their complaints, and
— that patients were significantly less active with physical exercise during their leisure time compared to the control group.

The videofilm showed:

— that the patients had a heavier work load than control subjects with regard to arm movements forwards and outwards
— that bending the head during work gave contradictory results, i.e. the patient group had slightly less strain while bending their heads than the control group
— that the method of recording identified the difference in work-load between the patient group and the control group and
— that it would be a suitable method for use in ergonomic investigations.

Conclusion

An outcome of this study was that the physiotherapists had demonstrated that they had developed a method which could facilitate:

— evaluation of ergonomic changes
— choices between different methods of production
— transfer to alternative duties on account of shoulder–neck strain
— investigations of occupational injuries and
— casual investigations and surveys in personnel health care.

A new support for better understanding of ergonomic problems had been introduced into the company and through this understanding an insight into the needs for improvement was established.

Shortly after this study was completed, the analysis system was further developed by the National Swedish Board of Occupational Safety and Health. The method which evolved is named VIRA (ASS undersokningsrapport 1983:10). This new system allowed the use of a computer rather than the previously used keypad and thereby saved considerable time.

Still further evolution of the system of analysis has recently been presented by Coggman & Coggman (1987). They introduced the idea that by connecting an angle-measuring device to an A/D converter it would be possible to continuously register the change in angles (10 times/second). In practice this allows an uninterrupted registration of the angles on the monitor, which can then be computer calculated with various degrees of resolution.

This new method has now been introduced to the physiotherapists in Ericsson, where it will be used extensively both in the educational programme and in ergonomic studies. Most jobs in the plant are short-cyclic, in a seated immobile working position and with relatively rapid, repetitive arm movements. It is in these jobs that the method can be used most successfully.

BIOFEEDBACK

Another instrument that has been used as a tool to evaluate workload on different individuals is biofeedback. The method of using biofeedback equipment to collect EMG data was first developed and introduced by two occupational physiotherapists in their attempt to determine whether armrests on chairs could relieve strain on the neck and shoulder (Norin & Seijmer-Andersson 1983).

The effect of armrests on neck and shoulder strain

The common opinion among staff involved in solving ergonomic problems was that armrests on chairs could prevent disorders in the neck and shoulder, and this was a very attractive thought. However, before such an opinion could be fully accepted, it was decided to carry out an evaluation. Three different jobs, representing sitting assembly work, were chosen to be investigated. Nine healthy women, aged between 25 and 41 years, were selected as subjects. They had all worked with the same task for more than one year. Before the measurements could be made, all subjects had to work with the armrests for one week so that they would become accustomed to the new work position.

Method

The biofeedback equipment was a Myometer 2 (SATT electronics), and since it only had one channel, only the activity in one muscle could be registered at a time. The muscle studied was the trapezius (Fig. 4.8). The EMG measurement was made during 25 minutes of work activity with the armrest in use and, after 20 minutes rest, a new measurement was taken without use of the armrest. The measurements started at the same time of the day for all subjects. An average value of the activity during the 25 minutes period of work was calculated in microvolts after monitoring readings every 15 seconds. Before and after each work period measured, the subject had to make three submaximal test contractions with the arm in a position of 90° forward flexion, semi-pronated and somewhat adducted (test 0 kg) whilst EMG activity was registered. The same test was performed with the subject holding a weight of 1 kg (test 1 kg). An average value in microvolts was estimated from these tests.

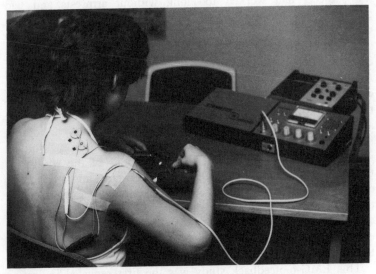

Fig. 4.8   Use of biofeedback during work activity.

Results

By determining the maximal torque (MVC) on each subject, the EMG measurement could be quantified according to the MVC. This MVC was calculated with the help of a calibrated dynamometer (PIAB) and biomechanical estimations. EMG was not registered while MVC was calculated.

By calculating the maximal torque, the magnitude of MVC and the percentage of MVC represented by the lifting of 1 kg and of 0 kg, the working values as a percentage of MVC could be quantified. In this way, any difference between work with and without armrests could be estimated. Both inter-individual and intra-individual comparisons could be determined.

Conclusion

It was clear from the results that the physiotherapists could not support the theory that the load on trapezius (neck–shoulder) decreased during work with armrests. In some situations, the armrests could even increase the load on the investigated muscle. Some theories to explain why the armrest did not give an unloading effect were proposed, for example: an armrest on the chair constituted a hindrance and could cause tension in the shoulders; the armrest might not provide an optimum position for the arms; or the subjects had worked too long without armrests and had developed an acquired work technique. The possibility that weightlifting might be used to increase MVC and hence decrease strain on neck and shoulder was considered. However, after searching the literature, there was hesitancy to adopt such a solution. A low MVC-level does not necessarily imply a poor static endurance (Persson & Kilbom 1985). Hansen also showed in 1967 that weightlifting only increases the isometric and dynamic strength, but not the isometric endurance. It was considered, therefore, that it is probably the static strain that causes disorders in this type of work. One of the conclusions of the study was therefore that 'microbreaks' were very important, and as a matter of urgency, different types of work break should be introduced in order to reduce the load on the shoulder muscles. As a consequence, instead of changing the design of the workplace, more emphasis was placed upon changing the work organization and on teaching a correct working technique.

This EMG-biofeedback study was the first reported indication that the physiotherapists in Ericsson ought to broaden their views on injurious work-load. It seemed evident that in order to contribute to the control or management of injuries in the workplace, the physiotherapist must examine the total working system: the individual and his working technique, the physical design of tools and workplace, the work organization, and finally the total psychosocial working environment.

REHABILITATION

The aim of rehabilitation is to assist individuals to return to work and become as independent as possible of their physical or psychological limitations. Within the Ericsson Company, the responsibility for the rehabilitation programme is divided between several categories of personnel: the individual, the employer, the four unions and the occupational health service (including the medical, technical and psychosocial departments). The rehabilitation programme includes medical treatment, which should commence as soon after injury as possible, and different activities designed to achieve an early return to work. As far as medical treatment is concerned, the occupational physiotherapy department primarily provides treatments of injuries closely related to the working station. Methods used today include acupuncture and transcutaneous electro nerve stimulation (TENS) for pain relief, mobilization of the spine and extremities through various manual techniques, and the use of sequence training and stretching to improve muscle functioning. Relaxation exercises are forming an increasing component of treatment.

Concomitantly with this treatment, a readjustment of the person's original workplace or his/her reallocation to another type of work form vital components of rehabilitation activities. An early attempt to return to some work while still being on sick leave is considered to be of the utmost importance. To this end, certain agreements have been made between the company and the social insurance, which permit an employee to return to his workplace on part or full-time work while receiving sick leave benefits, within a so-called 'work-training' programme. During that time, the individual can have the workplace adjusted to match his own ability and can also adjust himself to the new work.

Different programmes for patients with musculoskeletal disorders have been designed to restore the individual's capacity to adjust to a normal life. They have been in effect for several years. The occupational physiotherapist is involved in many rehabilitation activities in the company. Approximately 50% of the physiotherapist's total working time is spent on medical treatment and rehabilitation. Through regular contact with the patient and application of knowledge about the working environment, the physiotherapist often serves as a bridge between those two. The good relationship between the patient and the therapist increases the mutual confidence and subsequently, the possibilities for a successful result.

Training with biofeedback

Two particular studies exemplify the rehabilitation programme at the Ericsson Company. The first of these was an investigation into the value of training with biofeedback. Biofeedback equipment has been used as a training method for quite a long time. Good results had been reported from USA on people with tension headache. The results from the study reported earlier had also shown that a poor work technique could be one of the reasons for disorders in the neck and shoulder. With this background, the two occupational physiotherapists decided to evaluate the use of training with biofeedback (Norin & Seijmer-Andersson 1983).

Methods

The same measuring method was used as in the study to evaluate armrests, reported earlier. Ten subjects participated in the study, nine working in an office and one person in the workshop. All were patients attending the physiotherapy department. Their problems were subjectively regarded as being caused by an inadequate working technique. Initially, each subject received individual information about the investigation, its aim, design and likely effects. This was done in a quiet environment in the physiotherapy department. On that occasion, the subject was made familiar with the measuring and training equipment, which was applied and demonstrated.

As soon as possible (some days later), 25 minutes of the muscle activity of trapezius was recorded during work, through the use of a biofeedback. The subjects themselves specified which tasks caused the worst levels of pain according to their disorders. Jonsson et al (1981) recommended that the preliminary limit value for the average load level in a muscle should not exceed 10–14% of MVC during a 1 hour work period.

Immediately after the first measurement, the subjects had to start the biofeedback training. A threshold value could be set on the Myometer and the apparatus could be made silent during a muscle activity below a certain value. Every test person trained for 1 to 2 hours on this first occasion. The following day, the physiotherapist visited the subject in order to apply the electrodes and set the threshold value. During this training session, the subjects had to practise for 1 to 2 hours. After these two training sessions, a measurement was made during the next few days. The subjective opinion on the training was also registered for each subject.

Results

After having trained with biofeedback, five subjects were able to voluntarily decrease the amount of load on the trapezius muscle. Those subjects who had had a positive experience from the training gained the best results. The objective results of the measurements corresponded well with the subjects' own judgements.

Biofeedback training was found to be a good method by which to learn a correct work technique and thereby to enhance body awareness. This very awareness is in turn a prerequisite for a successful rehabilitation of patients in general, whether their complaints are of somatic or psychosomatic origin. The proportion of patients in the latter category has increased during the last couple of years. These employees require a completely new treatment approach, including stress management, relaxation exercises, physical fitness exercises. This treatment can be given either individually or in groups. Today, all of these techniques are included in the occupational physiotherapist's daily work programme.

BACKSCHOOL

Another example of an approach to rehabilitation at the Ericsson Company is the application of the Swedish Backschool. Dating back to the 70s, the Swedish Backschool has been used in the company in order to rehabilitate patients with back problems. During 1985, an evaluation of the effectiveness of this programme was completed (Norin & Johansson 1987).

A comparison of the backschool and the back fitness class

Many patients with more or less chronic back problems continuously visited the occupational health department in Ericsson's main factory and office. After a sick period of one month, some patients showed signs of chronic low back pain. It was decided, therefore, that a more effective care programme than the one in use at the time had to be offered to these patients. Supported by earlier experiences concerning education (Bergqvist-Ullman & Larsson 1977) and the positive effect of physical activity, a programme was commenced in 1980 in which back patients were treated without delay.

The backschool included an education programme according to a model which has been well evaluated (Zachrisson-Forsell 1981) and which was adjusted to the local conditions in the office and on the workshop floor. It involved four one hour sessions of information on paid time within a 2 week period. Each group consisted of approximately 10 people and 10 groups passed through the backschool each year.

The back fitness class could be described as a physical fitness class with musical accompaniment. Exercises that might strain the back had been excluded, and the stress level was decided from lesson to lesson depending on the nature and abilities of the group. Each back fitness class took place twice a week on paid working time and lasted for half on hour. Evaluation of initial data collected in a pilot study showed that the method was adequate but that the time factor needed to be very strictly controlled.

The aim of the backschool and the back fitness class was primarily to teach the low back pain (LBP) patient to lead a life which was as gentle to his back as possible. The aim was to change the patient's attitudes and behaviour in certain aspects such as experience of pain, ability to work, anxiety, physical activity and careful back behaviour. The goal with this present study was to determine the extent to which the person's way of life had actually changed as a result of exposure to the programme.

Material and methods

With the experience from the pilot study, it was decided to collect what was assumed to be relevant data before and after the backschool and before and after the back fitness class, by using a four piece questionnaire. The questions about pain and physical activity were based on Borg's pain scale (RPE) and Engström's assessment of physical activity.

Questionnaire No. 1 was answered at the commencememt of lesson No. 1 in the backschool, under the supervision of a physiotherapist. Questionnaire No. 2 was sent to each patient by post 4 weeks after the first lesson in the backschool. Questionnaire No. 3 was answered by the patient before the first lesson in the back fitness class, and Questionnaire No. 4 was sent to the patient 8 weeks after the first lesson in the backfitness class. Patients who did not return the questionnaire were reminded once or twice by telephone. The questionnaire was anonymous but was numbered, so that the patient could be identified through reference to a code. The received material was computerized at the Institute of Statistics, the University of Stockholm, where assistance with the programme design, the statistical information and the documentation was obtained.

The study included 166 consecutive patients who visited the Occupational Health Department during a 2 year period. Of these, 110 patients answered questionnaires No. 1 and 2 (giving a drop out of 37 people, or 25%). Thirty- nine patients answered questionnaires No. 3 and 4 (drop-out of 18 people, or 32%) and 20 of those only attended the back fitness, class. Consequently, the study included 130 individuals.

Results

A definite effect of backschool and back fitness classes was found to be a decrease in the sense of anxiety. Attendance at back fitness classes resulted in an increased level of physical activity and a possible decrease in experienced sense of pain.

All patients attended the backschool and the back fitness class on paid working time. The total cost for the back fitness class participants was considerably higher than for the patients in the backschool. In the light of these results, the back rehabilitation programme was subject to a critical review and revision. Today, the physical fitness programme is emphasized to a large extent and the backschool is used as a complementary form of rehabilitation.

The importance of re-evaluation of the physiotherapist's work was highlighted by this study. The value of constant critical reconsideration of ongoing programmes must be recognized, for a well-accepted and established programme does not necessarily give the optimal treatment over time.

CONCLUDING REMARKS

This chapter has illustrated the occupational physiotherapist's obvious role in an Industrial Health Department. To successfully live up to the expectations outlined, it is essential that the physiotherapist co-operates closely with other medical professionals, technicians and management. Finally, it is her duty to stay up-to-date in ergonomic research and to be prepared to re-evaluate her own work.

REFERENCES

Bergqvist-Ullman M, Larsson U 1977 Acute low back pain in industry. Thesis. Acta Ortop-Scand, Supplement 170: 8–102
Cardell H, Melin E 1981 A work symptom related investigation of neck–shoulder disorders and muscular loading factors among staff at the L. M. Ericsson Group. A method for developing the registration of work movements. Report from the Occupational Health Service, Ericsson Information Systems, Stockholm
Coggman L, Coggman I 1987 Vidareutveckling av VIRA-metoden genom automatisk vinkelavlasning. Arbetsmiljofonden
Engström L M Vuxnas motionsvanor IFR sid 38
Hansen J W 1967 Effect of dynamic training on the isometric endurance of the elbow flexors. Internationale Zeitschrift für angewandte Physiologie einschliesslich Arbeitsphysiologie 23: 367–375
Johansson M, Melin E 1973 The relationship between work-load disorders and the working situation at the main factory in 1972–73. Report from the Occupational Health Service, Ericsson Information Systems, Stockholm
Jonsson B, Ericsson B E, Hagberg M 1981 Elektromyografiska metoder for analys av belastningar pa enskilda muskler och muskulara uttrottningseffekter under langre tids arbete. Arbetarskyddsstyrelsen, undersokningsrapport 1981: 19
Norin K, Johansson H 1987 An evaluation of the back school and a physical fitness class at Ericsson Headquarters. Proceedings Tenth International Congress, WCPT, Sydney 821–824
Norin K, Seijmer-Andersson B 1983 Can elbow support relieve neck and shoulder load during sedentary assembly work—biofeedback study. Report from the Occupational Health Service, Ericsson Information Systems, Stockholm
Persson J, Kilbom Å 1985 Belastningsrelaterade besvar i nacke-skuldror. Arbetarskyddsstyrelsens undersokningsrapport 1985: 2
Reisig A, Seijmer-Andersson B 1981 Material handling in annealing. Report from the Occupational Health Service, Ericsson Information Systems, Stockholm
Zackrisson-Forsell M 1981 The back school. Spine 6: 104–106

5. Musculoskeletal complaints in workers engaged in repetitive work in fixed postures

B. McPhee

INTRODUCTION

Although occupational back pain is well known and generally accepted as a possible outcome of heavy, stressful work, there has been much less recognition of work-related neck and upper extremity disorders. While empirical evidence indicated that certain occupational groups were at higher risk of these disorders than others, until recently the conditions themselves were poorly understood, and research into their nature, causes and prevention proved difficult and inadequate. By the 1980s, however, there was a growing awareness by a number of researchers throughout the industrialized world that neck and upper extremity disorders were common and costly, not only in traditional areas of industry but increasingly in white collar work. Most notable was the growing incidence of the disorders in operators of visual display terminals (VDTs). With this awareness came an upsurge in research activity and the development of more effective preventive measures. Essential to prevention was the identification and control of factors considered necessary for the development of these disorders, and of primary importance was the application of ergonomic principles to the design of work and workplaces.

As could be expected, due to their knowledge and experience of musculoskeletal disorders, physiotherapists have been active in both research and prevention of these conditions in the workplace since the mid-1970s. This chapter gives an overview of this research and the physiotherapist's contribution to it.

RECOGNITION OF MUSCULOSKELETAL DISORDERS

In the simplest sense, musculoskeletal disorders are the effect of stresses on the body beyond its capacity to withstand them without

101

damage. This effect is usually referred to as strain and takes the form of a symptom or set of symptoms, including pain and often other forms of dysfunction. The stress may be physical and/or psychological. Physical stresses act on the soft and bony tissues of the body in different ways, depending on the health and resilience of the tissues, because of ageing and degeneration, previous injuries or strain, or congenital or acquired abnormalities; and depending on biomechanical factors which alter the way stresses are transmitted through the body. Psychological stresses may influence the way in which the strain manifests itself in different individuals. The interaction between physical and psychological factors is complex but always must be considered in the study of these conditions.

Descriptions of disorders in crafts and tradesmen, scribes and notaries can be found in early writings by Ramazzini (1713). From the 1920s to the 1960s, published papers described the clinical aspects of work-related disorders of the upper limbs and shoulder girdles.

By the middle of the 20th century, specific work-induced musculotendinous injuries, notably tenosynovitis and peritendinitis crepitans, were being recognized by the medical profession (Conn 1931, Thompson et al 1951, Smiley 1951, Howard 1937, 1938, Reed & Harcourt 1943) and in workers' compensation legislation in some industrialized countries (Conn 1931).

Conn (1931) ventured to suggest that the conditions appeared to increase in periods of spasmodic employment such as during the Great Depression, further confirming for him that the musculoskeletal system needed training to do certain types of arduous work. However, he had also noted that some older workers had low grade, chronic crepitus in flexor tendons of the wrist and that, where more than 30 to 40 movements of the fingers per minute were required, tenosynovitis crepitans was the norm rather than the exception. He also expressed the view that local anatomical considerations had an important bearing on aetiology.

Both Hunter (1959) and Ferguson (1967) described the perplexing problem of craft palsies or occupational cramps, with Hunter listing 49 different occupational groups in which the hands could be affected by such cramps. Recognized for over a hundred years and akin to writers' cramp, these conditions are a disturbance of function of the hands and/or arms associated with specific manipulative skills, and include visible spasm and impairment of co-ordination. Pain or discomfort may precede these symptoms and may continue to occur in some developed cases. The only treatment generally considered to be effective is the minimizing or avoidance of the actions known to precipitate the symptoms. Their exact aetiology and treatment are still the subject of considerable doubt.

Much work into the association between different types of work and complaints of musculoskeletal discomfort and occupational cramp was carried out in Australia by Ferguson (1967, 1971a, b, 1976), later in association with Duncan, a physiotherapist (Ferguson & Duncan 1972, 1974, 1976; Duncan & Ferguson 1974). In investigating an outbreak of unspecified upper limb injuries in 77 women working in an electronics factory, Ferguson (1971b) analysed injury records, examined some of those with symptoms and studied their tasks. He found that the injuries fell into two broad groups: well-defined clinical syndromes such as supraspinatus tendinitis and tennis elbow, and ill-defined symptoms complexes, with the latter group in the majority. For this reason, Ferguson broadened the scope of work-related musculoskeletal disorders of the upper extremities from simple tenosynovitis and peritendinitis crepitans to a wider and more complex set of conditions and coined the term Repetition Injuries to indicate what he believed to be their cause—repetitive manual work.

It was this term, later to be changed to Repetition Strain Injuries (RSI), which was used increasingly in Australia (NHMRC 1982) to describe pain and discomfort in the hands, arms, shoulders and necks of workers involved in repetitive, unvaried work and who were forced by their work and the workplace design to maintain awkward, fixed postures for long periods during the working day. In Japan, the study of a wide range of work-related neck and upper extremity disorders, known there as occupational cervicobrachial disorders (OCD), started in the late 1960s (Maeda et al 1982) in groups as diverse as cash register operators, industrial workers, film rollers, crèche attendants, nurses, keyboard operators, telephone operators and clerks writing with ball point pens (Komoike & Horiguchi 1971, Onishi et al 1973, Ohara et al 1976, Onishi et al 1976, Onishi et al 1977, Ono et al 1982, Nakaseko et al 1982, Maeda 1981, Maeda et al 1982).

A number of investigations of symptoms in the neck and upper extremities associated with work have also been undertaken in the Scandinavian countries in the last decade. Most have been concerned with musculoskeletal disorders in the arms and shoulders of workers in the manufacturing and construction industries.

Important studies in Finland have included literature reviews of occupational cervicobrachial syndrome (cervical, tension neck and thoracic outlet syndromes and humeral tendinitis) (Waris 1979); and of tenosynovitis (Kurppa et al 1979a, b). In the 1970s and 1980s, technology has enabled the mechanization and automation of much manufacturing and mining work, so decreasing the proportion of heavy work. Generally speaking, work has become progressively lighter but much remains repetitious and lacking in the variety of movements necessary for balanced, efficient musculoskeletal function.

Concomitantly, the rapid development of computer technology has led to widespread office automation so that much white collar work has taken on the nature of light process work. With these changes has come the realization that even light work may give rise to complaints if it is poorly designed and does not accommodate the capabilities and limitations of those engaged in it.

CLASSIFICATION OF DISORDERS AND NOMENCLATURE

A major problem with the study of neck and upper extremity disorders is the variety of names given to a very wide group of conditions. Even the diagnosis or classification of the disorders has been far from satisfactory, and evidence today suggests that many back disorders were either overlooked or wrongly diagnosed (Kelsey 1982, Bogduk & Marsland 1988). Nevertheless, the link between heavy work and musculoskeletal disorders was established.

While highlighting the need for more investigation of occupationally-related disorders, several reviewers have discussed the problems inherent in such data collection when different classifications, diagnoses and terminologies continue to exist (Luopajarvi et al 1979, Kuorinka & Koskinen 1979, Kuorinka & Viikari-Juntura 1982, Kuorinka 1983, Viikari-Juntura 1984).

In the researching of these disorders, the use of umbrella terms in various countries (OCD in Japan and other countries; Cumulative Trauma Disorder or CTD in the USA) has overcome, to a certain extent, the problem of lack of a standard nomenclature, definition and diagnosis. Only in Japan, and to some extent the Nordic countries, has there been a successful attempt to standardize these (Waris 1979, Waris et al 1979, Aoyama 1979, Maeda 1981, Maeda et al 1982). Another problem is that it is often difficult to distinguish complaints regarded as a normal part of life from more serious and potentially disabling conditions which may start with apparently trivial symptoms. Yet another difficulty is the lack of simple, reliable tests to measure these conditions quantitatively. The development of such tests remains unlikely while little or no objective evidence of some disorders exists (Wickström 1982, Hernberg 1984).

In Australia, for some years the term Repetition Strain Injuries or RSI was used to denote any one of a number of disorders. The use of this term has been discouraged recently in favour of the term Occupational Overuse Syndrome (NOHSC 1986a, b) and, to a lesser degree, others.

THE INCIDENCE OF MUSCULOSKELETAL COMPLAINTS ASSOCIATED WITH REPETITIVE WORK

The perceived increase in incidence of musculoskeletal disorders in those associated with repetitive activity prompted a number of researchers to focus their studies in this area. For example, in Finland, researchers examined the prevalence of tenosynovitis and other conditions in workers engaged in repetitive jobs (Luopajärvi et al 1979). In Sweden, Kvarnström (1983) examined the records of 11 000 factory workers and found that nearly 48% of all long-term absences (greater than 4 weeks) were due to musculoskeletal disorders. About two-thirds worked in heavy engineering and over one-third in light engineering, 20% being women. All subjects whose injuries were associated with heavy repetitive work had long-term sickness absences. Kvarnström found that the proportion of musculoskeletal disorders was twice as high in blue collar workers as in white collar workers. Other important findings were that:

— women suffered from the disorders 10 times more frequently than men
— young persons had significantly less sickness absence than older workers
— those reporting symptoms were more likely to work in a group piece rate system and be shift workers
— significantly more workers with symptoms than those without considered their work to be heavy, monotonous, stressful, detrimental to health and associated with heavy lifting and unsuitable work postures.

In other countries, also, the 1980s saw an upsurge of incidence in these complaints. For example, in Australia, an unprecedented number of musculoskeletal complaints was reported from the workforce between 1983 and 1986 (NOHSC 1985, 1986a,b, RSI Taskforce 1985, Hocking 1987). While many of the complaints occurred in workers in heavier manufacturing and industrial jobs, an increasing number of white collar workers also reported symptoms, some so severe that their ability to earn a living has been curtailed.

In white collar workers, particularly office workers performing keyboard tasks, the apparently increasing prevalence seems to be due to several factors:

1. The rapid introduction of computer technology without due regard for how human operators will work within such systems;
2. As a result of the above, the increasingly repetitive and fixed nature of tasks which were formerly more varied in terms of postures and movements
3. Increasing awareness by workers of occupational health and safety issues without the concomitant changes of attitudes required by planners and administrators to meet increasingly better standards in working conditions and services to workers.

The causes of the apparent increase in reporting, world-wide, of complaints in the neck and upper extremities of workers performing a variety of tasks is not understood fully. However, it is certain that managers and workers are more aware of the problems and more effective reporting systems have been established in the past 10 years.

Scientific evidence points to links between certain types of work and work factors, and the incidence of disorders. Most importantly, jobs involving highly repetitive movements, in fixed work postures, are considered to pose the highest risk.

The risk is further increased where force is a necessary component of the job and where work breaks are inadequate to allow recovery from fatigue.

Generally it appears that there is an increased risk of injury when:

— new demands are placed on the individual
— the individual habitually works beyond his/her capacity
— personal, social or environmental factors reduce the individual's tolerance to physical stress (McPhee 1980).

CAUSES OF MUSCULOSKELETAL DISORDERS IN THE WORKPLACE

The complexity of musculoskeletal disorders and their causes is well recognized. Even those conditions which arise directly from work may be influenced by personal and perhaps social factors which modify symptoms and how they are reported. Individuals exposed to hazards in the workplace react differently and this is no less true for reactions to stressful and/or repetitive movements and prolonged fixed postures. Notwithstanding this, it appears that the higher the levels of physical stress, the greater will be the numbers who succumb to injury.

The cause–effect relationship is subtler in light work than in heavy work and, although there has been considerable refinement of measurement techniques to identify and measure the outcome and to probe the possible causes, they are still insufficiently sensitive to establish beyond question what this relationship might be.

Complexity of risk factors

In mid-century, some authors speculated on the causes of musculoskeletal injuries in industries (Conn 1931, Howard 1937, 1938, Blood 1942, Flowerdew & Bode 1942, Reed & Harcourt 1943, Smiley 1951, Thompson et al 1951). The work factors listed as likely causes of the conditions described were:

— speed and intensity of muscle effort
— a single or persistent strain
— overuse
— unaccustomed work often occurring after a change of job or equipment, or returning from holidays
— infection
— trauma.

In 1971, a committee was formed in Japan to define OCD and outline its causative factors, clinical features, stages and the health services required to control the conditions (Aoyama et al 1979, Maeda et al 1982). Five main factors in the aetiology of the condition were identified:

a. dynamic and static muscle load
b. general muscle loading resulting from uncomfortable work postures

c. mental stress or severe tension
d. adverse environmental factors such as poor lighting, noise, uncomfortable temperatures
e. poor work organization.

The committee also described five detailed stages of the disorder.

Ferguson and Duncan (Ferguson & Duncan 1972, 1974, 1976; Duncan & Ferguson 1974) examined personality, social and work organization factors and associated medical conditions in relation to the aetiology of the disorders under investigation.

In 1972, Welch noted that symptoms in the upper limbs of manual workers were still causing concern and outlined several possible precipitating causes: movement—its force, direction, speed, frequency and number; and posture—of the body as a whole and of individual parts. He also speculated that predisposition could be an important aspect in the development of disorders in some workers while others remained unaffected. He took this argument further when in 1973 he advocated the use of the Hettinger apparatus to measure physiological predisposition to tenosynovitis (Welch 1973). However, subsequent research in Finland has disputed the validity of the test (Kuorinka et al 1981).

In Sweden, Kilbom et al (1984a,b 1986, Kilbom & Persson 1985) studied the relationship between risk factors and symptoms in female workers in an electronics factory. The study was in three parts. First it was demonstrated that there was a relationship between work technique, job experience and productivity, and early symptoms. One year later the number of women complaining of symptoms and symptom severity had increased (Kilbom et al 1984a). While productivity had increased 20%, sick leave had decreased by 4%. The results suggested that high static loading of muscles and short rest breaks were related to the development of symptoms. Significant symptom predictors were high individual productivity and previous sick leave. Factors related to symptom decrease were a change to a less repetitive job and high static muscle strength.

While these various studies of the possible effect of certain risk factors on the development of musculoskeletal injuries in general are of considerable value, much still needs to be learned before those concerned in prevention and treatment, including physiotherapists, can plan for effective management. This fact is highlighted by the comments of authors such as Viikari-Juntura (1984) who, after examining the literature on the aetiology, epidemiology and treatment of tenosynovitis, peritendinitis and tennis elbow, concluded that very little indisputable information existed on any aspect of these particular well-defined and described conditions.

The effect of load

The effect of load on the production of musculoskeletal injuries has also been the subject of inquiry. At work, static muscle loading may occur because of the prolonged maintenance of particular, and especially awkward, postures, or the need to stabilize or manipulate tools or controls. It may also be induced by concentration or working faster than a comfortable pace (Waersted et al 1986).

An early study (Carlsöo & Mayr 1974) showed that excessive loads were being placed on the shoulder and arm muscles of workers using pneumatic hammers and bolt guns. It was suggested that such loads over a period of time could lead to early degenerative changes in the musculoskeletal structures involved. In a study of telephonists, Ferguson (1976) concluded that the frequent complaints of discomfort, aching and other symptoms were due to static loads on joints and muscles resulting from the fixed forward bending postures determined by the nature of the design of the visual, auditory and manipulative tasks.

Some researchers through EMG and biochemical analysis have attempted to demonstrate direct connections between short-term and cumulative loading and the subsequent development of fatigue and other symptoms in specific jobs (Carlsöö & Mayr 1974, Herberts & Kadefors 1976, Herberts et al 1981, Hagberg 1981a,b,c 1982, Hagberg et al 1982, Jonsson 1982, Hagberg & Kvarnström 1984, Greico 1986, Valencia 1986). More detailed studies relating symptoms and work-load factors (Kuorinka & Koskinen 1979) revealed the contribution of specific factors such as cycle time, mode of control and number of pieces handled. A significant relationship between symptoms and number of pieces handled by manual workers in light industry was found.

In a recent study conducted by a Swedish physiotherapist, diffuse pain and discomfort were shown to arise from the maintenance of extreme flexion of the lower cervical/upper thoracic spine, similar to postures commonly adopted at work (Harms-Ringdahl 1986). It was suggested that these symptoms originated from the mechanical load on passive joint or spinal connective tissue structures rather than sustained muscle activity, and it is plausible that, with such symptoms, there is a neurological component.

Static muscle loading leads to more rapid fatigue than does dynamic muscle work, due to constriction of the circulation simultaneously with increased demands by the muscle for oxygen and nutrients and the need to disperse waste products resulting from the muscle activity. The relationship between the severity of symptoms and the degree of loading, commonly referred to as the dose–response relationship, is difficult to determine. It appears that the greater the physical load, i.e. the numbers and frequency of movements, and the force used to perform the task, the greater the risk of injury. However, there is no evidence to date that injury severity is directly related to the number and magnitude of load factors.

Psycho-social factors

Psychological and social factors affecting the development or prolongation of symptoms have been alluded to. It has been claimed that some of the psychological effects of repetitive work on individuals could be absenteeism, decreased job satisfaction, increased errors, signs of deteriorating mental health, such as anxiety, frustration, aggressiveness, irritability, tendency to depression and psychosomatic complaints, as well as pains in the neck, shoulders and arms (Weber 1981).

Ferguson (1976) noted that many cases of musculoskeletal injury in industry required long recovery periods. He felt malingering was unlikely as most workers needed to return to work for financial reasons, but suggested that in some cases there might have been some psychosocial reasons to prolong absence from work.

MUSCULOSKELETAL DISORDERS IN THE OFFICE WORKER

The incidence of musculoskeletal injuries in office workers has been a topic of growing concern for ergonomists in many countries, as well as for those concerned with their management. In the 1970s and early 1980s, for example, Swiss and Japanese researchers reported the results of studies of office workers (Hünting et al 1980a, Hünting et al 1980b, Maeda et al 1980, Hünting et al 1981,

Grandjean et al 1982a, Grandjean et al 1982b, Grandjean et al 1983a, b, Grandjean 1984a, b, Grandjean et al 1984, Läubli et al 1984, Läubli 1986). These reports heightened interest in the problems arising from light, highly repetitive manual jobs which required workers to sit in fixed postures for long periods. Many of the jobs studied involved the use of visual display terminals (VDTs) which were being introduced into workplaces all over the world. In addition to the widely publicized benefits, the computer revolution brought with it a number of concerns, one of which is the problem of deskilling and another, a much less publicized one, that of prolonged static work postures and highly repetitive movements.

Several studies of office workers showed that a large number of typists and VDT operators complained of pain in the neck, shoulders and arms, while these problems were relatively rare in 'traditional' office workers (Laübli et al 1984). In comparing symptoms of postural and visual fatigue in operators using VDTs or traditional office equipment, Laübli (1986) found a direct relationship between certain types of work and daily or occasional complaints of pain in the arms. Most interesting was the increasing of complaints associated with higher daily keystroke rates.

The factors contributing to musculoskeletal problems in this group of workers have been investigated in a number of studies. In Sweden, for example, 160 medical secretaries in a university were examined by physiotherapist Björkstén for musculoskeletal symptoms, particularly in the neck, shoulders and upper limbs (Björkstén 1984). The investigation identified three main factors associated with an apparently high prevalence (59%) of symptoms:

— poor ergonomic design of furniture and equipment
— lack of task variation, and
— insufficient rest breaks.

This study is described in greater detail in Chapter 7.

A study in Canada examined the workplace ergonomics of a group of 350 clerical workers doing routine office work (Webb et al 1984). The unprecedented number of complaints of musculos-keletal discomfort was shown to be related to the introduction of new office furniture.

Surveys of keyboard operators in Australian state government departments revealed that symptoms of repetition strain were common among the 466 keyboard operators engaged in data entry or word processing, with approximately half attributing their symptoms to their work (SA Health Commission 1984). Elements which were identified as having contributed to the symptoms were:

— the work (length of time spent on keyboard work without a break)
— percentage of day spent in keyboard work
— length of time in a keyboard job (work-load)
— the workplace (unsatisfactory ergonomics leading to poor workplace layout) and
— the work organization (limitations of training and supervision).

Similar conclusions regarding work organization were revealed by Bammer (1986a,b), who retrospectively investigated factors associated with the rapid rise in the numbers of reported complaints of injuries in keyboard workers at an Australian university in the period 1980 to 1984. She suggested that changes in work and management practices associated with the introduction of new VDT technology might account for such an increase.

A longitudinal study of the influence of age on health complaints in VDT operators was commenced in Singapore in 1980 (Ong & Phoon 1986). Results to date indicate that older operators have more health complaints, including visual fatigue and musculoskeletal ache, than younger operators. However, the majority of the older operators were working mothers so that the addition of domestic duties to the VDT work could have been responsible for the higher level of complaints.

Since 1980, a number of reviews and reports of studies into the health of office workers, particularly VDT operators, have been published by North American researchers (Dainoff 1982, 1984, Smith et al 1981, Stammerjohn et al 1981, Webb et al 1984, Springer 1982, Devolvé & Queinnec 1983). Much of this work has been concerned with visual and eye complaints. Musculoskeletal complaints were also of concern, while some researchers emphasized behavioural aspects, stress and other related issues. Both Dainoff (1982, 1984) and Smith et al (1981) expressed concern about the haphazard nature of the introduction of computer technology into workplaces and pointed out that, because of the anticipated exponential growth in the numbers of VDT operators during this decade, health complaints could pose a very large and expensive problem if they were not addressed immediately.

MECHANISM OF INJURY

While the links between certain types of work and symptoms in the neck and upper extremities have been established, the mechanism by which strain occurs is still unclear. Some researchers have, however, attempted to address this question.

Work-load

Extensive studies in poultry processing, garment making, automotive plants and medium-to-heavy industry have been undertaken in the USA (Armstrong & Chaffin 1979, Armstrong et al 1982, Armstrong et al 1984, Fine et al 1984, Silverstein et al 1984, 1987, Silverstein 1985. This group has tried to quantify work-load and its effects on workers in terms of musculoskeletal symptoms. It has also undertaken specific biomechanical studies and determined that the mechanism of injury appeared to be the overloading of tissues through excessive force, faulty work postures, repetitive movements and/or inadequate recovery periods. Excessive or premature degenerative changes in the joints and connective tissues also seemed to result from physically heavy work.

In the more easily recognizable conditions, such as tenosynovitis, tendinitis or bursitis, trauma to the respective tissues is believed to occur as the result of repeated or cumulative strain, such as occurs with light or forceful repetitive movements, setting up an inflammatory reaction within the tissues (Goldie 1964). As a secondary outcome of the inflammation of tendons, conditions such as traumatic carpal tunnel arise where the median nerve within the carpal tunnel at the wrist is compressed and neurogenic symptoms result (Armstrong & Chaffin 1979, Cannon et al 1981, Feldman et al 1983).

Muscle fatigue

Muscle fatigue is considered to be a function of static and dynamic loading on the muscle in relation to the maximum capacity of the muscle for contraction.

The relationship between work, fatigue and injury has been explored by a number of researchers. For example, Peres (1961) described injuries he believed were the result of chronic fatigue due to intense effort, monotony and the lack of variety in work. He emphasized the detrimental effects of static muscle load due to poor posture and recommended a preventive strategy based on redesign of work practices, early reporting of symptoms, redeployment and task alternation. Peres recognized that most cases occurred in women, and suggested that this was due to their weaker musculature and because more women were engaged in process work. He did point out, however, that men were not immune, and described similar conditions in male cane cutters, metal workers, milkers and carpenters.

In electromyographic studies Herberts & Kadefors (1976) and Herberts et al (1981) in Sweden demonstrated fatigue in the shoulder muscles of welders, thereby tending to confirm the belief that fatigue was an important factor in the aetiology of the shoulder pain commonly experienced by older welders.

Both Jonsson and Hagberg investigated objective measures of local muscle activity, fatigue and injury (Hagberg 1981a,b,c, 1984, Hagberg et al 1982, Jonsson 1982), their research being based on the hypothesis that fatigue was a precursor to many of the symptoms of neck, shoulder and arm pain currently occurring in workers. Studies of vocational electromyography (EMG) and serum creatine kinase (SCK) levels in people doing a variety of tasks carried out by Hagberg et al (1982) revealed that so-called light work, such as that done by cash register operators, led to significant changes in both EMG and SCK in local muscles. On the other hand, heavy cardiovascular work (bicycle ergometry) did not lead to such changes. In addition, local muscle endurance testing was undertaken and it was found that recovery took more than a day and, in some cases, up to 10 days. The lack of sufficiently sensitive measuring devices in the past has meant that the differences between local muscle fatigue and general physiological fatigue have not been able to be studied with such accuracy. This research helps to explain the possible mechanisms for local muscle fatigue which may lead to injury. In considering the relationships between load, the development of fatigue and injury, it is apparent that the quality and frequency of rest pauses need to be considered along with the level, duration and type of muscle work (Rohmert 1973a, b) and the capacity of the muscle for contraction.

MANAGEMENT

Acknowledgement of the incidence and problems of work-related musculoskeletal disorders demands that attention be given to the development of appropriate management approaches. In many research reports, the medical conditions have been described with care but their prevention in the workplace seems to have been considered to be secondary to their identification and treatment.

Work-related musculoskeletal disorders of the upper extremities and neck in Australia were first described by Perrott (1961), who was also concerned about prevention. Using a biomechanical model of injury and its prevention, Perrott described how unnecessary movement, shear strain, torsion and muscle imbalance could be minimized.

Ferguson (1967) supported Perrott's views and advocated preventive measures, particularly selection, training, education and supervision of workers; the reduction or variation in work load; and the application of ergonomics in workplace layout and work design.

A number of authors, concerned to apply the ergonomic principles of prevention in this area, have discussed the factors to be considered as well as measures which might be implemented. Van Wely was one of the first of such authors and, in 1970, he reported that a team of health and safety professionals demonstrated that they could predict, with reasonable accuracy, which tasks and work postures would lead to symptoms in operators and what parts of the worker's body would be affected. Van Wely (1970), in suggesting how these disorders may have been prevented, emphasized two approaches: the ergonomic design of tools, furniture and equipment; and the thorough training of workers in correct postures and work techniques.

Factors which have been listed as needing consideration when determining a preventive strategy for musculoskeletal disorder include the following (McPhee 1987):

1. External load factors (task and workplace design and work organization) which are required by the task:
   — number of movements
   — static muscle work
   — force
   — work postures determined by equipment and furniture
   — time worked without a break.
2. Factors which influence load but which may vary between individuals:
   — work postures adopted
   — unnecessary static muscle used
   — unnecessary force used

— number and duration of pauses taken
— speed and accuracy of movements.
3. Factors which alter the individual's response to a particular load (workplace, individual and social factors):
— age
— gender
— physical capabilities
— environmental factors such as noise and other contaminants
— time worked on repetitive tasks and job experience
— psychosocial variables.

Pre-employment screening

Susceptibility to strain appears to be a continuum, with the highly susceptible at one end and the highly resilient at the other. If so, there is an argument for screening out susceptible individuals before permitting them to work at jobs known to cause symptoms, but this is not easy, nor is it usually acceptable. For screening to be successful, there must be some understanding of why some people are resilient and others are not. A number of anatomical, physiological and psychological factors probably influence this resilience. However, much more evidence on the contribution of individual factors to musculoskeletal disorders is needed before it can be determined which people may be at greater risk. Some work in this area has been reported and the development of a screening procedure for occupational health professionals has been described by Waris (1979) and Waris et al (1979).

PREVENTION

Work breaks

Focusing upon the need for periodic rest from repetitive activity, Pulket & Kogi (1984) studied the 'free break' system in Thailand. They found that for a variety of reasons, most operators worked much longer than advisable without a break. Moreover, most operators continued to work when they felt the urge to rest. By comparison, complaints of fatigue in operators working in the 'fixed break' system were much fewer. Apart from more encouragement for operators to take breaks, ergonomic changes in the workplaces were also considered necessary.

Functional capacity assessment

The mismatch between the demands of the job and the worker's capacity at any particular time to undertake his/her work safely implies that physiotherapists must appreciate in some detail the demands of each task and the capabilities of individual workers, understanding that both are likely to change over time. Defining relevant worker capabilities and task characteristics is not easy and ideally requires pre-employment and periodic worker assessments and routine task analysis, as described in Chapter 3.

Intervention

Despite the problems inherent in studying these disorders, it is important to remember that most of them appear to be preventable as some researchers in Norway have shown (Westgaard & Aaras 1984, 1985). In Finland, a physiotherapist has reported on an intervention study which encompassed ergonomic improvements and health education, including the optimum use of furniture and equipment and why this is important, and physical activity in bank data entry operators (Kukkonen et al 1983). Results showed that the effects of the intervention were positive, with a significant decrease in signs and symptoms of musculoskeletal disorders occurring in the study group when compared with controls.

Intervention procedures for those who had developed musculoskeletal injuries were also examined by Ferguson & Duncan (1976), who reported that with physiotherapy, improvements occurred in subjects over a year. While they found it difficult to determine which aspects of the intervention by the physiotherapist had been beneficial, they confirmed, nonetheless, that the benefits were measurable both objectively and subjectively.

METHODS USED TO STUDY WORK-RELATED MUSCULOSKELETAL DISORDERS

Musculoskeletal disorders are studied in a variety of ways. In the laboratory, well-controlled experiments have been conducted to attempt to quantify load and outcomes, such as fatigue, through biomechanical modelling and calculations, EMG, performance of simulated tasks over set time periods, self-rating of effort, recording of heart and respiration rates and with the use of a variety of techniques and instruments to record and analyse postures and movements. Information from such studies is useful as a guide to how certain work may affect performance or lead to fatigue or even strain. However, for more directly applicable data, research in the workplace is necessary. In the workplace it is more difficult to measure muscle work directly, particularly when it involves fine movements of the hands and fingers and involves fixed postures. Most methods currently used in industry have been developed for the specific purpose of measuring heavy jobs and usually need modification and perhaps validation to be used in other ways (Karhu et al 1977, Karhu et al 1981, Corlett & Bishop 1976, Corlett et al 1979, Corlett 1983, Armstrong 1985, 1986).

The scientific study of work-related disorders of the locomotor system has developed comparatively recently. To begin with, researchers such as Lawrence (1955, 1961) and Lawrence & Aitken-Swan (1952) investigated straightforward, readily diagnosable rheumatic conditions associated with heavy work. Because of the lack of sufficiently sensitive measurement techniques, their methods of investigation were crude, usually with no attempt made to quantify the workload or identify the mechanisms of injury.

Generally speaking, given the demands of work and the need to minimise interference of workers while they perform their tasks, the simpler the methods of recording various parameters the more practically useful they are. For this reason and because, in some cases, sufficiently sophisticated recording and analysis techniques of work movements and postures have yet to be devised, much information about human physical performance in the workplace is basic. However, despite this, it has been possible to make comprehensive recommendations about the suitability of work for different groups of workers, and to identify risk factors for musculoskeletal disorders for the purposes of prevention.

Movement analysis

As outlined in Chapter 4, specific techniques such as VIRA (Persson & Kilbom 1983) developed in Sweden, use video recordings and templates on the video screen to define and quantify movements (especially of the neck and upper limbs) of workers engaged in fine manipulative tasks. Information on postures and movements from the video is keyed directly into a computer and analysis is carried out by a specially designed computer program. A similar method is currently being developed at the University of Melbourne (Green et al 1987). Instead of a template, it uses luminous markers on key anatomical points which are read, recorded and analysed directly by the computer. The CODA-3, described in Chapter 2, also provides an immediate, computerized 30 motion analysis.

Measurement of work-load

In the quantification of load at work, indirect measures such as production rates, the amount of force required or the number of movements made, are now commonly used. As early as 1973, for instance, Chaffin demonstrated that fatigue resulting from sustained or repeated contractions led to a measurable decrement in performance as well as various discomfort states (Chaffin 1973). However, the direct quantification of physical load, particularly muscle load, on individuals at work has proved most difficult.

Epidemiology

Another approach in the study of these disorders is the use of epidemiological techniques which have become increasingly sophisticated with the aid of computers. Given that the magnitude of risk is sufficient and the group being examined is large enough, jobs with higher than expected risks of disorders can be identified. However, with disorders which are common in the population as a whole, it may be difficult to determine the contribution made by occupation, as opposed to that made by non-work factors. Demonstrating the link between common disorders and work is often quite difficult, especially when a number of interacting risk factors are present (Hernberg 1984).

In the epidemiology of occupational disorders, one must examine the so called 'determinants' or causes of the disorders, as well as the 'outcomes' or the disorders themselves. This is a reasonably satisfactory approach as long as the mechanisms by which the disorders occur can be described in some way. Unfortunately, with many musculoskeletal disorders, these are not straightforward as there is no universally accepted explanation for how they occur.

However, some progress has been made in this area in the last 10 years. The interaction may be illustrated in the following way:

STRESS ... THE MUSCULOSKELETAL ... STRAIN
SYSTEM

or

DETERMINANTS ... MECHANISMS OF ... OUTCOME
INJURY

| (Physical and psychological stress factors) | (Patho-mechanics) | (Pain, dysfunction) |

Therefore, the main problems with studying work-related musculoskeletal disorders epidemiologically are associated with the:

1. measurement of *determinants* (causes) or exposure to risk factors within and outside the workplace
2. understanding the *mechanisms of injury* and
3. delineating the *outcome*, which in this case is symptoms, usually pain, sometimes accompanied by other forms of dysfunction such as weakness or stiffness.

Physiotherapists working in the field of ergonomics have the appropriate background necessary for involvement in research studies concerned with such epidemiological investigations, since they have a clear appreciation for causes, mechanisms and outcomes of injury. An epidemiological study carried out in Australia by a team of physiotherapists provides the background for a discussion of some of the problems associated with this type of research. That study is outlined below.

An epidemiological study of neck and upper extremity disorders in keyboard workers

This study, conducted by a team of physiotherapists of which the author was the principal investigator, within one branch of a government department in Sydney, was initiated to investigate the reasons for increasing reports of work-related neck and upper extremity disorders (commonly referred to at that time in Australia as Repetition Strain Injuries or 'RSI') in dedicated keyboard operators involved in data entry tasks.

The study as a whole aimed at answering a wide range of general questions of particular interest to physiotherapists in ergonomics and occupational health about the prevalence of symptoms in the neck and upper extremities and other parts of the body and their relationship to work postures and techniques in those working in the branch under study. It was conducted over a 2- year period from January 1984 to May 1986 and consisted of three stages: an initial biographic questionnaire (referred to as the BIOQ) administered early in 1984; checklists of ergonomic factors in the workplace and work postures and movements, administered later in that year; and a self-administered questionnaire (referred to as the SAQ), accompanied by an interview and physical examination, all of which were administered at the same visit 2 years later. As the primary research methods used were developed specifically for this project, it was treated as an elaborate pilot study. This enabled the gathering of some important information and testing of the method at the same time.

The first part of this study was directed towards resolving the question: is there a difference in the occurrence of these complaints between workers engaged in high intensity keyboard work and those doing routine clerical work? To answer the question, information on a range of personal and work variables was collected. Some methodological issues regarding the use of certain types of data-gathering techniques were also addressed.

Subjects and methods

The keyboard operators, who were all female, became the study group, while the 'controls' were all non-keyboard operators such as clerical assistants, supervisors and administrators and pharmacists, both female and male. Keyboard operators were identified with information from two sources: their classification as Data Processing Operators (DPOs) and those who spent more than 4 hours keying per day on average. Of the 295 staff in the branch, 243 (82.4%) consented to take part: 126 keyboard operators and 117 non keyboard operators, of whom 32 were male. Because of significantly different personal and demographic characteristics of males and females in the study, males have not been included in this summary of findings.

Symptoms of pain, ache or discomfort in the previous 4 weeks, as reported by the subject, were used as the outcome variable under study, as this approach had been successful in several projects previously reported. These symptoms were marked on a body chart by the subject in a self-administered questionnaire and at interview by an interviewer on a similar body chart. No attempt was made to diagnose the conditions.

The severity of the reported symptoms and their impact on the individual were determined by interview with questions on whether the subject had experienced any problems with three categories of activities: work, activities of daily living and leisure-time pursuits. Four levels of disruption emerged: none, mild (difficulty with the activity but nothing more), moderate (need to modify activity or how it was done) and severe (activity had to be stopped).

An attempt was made also to identify and investigate the influence of the most commonly cited work and personal variables believed by the subjects to contribute to the occurrence of these disorders.

In addition to analysis of selected data, some methodological issues were addressed such as the difference in reporting of symptoms at interview and in a self-administered questionnaire; the usefulness of checklists in gathering data on ergonomics and work techniques and postures; and the benefits and drawbacks of using a standardized physical assessment to determine physical signs and symptoms of neck and upper extremity disorders.

Other information on the work and how it was done, the workplace and work organization, and the provision of workers' compensation for 'RSI' in the branch, was also collected.

Results

The main finding from this study is straightforward: the keyboard operators reported significantly more pain, ache or discomfort in the neck and/or upper extremities than clerical workers ($p < 0.01$) in the previous 4 weeks, even when major work and personal variables were taken into account. 61% of all female subjects reported symptoms in these body regions. The most frequently reported anatomical areas with symptoms were the shoulders, the upper trapezius region of the neck, the forearms and the hands, with differences being highly significant between keyboard operators and non-operators, particularly in the shoulders (see Fig. 5.1).

Other variables found to be associated with complaints to a significant degree were lack of job satisfaction ($p < 0.05$) and working a regular 9-day fortnight, i.e. working longer hours for nine days and having the 10th day free ($p < 0.05$).

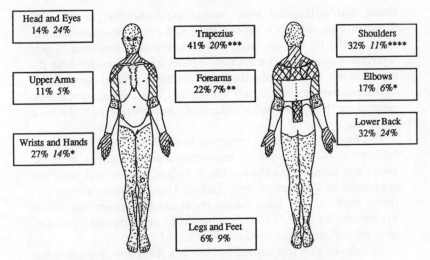

Fig. 5.1 Distribution of complaints recorded by 212 female keyboard operators. The level of significance in the difference between keyboard operators and non-keyboard operators is shown by:

*   p <0.05
**   p <0.01
***   p <0.005
****   p <0.001

NB. The first percentage in the box refers to keyboard operators while the second percentage refers to clerical workers.

On the whole, workers' compensation claims for 'RSI' by the study group reflected the neck and upper extremity symptoms reported and the impact they had on the individual, but there was a wide range of symptom severity leading to a claim.

Nearly 29% of all female subjects reported low-back pain, ache or discomfort. Although the differences between the two groups were not significant, the generally higher than expected level of low-back symptoms in a relatively young group of workers does tend to confirm other research findings which have indicated that these symptoms are common in sedentary workers.

There appeared to be no major differences between those who left the study and those who stayed, particularly in the important areas of age, job classification, workers' compensation claims for 'RSI' and reported symptoms.

Discussion

Because the study was conducted over a 2-year period, the expectation that differential losses would occur because of the high turnover rate, especially among keyboard operators, was realized. As a result, by the last stage, the investigation was of a largely 'survivor' population. Such a situation has implications for both the experiencing and the reporting of symptoms related to work, as well as variables such as job satisfaction. Therefore, information gleaned on those who had left the study was considered to be most important.

The finding that factors reflecting both physical and psychological aspects of work and its organization are associated with the symptoms supports the theory that their development and reporting are related to a variety of work factors. Unfortunately, a cross-sectional study of this kind cannot conclusively support any causal hypothesis. As regards the contribution of personal and social factors, no significant associations were found.

As this analysis was carried out on data from two cross-sectional studies, 2 years apart, few conclusions can be drawn from the results without further analysis, regarding the reasons why some subjects claimed workers' compensation for 'RSI' and others did not. However, there was some evidence that the disruptiveness of the symptoms related more to whether or not the individual had been diagnosed as having 'RSI', and the approach that had been taken in managing the disorder, than to work-load factors. The iatrogenic nature of symptoms being classified as 'RSI' therefore should be of great concern. Consideration must be given to developing strategies for the most effective prevention and management of musculoskeletal disorders in the workplace if such problems are to be avoided in the future.

As in all research of work-related musculoskeletal disorders, a number of problems were encountered in the design and analysis aspects of this study. However, unlike most similar projects, it was possible to study all employees in one branch, rather than just those who had reported symptoms, and to reduce the effects of misclassification of workers as keyboard operators. In addition, given the unvaried nature of the job and uniform configuration of the equipment used, a fairly accurate estimate of the minimum work-load for each individual keyboard operator could be made.

As physiotherapists in ergonomics and occupational health are likely to be involved in other studies of this nature, some comments on problems encountered in this study could be of value to future researchers. These problems arose largely from three sources:

— The lack of a 'hard' outcome variable, the use of reported symptoms being the only feasible alternative for this study
— The complex and largely unexplored nature of conditions labelled as 'RSI' in Australia and work-related musculoskeletal symptoms generally
— The lack of suitable techniques for recording and analysing work postures and movements, particularly in fixed, highly repetitive manual tasks.

The first problem was addressed by accompanying the questionnaire and interview with a physical assessment in which the assessor was given no information on reported symptoms. Future analysis of these data should reveal more about the relationship between reported symptoms and musculoskeletal dysfunction, as well as providing more objective information on the symptoms.

The second problem arose from the fact that 'RSI' appears to have been as much a social as a health phenomenon and as such, any investigation of it required a broad approach. This necessitated a wide range of questions with little opportunity to explore any area in depth. The one area in which some depth was attempted (leisure activities and hobbies) proved very difficult to code and analyse.

One aspect, job dissatisfaction, was investigated in greater depth in the second questionnaire. The results of this future analysis may pinpoint specific areas of dissatisfaction related to the reporting of symptoms and the relationship, if any, with claims for 'RSI'.

In 1983, the lack of information on a wide range of factors which may have been related to symptoms and claims for 'RSI' meant that many questions were framed in very simplistic terms and lack of association in this study does not mean that their further investigation is not warranted.

The third problem area was the development of a simple, reliable method for recording and analysing details of work postures and movements in sedentary jobs. Such information is necessary if the link between symptoms in the neck, upper trunk and upper extremities and particular aspects of the task is to be made. The checklist developed for this study was difficult to use, code and analyse and therefore could not be readily adapted for other investigations. However, it did encourage very close and systematic observation of general sitting posture, the posture and movements of the upper trunk, shoulders, arms and hands, and the careful recording of observations. Through this process, it was possible to identify individuals by the posture and movements of their hands, arms and shoulders and by their keying technique. It became obvious very quickly that despite an apparently uniform work-load, the actual load imposed on the musculoskeletal system of each individual was different. It therefore can be concluded, among keyboard operators at least, that analysing the work as it is performed by one or two individuals may not be sufficient to determine why some people develop symptoms and others do not.

From the work being done in Sweden and Australia in the development of video/computer analysis of work postures and movements, it would appear that this method is likely to be more efficient and accurate in recording such information, especially in sedentary work.

CONCLUDING REMARKS

Much is now known about the relationship between the occupational loading of the musculoskeletal system and the development of postural discomfort and pain. Most importantly, it appears, from the investigations carried out to date, that such conditions arise from a range of factors, both physical and psychological, and may be exacerbated by social factors. Their occurrence appears to be predictable, given certain combinations of these factors, and, therefore, theoretically at least, they should be preventable in the workplace. However, the mechanisms by which such symptoms develop into pathological conditions, requiring treatment and other action to reverse, is still very poorly understood.

The contribution of physiotherapists to knowledge in these areas has been considerable in several countries. However, as in the past, it is still possible for work-related musculoskeletal disorders to be overlooked, underestimated in their impact, or over-simplified in their diagnosis. Physiotherapists have developed a considerable body of knowledge and experience in working with these conditions and, with many questions still remaining to be answered, it is necessary, if such disorders are to be controlled in the future, that they publish and publicize their findings as widely and as frequently as possible.

REFERENCES

Aoyama H, Ohara H, Oze Y, Itani T 1979 Recent trends in research in occupational cervical disorder. Journal of Human Ergology 8: 39–45

Armstrong T J, Chaffin D B 1979 Carpal tunnel syndrome and selected personal attributes. Journal of Occupational Medicine 21: 481–486

Armstong T J, Foulke J, Joseph B, Goldstein S 19S2 Investigation of cumulative trauma disorders in a poultry processing plant. American Industrial Hygiene Association Journal 43: 103–116

Armstrong T J, Joseph B, Woolley C 1984 Analysis of jobs for control of upper extremity cumulative trauma disorders. Proceedings of the 1984 International Conference on Occupational Ergonomics, Toronto, pp 416–420

Armstrong T J 1985 Upper extremity posture: definition, measurement and control. Proceedings of the International Ergonomics Symposium: The Ergononics of Working Postures: Models, Methods and Cases, Zadar

Armstrong T J 1986 upper extremity posture: definition, measurement and control. In: Wilson, J, Corrlett E N and Manenica I (eds) Ergonomics of working postures: models, methods and cases. Taylor and Francis, London, pp 59–73

Bammer G 1986a VDUs and musculoskeletal problems at the Australian National University—a case study. Proceedings of the International Scientific Conference on Work with Display Units, Stockholm, pp 243–246

Bammer G 1988b Musculoskeletal problems associated with VDU use at the Australian National University—a case study of changes in work practices. In: Karwowski W (ed) Trends in ergonomics/human factors III. Elsevier Science Publishers B V, Amsterdam, pp 285–293

Björkstén M 1984 Musculoskeletal disorders among medical secretaries. Abstracts of the XXI International Occupational Health Congress, Dublin, p 31

Blood W 1942 Tenosynovitis in industrial workers. British Medical Journal 2: 468

Bogduk N, Marsland A 1988 The cervical zygapophysial joints as a source of neck pain. Spine 6: 610–617

Cannon L J, Bernacki E K, Walter S D 1981 Personal and occupational factors associated with carpal tunnel syndrome. Journal of Occupational Medicine 23: 255–258

Carlsöö S, Mayr J 1974 A study of the load on joints and muscles in work with pneumatic hammer and bolt gun. Scandinavian Journal of Work Environment and Health 11: 32–38

Chaffin D B 1973 Localized nuscle fatigue–definition and measurement. Journal of Occupational Medicine 15: 346–354

Conn H R 1031 Tenosynovitis. Ohio State Medical Journal 27: 713–716

Corlett E N, Bishop R P 1976 A technique for assessing postural discomfort. Ergonomics 2: 175–182

Corlett E N, Madeley S J, Manenica I 1979 Posture targetting: A technique for recording working postures. Ergonomics 3: 357–366

Corlett E N 1983 Analysis and evaluation of working posture. In: Kvalseth T O (ed) Ergonomics of workstation design. Butterworths, London, pp 1–18

Dainoff M J 1982 Occupational stress factors in visual display terminal (VDT) operation: a review of empirical research. Behaviour and Information Technology 1: 141–176

Dainoff M 1984 Ergonomics of office automation—a conceptual overview. Proceedings of the 1984 International Conference on Occupational Ergonomics, Toronto, pp 72–80.

Devolvé N, Queinnec Y 1983 Operator's activities at CRT terminals: a behavioural approach. Ergonomics 26: 329–340

Duncan J, Ferguson D 1974 Keyboard operating posture and symptoms in operating. Ergonomics 17: 651–662

128   ERGONOMICS

Feldman R G, Goldman R, Keyserling W M 1983 Peripheral nerve entrapment syndromes and ergonomic factors. American Journal of Industrial Medicine 4: 661–681

Ferguson D A 1967 Report on health survey of telegraph officers. School of Public Health and Tropical Medicine, University of Sydney

Ferguson D A 1971a Repetition injuries in process workers. Medical Journal of Australia 2: 408–412

Ferguson D A 1971b An Australian study of telegraphists' cramp. British Journal of Industrial Medicine 28: 280–285

Ferguson D A 1974 Occupational fatigue. Bulletin of the Postgraduate Committee in Medicine, University of Sydney 30: 138–147

Ferguson D A 1976 Posture, aching and body build in telephonists. Journal of Human Ergology 5: 183–186

Ferguson D A, Duncan J 1972 A study of the effect of equipment design on posture. Scientific Proceedings of the Australian and New Zealand Society of Occupational Medicine, Melbourne, pp 56–60

Ferguson D A, Duncan J 1974 Keyboard design and operating posture. Ergonomics 17: 731–744

Ferguson D A, Duncan J 1976 A trial of physiotherapy for symptoms in keyboard operating. Australian Journal of Physiotherapy 22: 61–72

Fine L J, Silverstein B A, Armstrong T J, Anderson C A 1984 An alternative way of detecting cumulative trauma disorders of the upper extremities in the workplace. Proceedings of the 1984 International Conference on Occupational Ergonomics, Toronto, pp 425–429

Flowerdew R E, Bode O B 1942 Tenosynovitis in untrained farm workers. Letter to the Editor. British Medical Journal 2: 367

Goldie I 1964 Epicondylitis lateralis humeri. A pathogenetical study. Acta Chirurgica Scandinavica Suppl 339: 43–47

Grandjean E, Hünting W, Nishiyama K 1982a Preferred VDT workstation setting, body posture and physical impairments. Journal of Human Ergology 11: 45–54

Grandjean E, Nishiyama, Hünting W, Piderman M 1982b A laboratory study on preferred and imposed settings of a VDT workstation. Behaviour and Information Technology 1: 289–304

Grandjean E, Hünting, Maeda K, Läubli T 1983a Constrained postures at office workstations. In: Kvalseth T O (ed) Ergonomics of workstation design. Butterworths, London, pp 19–27

Grandjean E, Hünting W, Piderman M 1983b VDT workstation design: preferred settings and their effects. Human Factors 25: 161–175

Grandjean E 1984a Postural problems at office machine workstations. In: Grandjean E (ed) Ergonomics and health in modern offices. Taylor and Francis, London, pp 445–455

Grandjean E 1984b Postures and the design of VDT workstations. Behaviour and Information Technology 3: 301–311

Grandjean E, Hünting, Nishiyama K 1984 Preferred VDT workstation design, body posture and physical impairments. Applied Ergonomics 15: 99–104

Green R A, Briggs C A, Wrigley T U et al 1987 Application of an objective, computerized video image processing system for the assessment of sitting posture among keyboard operators. Proceedings of the 24th Annual Conference of the Ergonomics Society of Australia, Melbourne, pp 184–195

Grieco A 1986 Sitting posture: an old problem and a new one. Ergonomics 29: 345–362

Hagberg M 1981a On evaluation of local muscular load and fatigue by electromyography. Arbete och Halsa 24: 552

Hagberg M 1981b Electromyographic signs of shoulder muscular fatigue in two elevated arm positions. American Journal of Physical Medicine 60: 111–121

Hagberg M 1981c Muscular endurance and surface electromyogram in isometric and dynamic exercise. Journal of Applied Physiology 51: 1–7

Hagberg M 1982 Local shoulder muscular strain—symptoms and disorders. Journal of Human Ergology 11: 99–108

Hagberg M, Michaelson G, Ortelius A 1982 Serum creatine kinase as an indicator of local muscle strain in experimental and occupational work. International Archives of Occupational and Environmental Health 50: 377–388

Hagberg M 1984 Delayed effects on muscular endurance, electromyography, creatine kinase and shoulder discomfort in lifting tasks. Abstracts of the XXI International Occupational Health Congress, Dublin, p 366

Hagberg M, Kvarnström S 1984 Assessment of industrial myofascial shoulder pain by muscular endurance and EMG fatigue studies. Abstacts of the XXI International Occupational Health Congress, Dublin, p 365

Harms-Ringdahl K 1986 On assessment of shoulder exercise and load-elicited pain in the cervial spine. Scandinavian Journal of Rehabiltation Medicine Suppl 14

Herberts P, Kadefors R 1976 A study of painful shoulders in welders. Acta Orthopaedica Scandinavica 47: 381–387

Herberts P, Kadefors R, Andersson G, Petersen I 1981 Shoulder pain in industry: an epidemiological study on welders. Acta Orthopaedica Scandinavica 52: 299–306

Hernberg S 1984 Work-related diseases—some problems in study design. Scandinavian Journal of Work Environment and Health 10: 367–372

Hocking B 1987 Epidemiological aspects of 'repetition strain injury', in Telecom Australia. Medical Journal of Australia 147: 218–222

Howard N J 1937 Peritendinitis crepitans. A muscle-effort syndrome. Journal of Bone and Joint Surgery 19: 447–459

Howard N J 1938 A new concept of tenosynovitis and the pathology of physiologic effort. American Journal of Surgery 42: 723–730

Hunter D 1959 Health industry, 1st edn, Penguin, Harmondsworth, pp 230–234

Hünting W, Grandjean E, Maeda K 1980a Constrained postures in accounting machine operators. Applied Ergonomics 11: 145–149

Hünting W, Läubli T, Grandjean E 1980b Constrained postures of VDU operations. In: Grandjean E, Vigliani E (eds) Ergonomic aspects of visual display terminals. Taylor and Francis, London, pp 175–184

Hünting W, Läubli T, Grandjean E 1981 Postural and visual loads at VDT workplaces I. Constrained postures. Ergonomics 24: 917–931

Jonsson B 1982 Measurement and evaluation of local muscular strain in the shoulder during constrained work. Journal of Human Ergology 11: 73–88

Karhu O, Kansi P, Kuorinka I 1977 Correcting work postures in industry: A practical method for analysis. Applied Ergonomics 8: 199–201

Karhu O, Harkonen R, Sorvali P, Vepsalainen P 1981 Observing working postures in industry: examples of OWAS application. Applied Ergonomics 12: 13–17

Kelsey J L 1982 Monographs in epidemiology and biostatistics, Vol 3. Epidemiology of musculoskeletal disorders. Oxford University Press, New York, pp 145–167

Kilom Å, Lagerlof, Liew M, Broberg E 1984a An ergonomic study of notified cases of occupational musculoskeletal disease. Proceedings of the 1984 International Conference on Occupational Ergonomics, Toronto, pp 256–260

Kilbom Å, Persson J, Jonsson B 1984b Risk factors for cervicobrachial disorders—a 2-year follow-up study. Abstracts of the XXI International Occupational Health Congress, Dublin, p 362

Kilbom Å, Persson J 1985 Low capacity of the shoulder muscles as a risk factor for occupational cervicobrachial disorders. In: Brown I, Goldsmith R, Coombes K, Sinclair M (eds) Proceedings of the 9th Congress of the

International Ergonomics Association, Bournemouth pp 553–555

Kilbom Å, Persson J, Jonsson B G 1986 Disorders of the cervicobrachial region among female workers in the electronics industry. International Journal of Industrial Ergonomics 1: 37–47

Komoike Y, Horiguchi S 1971 Fatigue assessment on key punch operators, typists and others. Ergonomics 14: 101–109

Kukkonen R, Luopajärvi T, Riihimaki V 1983 Prevention of fatigue among data entry operators. In: Kvalseth T O (ed) Ergonomics of workstation design. Butterworths, London, pp 28–34

Kuorinka I, Koskinen P 1979 Occupational rheumatic diseases and upper limb strain in manual jobs in a light mechanical industry. Scandinavian Journal of Work Environment and Health 5 (Suppl 3): 39–47

Kuorinka I, Videman T, Lepisto M 1981 Reliability of a vibration test in screening for predisposition to tenosynovitis. European Journal of Applied Physiology 47: 365–376

Kuorinka I, Viikari-Juntura E 1982 Prevalence of neck and upper limb disorders (NLD) and work-load in different occupational groups. Problems in classification and diagnosis. Journal of Human Ergology 11: 65–72

Kuorinka I 1983 Subjective discomfort in a simulated repetitive task. Ergonomics 28: 108–1101

Kurppa K, Waris P, Rokkanen P 1979a Tennis elbow: lateral elbow pain syndrome. Scandinavian Journal of Work Environment and Health 5 (suppl 3): 15–18

Kurppa K, Waris P, Rokkanen P 1979b Peritendinitis and tenosynovitis: a review. Scandinavian Journal of Work Environment and Health 5 (suppl 3): 19–24

Kvarnström S 1983 Occurrence of musculoskeletal disorders in manufacturing industry, with special attention to occupational shoulder disorders. Scandinavian Journal of Rehabilitation Medicine suppl 8: 1–114

Läubli T, Thomas C, Zeier H 1984 Causative factors of visual and postural problems in VDT work. Abstracts of the XXI International Occupational Health Congress, Dublin, p 35

Läubli T 1986 Review on working conditions and postural discomfort in VDT work. Abstracts of the International Scientific Conference on Work with Display Units, Stockholm pp 3–6

Lawrence J S Aitken-Swan 1952 Rheumatism in coal miners I: Rheumatic complaints. British Journal of Industrial Medicine 9: 1–18

Lawrence J S 1955 Rheumatism in coal miners III: Occupational factors. British Journal of Industrial Medicine 12: 249–261

Lawrence J S 1961 Rheumatism in cotton operatives. British Journal of Industrial Medicine 18: 270–276

Luopajärvi T, Kuorinka I, Virolainen M, Holmberg M 1979 Prevalence of tenosynovitis and other injuries of the upper extremities in repetitive work. Scandinavian Journal of Work Environment and Health 5 (suppl 3): 48–55

McPhee B J 1880 Tenosynovitis–the physiotherapists' viewpoint. Proceedings of the 20th NSW Industrial Safety Convention and Exhibition, pp 15–19

McPhee B 1987 Work-related musculoskeletal disorders of the neck and upper extremities in workers engaged in light, highly repetitive work. In: Osterholz U, Karmaus W, Hullman B Ritz B (eds) Proceedings of an International Symposium: Work-Related Musculoskeletal Disorders, Bonn, pp 244–258

Maeda K, Hünting W, Grandjean E 1980 Localized fatigue in accounting machine operators. Journal of Occupational Medicine 22: 810–816

Maeda K 1981 Concept and criteria of occupational cervicobrachial disorder in Japan. Proceedings of the Seminar on Ergonomics and Repetitive Tasks, Nordic Council of Ministers, Helsinki (Unpublished)

Maeda K, Horoguchi S, Hosokawa M 1982 History of the studies on occupational cervicobrachial disorder in Japan and remaining problems. Journal of Human Ergology 11: 17–29

Nakaseko M, Tokunaga R, Hosokawa M 1982 History of occupational cervicobrachial disorder in Japan. Journal of Human Ergology 11: 7–16

National Health and Medical Research Council—NH&MRC 1982 Approved occupational health guide. Repetition strain injuries. Commonwealth Department of Health

National Occupational Health and Safety Commission—NOHSC 1985 Interim Report of the RSI Committee. AGPS, Canberra

National Occupational Health and Safety Commission—NOHSC 1986a Repetition strain injury. A report and model code of practice. AGPS, Canberra

National Occupational Health and Safety Commission 1986b The prevention and management of occupational overuse syndrome. General Code of Practice, NOHSC, Sydney.

Ohara H, Nakagiri S, Itani T et al 1978 Occupational health hazards resulting from elevated work-rate situations. Journal of Human Ergology 5: 173–182

Ong C N, Phoon W O 1986 Influence of age on VDU work. Abstracts of the International Scientific Conference on Work with Display Units, Stockholm, pp 17–20

Onishi N, Nomura H, Sakal K 1973 Fatigue and strength of upper limb muscles of flight reservation system operators. Journal of Human Ergology 2: 133–141

Onishi N, Nomura H, Sakai K et al 1976 Shoulder muscle tenderness and physical features of female industrial workers. Journal of Human Ergology 5: 87–102

Onishi N Sakai K, Itani T, Shindo 11 1977 Muscle load and fatigue of film rolling workers. Journal of Human Ergology 8: 179–186

Ono Y, Masuda K, Iwata M et al 1982 Fatigue and health problems of workers in a home for mentally and physically handicapped persons. Proceedings of the 8th International Association Congress, Tokyo, pp 158–159

Peres N J C 1961 Process work without strain. Australian Factory pp 1–12, July, Tait, Sydney. Also published in 1964 in; Human factors in Industrial strains. Tait, Sydney pp 59–81

Perrot J W 1961 Anatomical factors in occupational trauma. Medical Journal of Australia 1: 73–82

Persson J, Kilbom Å 1983 VIRA—en enkel videofilmtecknik for registrering och analys av arbetsstallninger och rorelser. Undersokningrapport 1983: 10. Arbetarskyddsstyrelsen, Stockhohm

Pulket C, Kogi K 1984 Fatigue of visual display unit operators in the free break system. Abstracts of the XXI International Occupational Health Congress, Dublin, p 364

Ramazzini B 1713 De Morbis Artificum (Diseases of workers). Translated by Wright W C, pp 15,21,23. University of Chicago Press, Chicago, 1940

Reed J V Harcourt A K 1943 Tenosynovitis: an industrial disability. American Journal of Surgery 62: 392–396

Repetition Stain Injuries (RSI) Taskforce 1985 Repetition strain injuries in the Australian Public Service. Taskforce Report, AGPS, Canberra

Rohmert W 1973a Problems in determining rest allowances I. Applied Ergonomics 4: 91–95

Rohmert W 1973b Problems of determining rest allowances II. Applied Ergonomics 4: 158–162

Silverstein B A, Fine L J, Armstrong T J, Joseph B 1984 The effect of forceful and repetitive work on the upper extremity. Proceedings of the 1984 International Conference on Ergonomics, Toronto, p 351

Silverstein B A 1985 The prevalence of upper extremity cumulative trauma disorders in industry. A Dissertation. Occupational Health and Safety Engineering, University of Michigan

Silverstein B A, Fine L J, Armstrong T J 1987 Occupational factors and carpal tunnel syndrome. American Journal of Industrial Medicine 11: 343–358

Smiley J A 1951 The hazards of rope making. British Journal of Industrial Medicine 8: 265–270

Smith M J, Cohen B G F, Stanunerjohn L W 1981 An investigation of health complaints and job stress in video display operations. Human Factors 23: 387–400

South Australian Health Commission 1984 Repetition strain symptoms and working conditions among keyboard workers engaged in data entry or word processing in the South Australian Public Service (a report). SA Health Commission

Springer T 1982 VDT workstations—comparative evaluation of alternatives. Applied Ergonomics 13: 211–212

Stammerjohn L W, Smith M J, Cohen B G F 1981 Evaluation of work-station design factors in VDT operations. Human Factors 23: 401–412

Thompson A R, Plewes L W, Shaw E G 1951 Peritendinitis crepitans and simple tenosynovitis: a clinical study of 544 cases in industry. British Journal of Industrial Medicne 8: 150– 160

Valencia F 1986 Local nuscle fatigue. Medical Journal of Australia 145: 327–330

Van Wely P 1970 Design and disease. Applied Ergonomics 1: 262–269

Viikari-Juntura E 1984 Tenosynovitis, peritendinitis and the tennis elbow syndrome. Scandinavian Journal of Work Environment and Health 10: 443–449

Waersted M, Bjørklund R, Westgaard R H 1986 Generation of muscle tension related to a demand of contiuing attention. Unpublished abstract of a paper presented at the International Scientific Conference on Work with Display Units, Stockholm

Waris P 1979 Occupational cervicobrachial syndromes. Scandinavian Journal of Work Environment and Health 5 (suppl 3): 3–14

Waris P, Kuorinka I, Kurppa K et al 1979 Epidemiologic screening of occupational neck and upper limb disorders. Scandinavian Journal of Work Environment and Health, 5 (suppl 3): 25–38

Webb R D G, Tack D, McIlroy W E 1984 Assessment of musculoskeletal discomfort in a large clerical office: a case study. Procecdings of the 1984 International Conference on Occupational Ergonomics, Toronto, pp 392–396

Weber A 1981 Reactions to repetitive tasks. Proceedings of the Seminar on Ergonomics and Repetitive Tasks, Nordic Council of Ministers, Helsinki (Unpublished)

Welch R 1972 The ergonometrics of tenosynovitis. Proceedings of a Seminar on Occupational Injuries conducted by the Royal Australasian College of Surgeons, Melbourne, pp 145–147

Welch R 1973 The measurement of physiological predisposition to tenosynovitis. Ergonomics 16: 665–668

Westgaard R H, Aaras A 1984 Postural muscle strain as a causal factor in the development of musculo-skeletal illnesses. Applied Ergonomics 15: 162–174

Westgaard R H, Aarås A 1985 The effect of improved workplace design on the development of work-related musculoskeletal illnesses. Applied Ergonomics 16: 91–97

Wickstrom G 1982 Drawbacks in clinical diagnoses in epidemiological research on work-related musculoskeletal morbidity. Scandinavian Journal of Work Environment and Health 8 (suppl 1): 97–99

6. Neck and shoulder load and load-elicited pain in sitting work postures

K. Harms-Ringdahl and K. Schüldt

INTRODUCTION

Load-elicited pain or discomfort in the neck and/or shoulder region associated with prolonged work in sitting postures is an increasing problem with which physiotherapists involved in occupational health care or vocational rehabilitation must cope. The introduction of ergonomic measures, changes in work organization, training in the use of load-reducing-work postures and movements and the frequent use of micropauses are some of the methods used to reduce pain and to increase function. Which particular measure is of major importance often has to be decided for each individual by the physiotherapist after a careful analysis of the work tasks, postures and movements. Further, if ergonomic measures are to be of help they often require individual training supervised by a physiotherapist, often in a realistic work situation. This chapter presents a theoretical basis developed from studies which were concerned with neck and shoulder load and load-reducing measures.

THE DEMANDS OF SITTING WORK POSTURES

Work tasks nowadays require various specialized skills, of which rapid performance is one. There is also a tendency towards specialization in movement patterns. Sitting work postures are often used when the hands are employed for a considerable part of the working day, and often there are additional high demands on vision: for example, for close reading or for seeing in detail the objects being handled. The sizes and positions of the work objects, as well as lighting conditions, often govern neck, arm and hand movements and positions and thus muscle tension levels. Traditionally, sitting work—unlike standing—was looked upon as light work, since sitting work made lesser demands on such features as lifting capacity and respiratory–circulatory function. But recent research has shown that the way in which many sitting work tasks are organized often entails the maintenance of static neck, arm and hand positions or demands monotonous, repetitive movements, so inducing sustained muscle work.

NECK AND SHOULDER LOAD—CHARACTERISTICS AND CONCERNS

One way of defining mechanical load—thus not taking circulatory load into account—is to use the concept of *load moment of force* about a defined axis. This is expressed in Newtonmetres (Nm) (Fig. 6.1). Usually an induced load moment is counteracted by *muscle activity* causing a muscular moment. The complexity of the anatomy makes calculation of the muscular forces in the cervical spine complicated, but muscle activity levels in different work postures can be recorded with electromyography (EMG), which reflects the muscle load and allows comparisons between different movements or postures.

However, a load moment, if applied at the limit of a motion range, can also be counteracted by *passive soft tissues structures*, such as ligaments, joint capsules and muscular connective tissue. In such circumstances, the muscular activity can be low despite a high induced load moment.

One method of analysing the load moment in ergonomics in a given posture is to use calculations of moment arm lengths from photos or video displays (Fig. 6.1) combined with body segment parameters, burden weights and other external forces acting on the

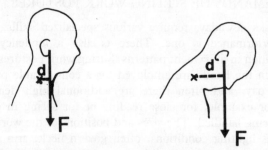

Fig. 6.1 Gravity force (F) induced by the weight of the head-and-neck and its moment arm (d) about the bilateral axis of lower-cervical-upper-thoracic motion segment (C7–T1). The load moment (Nm; F × d) of C7–T1 increases with increased neck flexion (left, neutral position compared to right, much flexed).

body. In this way, the induced load moment about the shoulder joint or cervical spine axis can be calculated (Harms-Ringdahl et al 1986b).

However, the induced load moments only partly reflect the joint compressive and shear forces and the load on the different neck structures: neck muscle activity due to arm work is not taken into account. Neck and shoulder muscle activity levels are influenced in a complicated way by the load moment induced by the arms; by forces applied at, and weights held in the hands; and by the moment induced by the weight of the head and neck. In addition, demands on precision, speed and concentration, which raise the psychological stress level, add further muscle activity to that induced by the load moments.

Level of load considered as 'high' or 'low' depends on the load duration and on repetitiveness. To assess the magnitude of the induced load moment, its relation to the maximum muscular moment (strength) about a joint axis at a given joint angle can be calculated. This relationship is termed the Muscular Strength Utilization Ratio (MUR). The possible portion of the counteracting moment caused by passive joint structures is ignored. The proportion of neck muscle strength required to counteract the load moment induced by the weight of the head and neck varies with neck angle (Harms-Ringdahl & Schüldt 1988) (Fig. 6.2). Thus, in a neutral, vertical position, approximately 2% of the maximum muscular strength has to be used. In the slightly flexed neck position, 10% is used and in a much flexed position, 17%. Assessments of neck and shoulder muscular activity levels in relation to fatigue can be recorded with EMG (Jonsson 1978, 1982; Hagberg 1981 a, b; Petrofsky & Phillips 1982). 2 to 5 % of a maximum voluntary contraction (MVC) in the upper trapezius causes signs of fatigue if maintained for an hour, and this contraction level is easily reached by arm flexion or abduction even without loading the hand. Since many shoulder muscles act to stabilize the shoulder girdle joints, arm work which might seem dynamic might entail static shoulder muscle activity as well. The possibilities of allowing micropauses, described as very short but frequently repeated pauses with no muscle activity, are of importance for muscle performance and influence the assessment of muscular load over the work day.

For assessing the occurrence of extreme positions in different work postures, recordings of neck position in relation to adjacent body segments can be compared with the voluntary motion range (Fig. 6.3) (Harms-Ringdahl et al 1986b). But the analysis of the

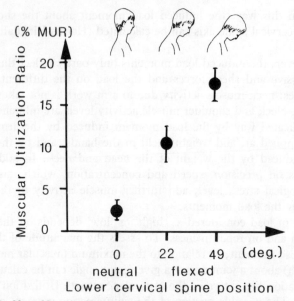

Fig. 6.2 Mean Muscular Utilization Ratios (% MUR) between load moment induced by gravitational forces of head-and-neck and muscular moment about bilateral motion axis of C7–T1 (*y*-axis). Lower cervical spine positions (*x*-axis): neutral, slightly and much flexed. Vertical bars: 95% confidence intervals (n=10).

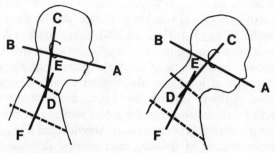

Fig. 6.3 Construction lines for determination of cervical spine position in relation to thoracic spine and head.
AB: nose/upper lip junction—motion axis of Occ-C1.
CD: motion axes of Occ-C1—C7-T1.
EF: motion axes of C7-T1—T5-T6.
Angle between AB and AC: degree of flexion/extension of Occ-C1.
Angle between CD and EF: degree of flexion/extension of C7-T1.
Left: upper- and lower-cervical spine in neutral position
Right: upper-cervical spine extended, lower-cervical spine flexed.

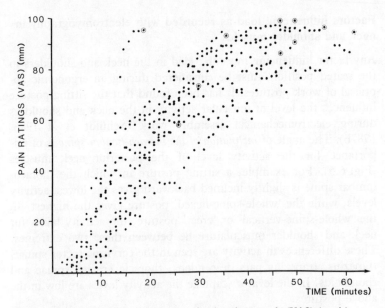

Fig. 6.4 Intensity of pain ratings on a visual analogue scale (VAS) (y-axis) during provocation induced by maintained full flexion of head-and-neck in 10 healthy female subjects (time: x-axis). Last assessment before discontinuing provocation: circled dot. (From Harms-Ringdahl & Ekholm, Scandinavian Journal of Rehabilitation Medicine 1986).

load caused by connective tissue tension in extreme neck positions is complicated.

Maintained extreme cervical spine flexion or extension, where no or very little EMG activity is recorded and where the load moment is counteracted by the passive structures, causes pain within 15 minutes even in healthy subjects (Fig. 6.4) (Harms-Ringdahl & Ekholm 1986). However, discomfort can also be perceived after frequently performed, short neck rotations to extreme positions, such as occur in fork-lift truck driving (Eklund 1986).

To analyse *load dosage*, not only must load moments, muscle activity and the occurrence of extreme positions be taken into account, but also time studies are needed, where the time taken for performance of activities under different loads is recorded and the variation in positions and movements is included.

Assessments of perceived discomfort and pain, when carefully performed, are useful for evaluating the effectiveness of certain ergonomic measures used to prevent fatigue or extreme positions in the neck and shoulder region.

Factors influencing load as recorded with electromyography in neck and shoulder muscles

Any factor influencing muscular load in the neck and shoulders in the seated position must be considered during an ergonomic appraisal of work postures. It has been found that the sitting posture influences the level of muscular activity in the neck and shoulders during electromechanical assembly work (Schüldt et al 1986, 1987b). The angle of *inclination of the thoraco-lumbar spine* is of importance for the activity level of the posterior neck muscles (Fig. 6.5). For example, a sitting posture in which the thoraco-lumbar spine is slightly inclined backward gives the lowest activity levels, while the 'whole-spine-flexed' posture gives the highest. In the 'whole-spine-vertical' or 'erect' posture, the activity levels for neck and shoulder musculature lie between these two extremes. These differences in activity are seen in the cervical erector spinae/trapezius, trapezius pars descendens, thoracic erector spinae and rhomboids. In the levator scapulae the activity levels are low in the above postures.

It is thus possible to reduce neck and shoulder muscular activity significantly during the performance of certain tasks by choosing a sitting posture with the trunk slightly inclined backward. This finding tallies with the results of studies of rated preferred sitting posture described by Grandjean et al (1982, 1983). However, this backwardly inclined posture generally requires that the work object be raised from a horizontal surface, for instance by using a sloping desk or an angled attachment frame.

If a backward-inclined posture is not feasible for a particular work situation, a 'vertical' posture is the second preferred option. A third choice could be a posture in which normal spinal curvature is maintained but the body is inclined forward through hip flexion.

What then is the effect of the *cervical spine position* on posterior neck muscular activity? The incidence of neck complaints seems in some studies to be related to the degree of forward flexion of the neck during work (Tichauer 1968a, Chaffin 1973, Ferguson 1976, Hünting et al 1980). Postures in which the neck is flexed increase the load moment of the cervical spine. The more the head is tilted, the earlier fatigue will develop in the neck extensors (Chaffin 1973). When the cervical spine is in a 'vertical' alignment, rather than in the flexed postures in which the thoraco-lumbar spine is slightly inclined backward or the whole spine is held in the 'vertical' erect position (Fig. 6.5), there are lower muscle activity levels in the cer-

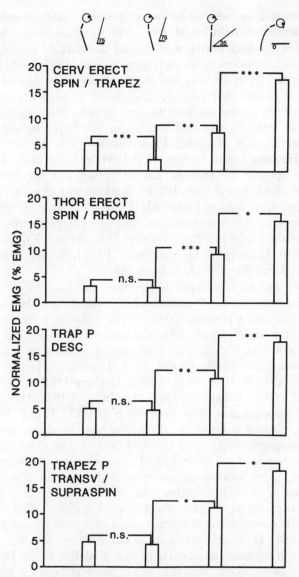

Fig. 6.5 Comparisons between four different sitting postures: trunk slightly inclined backward and cervical spine flexed and neutral, whole spine vertical and straight, and whole spine flexed (as indicated above columns).

Levels of muscular activity (means) expressed as % EMG. Muscles: cervical erector spinae covered by trapezius (n = 10), thoracic erector spinae covered by rhomboids (n = 10), trapezius pars descendens (n = 10) and trapezius pars transversa covering supraspinatus (n = 9).

Student's t test for paired observations are used.

*** = p<0.001, ** = 0.001<p≤0.01, * = 0.01<p≤0.05, n.s. = p>0.05, not significant.

vical erector spinae, while other posterior neck muscles are uninfluenced (Schüldt et al 1986, 1987b). Unnecessary forward flexion of the neck during work should therefore be avoided.

Another important factor increasing the static level of activity and thereby fatigue in the neck and shoulder muscles is *the load caused by the arms and their position*, transmitted through the shoulder girdle. Work carried out with the arms in abduction rather than by the side leads to increased activity in the trapezius and other shoulder muscles (Tichauer 1966, Chaffin 1973, Herberts et al 1980, Hagberg 1981a, Sigholm et al 1984) and also in the cervical erector spinae, the thoracic erector spinae and the rhomboid muscles (Schüldt et al 1986, 1987b). Working with more elevated or advanced arms induces higher EMG levels and signs of fatigue in the trapezius pars descendens, thoracic erector spinae, rhomboids and shoulder joint muscles (Herberts & Kadefors 1976, Herberts et al 1980, Hagberg 1981a, Sigholm et al 1984, Schüldt et al 1986, 1987b, Harms-Ringdahl & Ekholm 1987).

Other factors considered to increase the load on neck and shoulder muscles include excessive horizontal distance between the *work object* and a plumbline through the shoulder, a high position of the work object, a high work table surface, the weight and design of the tool, and other external forces acting on the arms and hands (Tichauer 1966, 1968b, Chaffin 1973, Jonsson & Hagberg 1974, Bjelle et al 1979, Herberts et al 1980, Hagberg 1981b, Onishi et al 1982, Kadefors & Petersén 1982, Sigholm et al 1984, Habes et al 1985 Arborelius et al 1986, Svensson et al 1987, Bendix 1987).

Poor *working technique* during sitting work is a risk factor for developing symptoms from the neck and shoulder: for instance, symptoms are related to time spent in neck flexion, shoulder elevation or upper arm abduction or total duration of arm activity (Kilbom et al 1986). Further, the endurance time in a posture depends partly on the person's muscular condition. With efficient muscular co-ordination, a posture could thus be maintained longer (Dul 1986). However, no amount of skill prevents muscular fatigue in the supraspinatus muscle (Herberts & Kadefors 1976). The duration of each contraction, that is the interval between muscular relaxation periods, is considered to be very important for muscular fatigue (Rohmert 1960, Jonsson 1978, Hagberg & Sundelin 1986). With micropauses, there is less perceived fatigue during repetitive work than when the same amount of work is performed without pauses.

The activity level in the neck and shoulder muscles during arm work movements is generally higher than when the arm is kept still (Schüldt et al 1987a, b). Thus, continuous dynamic arm movements entail no decrease to zero activity, so there is no intermittent relaxation of the neck and shoulder muscles. Rather, the movement activity is added to the static level. The case is similar for the upper part of the trapezius (Jonsson 1982, Christensen 1986). Hagberg's (1981b) work on elbow flexors shows similar endurance times and fatigue effects when comparing sustained isometric exertions and dynamic exertions.

Load-reducing measures

By adopting these *ergonomic guidelines on sitting postures* it might be possible not only to reduce the level of activity in neck and shoulder muscles to recommended levels (Jonsson 1978, 1982), but also hopefully, to reduce the incidence of muscular pain during sitting work. These conclusions about sitting postures can also be used for individual ergonomic advice and re-training for patients with load-elicited pain in the neck and shoulder region.

Another way of reducing muscle activity levels is by using *ergonomic aids*.

Opinions differ as to the value of *elbow support* in reducing neck-and-shoulder muscle load during sitting work (Lundervold 1951, Carlsöö 1972, Chaffin 1973, Andersson & Örtengren 1974, Grandjean 1988). Hünting et al (1981) found that when hands and arms are frequently supported during the work there is less pain in neck, shoulder and arms. A study of female electromechanical assembly workers by Schüldt et al (1987a) showed that elbow support reduces the activity in the trapezius, thoracic erector spinae and rhomboid muscles in both the 'whole spine flexed' and the 'whole spine vertical' postures. Of course the load-reducing effect of elbow support operates only when the elbow remains on the support plate.

Another ergonomic aid is an *arm suspension* device, the 'arm balancer' (Mabs Int AB, Norrköping, Sweden). This provides an adjustable but constant suspending force however much cord is drawn out of it, and it therefore gives a continuous reducing effect on muscle activity.

The reduction in muscle activity achieved by arm suspension is largely similar to that given by elbow support in the postures mentioned. Suspension also offloads the cervical erector spinae. In the posture with the trunk slightly inclined backward, it gives a reduction in the upper portion of the trapezius. If the hand must cover

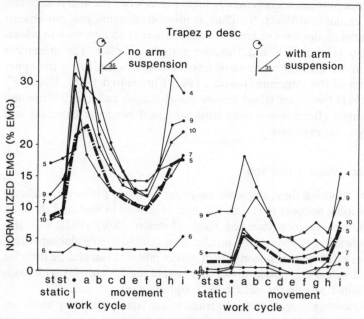

Fig. 6.6 Effect on muscle activity of arm suspension compared to no suspension (% EMG, vertical axis) in trapezius pars descendens during a simulated work cycle (horizontal axis). Work cycle consists of a static phase (*st*) followed by a movement phase pointing a soldering pen at dots on the work object (*a-i*). Sitting posture vertical and straight. Thick segmented line indicates means. Numerals at beginning and end of curve indicate each subject.

a large work area, arm suspension is probably better than elbow support since it can diminish muscular activity regardless of forearm and elbow position (Fig. 6.6).

A reduction in the level of activity in neck and shoulder muscles can be obtained with either aid: both seem to be appropriate preventive measures for reducing neck and shoulder muscular load in sitting assembly work, and their use may possibly reduce load levels below those of pain generation (Arborelius & Harms-Ringdahl 1986, Harms-Ringdahl & Arborelius 1987).

A large group of patients experiences easily elicited, load-dependent nape pain due to such factors as degenerative changes in the cervical spine structures. Since arm and hand loading is transmitted to the cervical spine structures via the shoulder girdle suspending muscles, these patients too may usefully learn to unload the cervical spine by working with an elbow support or arm balancer.

Factors influencing load in passive joint structures provoking load-elicited pain

Ergonomic measures aiming at reducing muscle activity do not, however, necessarily decrease the risk in those working postures where the cervical spine is at the limit of the motion range (i.e. in an extreme position of a joint or joints). If, in spite of a sloping desk, the distance to the work object requires maintained flexion of the upper and/or lower cervical spine, load-elicited pain can be provoked, as shown in Figures 6.4 and 6.7. Such pain can last for several days after the provocation (Harms-Ringdahl & Ekholm 1986) despite very low or no muscle activity during the provocation. Thus, even postures with a slightly backward-inclined thoraco-lumbar spine and very low neck muscle activity, entail neck flexion and a risk of adopting extreme positions (Harms-Ringdahl et al 1986b). Muscular activity due to arm work adds to the load on the cervical spine (Harms-Ringdahl & Ekholm 1986).

Perceived pain induced by extreme joint position is related to the magnitude of the load moment and its duration (Harms-Ringdahl et al 1986a), but the time course differs depending on the structures loaded and their moment arms (Harms-Ringdahl et al 1983, 1986a, Harms-Ringdahl & Ekholm 1986). As the load moment about the bilateral axis of the lower cervical spine (C7) in full flexion is about

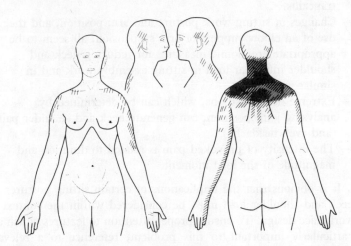

Fig. 6.7 Localization of pain just before discontinuation of maintained extreme flexion position in the lower-cervical-upper-thoracic-spine. Areas of pain of 10 subjects are superimposed (From Harms-Ringdahl & Ekholm, Scandinavian Journal of Rehabilitation Medicine 1986).

3.5 times that in a vertical position (Harms- Ringdahl et al 1986b) (Fig. 6.1), an upright, neutral position—if this can be adopted— decreases not only the muscular load as already mentioned, but also the connective tissue load.

Extreme positions seem to be caused not only by the work environment, but also by postural habits and a lack of posture consciousness. Individual instructions and training of working technique in real work environments are important.

SUMMARY

Results of the studies referred to within this chapter emphasize a number of important points about neck and shoulder load during sitting.

— A sitting work posture with the trunk slightly inclined backward and neck vertical demands the lowest muscle activity levels.
— A flexed neck is associated with higher activity in the cervical erector spinae than is a vertical neck.
— Work with the arm in abduction produces high neck muscle activity.
— Work with the hand higher and more distant compared to lower and nearer to the body places a higher load on the trapezius.
— Changes in sitting work posture and arm position, and the use of an elbow support or arm suspension, all seem to be appropriate ergonomic measures for reducing neck and shoulder muscular load in sitting assembly work and in similar work tasks.
— Extreme neck positions, which can be determined by analysing joint position, can generate neck and shoulder pain (and even headache).
— The intensity of provoked pain is related to duration and magnitude of the load moment.

It is obvious that the implications of certain sitting postures on neck and shoulder load must be considered within the context of workplace design. To ensure proper attention to features which are particularly important to this problem, reference to a relevant workplace checklist could offer appropriate guidance. The following list provides an example of such an approach.

Workplace checklist

— What is the thoraco-lumbar position?
— What are the upper and lower cervical spine positions (in relation to the vertical as well as to the adjacent body segments)?
— What are the arm and hand positions?
— For how long are the positions maintained?
— What work movements are being performed in what movement sectors?
— How repetitive are the movements?
— What are the weights of the objects being handled and the forces required?
— What are the possibilities for load-reducing measures?
— What are the possibilities for variation in postures and movements?
— What other muscle-activity-increasing factors such as poor lighting conditions or psychological stress may there be?

CONCLUDING REMARKS

The prevalence of load-elicited pain in sitting work postures makes a study of factors relating to neck and shoulder essential for ergonomists in their evaluation of the workplace. As this chapter has demonstrated, physiotherapists can play an important role in prevention by their involvement in the research which is so vital if the influence of load on muscle activity is to be properly appreciated. Only then can appropriate measures be taken to ensure that optimum conditions are applied for a particular task in the seated position.

REFERNCES

Andersson B J G, Ortengren R 1974 Lumbar disc pressure and myoelectric back muscle activity during sitting. III. Studies on a wheelchair. Scandinavian Journal of Rehabilitation Medicine 6: 122–127
Arborelius U P, Ekholm J, Nisell R, Németh G, Svensson O 1986 Shoulder load during machine milking. An electromyographic and biomechanical study. Ergonomics 29: 1591–1607
Arborelius U P, Harms-Ringdahl K 1986 The results from a full-scale field test of an arm suspension balancer. In: Proceedings of the International Scientific Conference on Work With Display Units, Part 1, pp 329–332, Stockholm
Bendix T 1987 Adjustment of the seated workplace—with special reference to heights and inclinations of seat and table. Danish Medical Bulletin 34: 125–139

Bjelle A, Hagberg M, Michaelsson G 1979 Clinical and ergonomic factors in prolonged shoulder pain among industrial workers. Scandinavian Journal of Work Environment and Health 5: 205–210

Carlsöö S 1972 How man moves. Heinemann, London

Chaffin D B 1973 Localized muscle fatigue—definition and measurement. Journal of Occupational Medicine 15: 346–354

Christensen H 1986 Muscle activity and fatigue in shoulder muscles of assembly-plant employees. Scandinavian Journal of Work and Environment Health 12: 582–587

Dul J 1986 Muscular coordination in working postures. In: Corlett N, Wilson J, Manenica I (eds) The ergonomics of working postures. Taylor & Francis, London, pp 115–125

Eklund J 1986 Industrial seating and spinal loading. Thesis. University of Nottingham, England

Ferguson D 1976 Posture, aching and body build in telephonists. Journal of Human Ergology 5: 183–186

Grandjean E, Hünting W, Nisihiyama K 1982 Preferred VDT work station settings, body posture and physical impairments. Journal of Human Ergology 11: 45–53

Grandjean E, Hünting W, Pidermann M 1983 VDT work station design: Preferred settings and their effects. Human Factors 25: 161–175

Grandjean E 1988 Fitting the task to the man. Taylor and Francis, London

Habes D, Carlson W, Badger D 1985 Muscle fatigue associated with repetitive arm lifts: effects of height, weight and reach. Ergonomics 28: 471–488

Hagberg M 1981a Electromyographic signs of shoulder muscular fatigue in two elevated arm positions. American Journal of Physical Medicine 60: 111–112

Hagberg M 1981b Workload and fatigue in repetitive arm elevations. Ergonomics 24: 543–555

Hagberg M, Sundelin G 1986 Discomfort and load on the upper trapezius muscle when operating a wordprocessor. Ergonomics 29: 1637–1645

Harms-Ringdahl K, Brodin H, Eklund L, Borg G 1983 Discomfort and pain from loaded passive joint structures. Scandinavian Journal of Rehabilitation Medicine 15: 205–211

Harms-Ringdahl K, Carlsson A M, Ekholm J, Raustorp A, Svensson T, Toresson H-G 1986a Pain assessment with different intensity scales in response to loading of joint structures. Pain 27: 401–411

Harms-Ringdahl K, Ekholm J 1986 Intensity and character of pain and muscular activity levels elicited by maintained extreme flexion position of the lower-cervical-upper-thoracic spine. Scandinavian Journal of Rehabilitation Medicine 18: 117–126

Harms-Ringdahl K, Ekholm J, Schüldt K, Németh G, Arborelius U P 1986b Load moments and myoelectric activity when the cervical spine is held in full flexion and extension. Ergonomics 29: 1539–1552

Harms-Ringdahl K, Ekholm J 1987 Influence of arm position on neck muscular activity levels during flexion–extension movements of the cervical spine. In: Jonsson B (ed) Biomechanics X-A, Human Kinetics Publishers, Champaign, pp 249–254

Harms-Ringdahl K, Arborelius U P 1987 One-year follow-up after introduction of arm suspension at an electronics plant. In: Proceedings of the Xth International Congress of World Confederation for Physical Therapy, Sydney, pp 69–73

Harms-Ringdahl K, Schüldt K 1988 Maximum neck extension strength and relative neck muscular load in different cervical spine positions. Clinical Biomechanics 4: 17–24

Herberts P, Kadefors R 1976 A study of painful shoulder in welders. Acta Orthopedica Scandinavica 47: 381–387

Herberts P, Kadefors R, Broman H 1980 Arm positioning in manual tasks. An electromyographic study of localized muscle fatigue. Ergonomics 23: 655–665

Hünting W, Grandjean E, Maeda K 1980 Constrained postures in accounting machine operators. Applied Ergonomics 11: 145–149

Hünting W, Läubli T, Grandjean E 1981 Postural and visual load at VDT workplaces. I. Constrained postures. Ergonomics 24: 917–931

Jonsson B, Hagberg M 1974 The effect of different working heights on the deltoid muscle. Scandinavian Journal of Rehabilitation Medicine (suppl 3), pp 26–32

Jonsson B 1978 Kinesiology with special reference to electromyographic kinesiology. In: Cobb W, van Duijin H (eds) Contemporary clinical neurophysiology (suppl 34). Elsevier, Amsterdam, pp 417–428

Jonsson B 1982 Measurement and evaluation of local muscular strain in the shoulder during constrained work. Journal of Human Ergology 11: 73–88

Kadefors R, Petersén I 1982 Electromyographic studies of muscle strain in industrial work. In: Buser P A, Cobb W A, Okuma T (eds) Electroencephalography and Clinical Neurophysiology (suppl 36). Elsevier, Amsterdam, pp 750–758

Kilbom Å, Persson I, Jonsson B G 1986 Disorders of the cervicobrachial region among female workers in the electronics industry. International Journal of Industrial Ergonomics 1: 37–47

Lundervold A 1951 Electromyographic investigations during sedentary work. British Journal of Physical Medicine 14: 32–36, 1951

Onishi N, Sakai K, Kogi K 1982 Arm and shoulder muscle load in various keyboard operating jobs of women. Journal of Human Ergology 11: 88–97

Petrofsky J C, Phillips C A 1982 The strength–endurance relationship in skeletal muscle: Its application to helmet design. Aviation, Space and Environmental Medicine 53: 365–369

Rohmert W 1960 Ermittlung von Erholungspausen für Statische Arbeit des Menschen. Internationale Zeitung Angew Physiology und Arbeitsphysiology 18: 123–164

Schüldt K, Ekholm J, Harms-Ringdahl K, Németh G, Arborelius U P 1986 Effects of changes in sitting work posture on static neck and shoulder muscle activity. Ergonomics 29: 1525–1537

Schüldt K, Ekholm J, Harms-Ringdahl K, Németh G, Arborelius U P 1987a Effects of arm support or suspension on neck and shoulder muscle activity during sedentary work. Scandinavian Journal of Rehabilitation Medicine 19: 77–84

Schüldt K, Ekholm J, Harms-Ringdahl K, Arborelius U P, Németh G 1987b Influence of sitting postures on neck and shoulder EMG during arm-hand work movements. Clinical Biomechanics 2: 126–139

Sigholm G, Herberts P, Almström C, Kadefors R 1984 Electromyographic analyses of shoulder muscle load. Journal of Orthopedic Research 1: 379–386

Svensson O K, Arborelius U P, Ekholm J 1987 Relative mechanical load on shoulder and elbow muscles during standing manual materials handling. A study of packing work. Scandinavian Journal of Rehabilitation Medicine 19: 169–178

Tichauer E R 1966 Some aspects of stress on forearm and hand in industry. Journal of Occupational Medicine 8: 63–71

Tichauer E R 1968a Industrial engineering in the rehabilitation of the handicapped. Journal of Industrial Engineering 19: 96–104

Tichauer E R 1968b Electromyographic kinesiology in the analysis of work situations and hand tools. In: Proceedings of the First International Congress of Electromyographic Kinesiology, Montreal, 1968, p 197. Published in Electromyography (suppl 1) vol 8, 1968

7. Design for prevention of work-related musculoskeletal disorders

L. Karlqvist and M. G. Björkstén

INTRODUCTION

Work environment issues have a long tradition in Sweden. As early as 1889, the Parliament passed the Occupational Hazards Act and three labour inspectors were appointed. Today, the National Board of Occupational Safety and Health is the central administrative authority with the Inspectorate. Research is carried out within the National Institute of Health and in many University departments all over Sweden (Arbetarskyddsstyrelsen 1986).

The legislation of 1978 now forms the basis also for the field work. According to the Work Environment Act, all workers have the right to belong to a centre of Occupational Health. In these centres there is a team consisting of doctors, engineers, nurses, social workers or psychologists and physiotherapists working together (SAF, LO, PTK, 1979).

The preventative role of industrial physiotherapists in Sweden began when, as professionals, they were allowed to investigate workplaces. Now, as a member of the team, physiotherapists are able to identify risk factors already in the workplace layout and examine working technique, task design and work organization. Prevention may be 'primary', when the design is still on the drawing board. Most frequently, however, problems which need solving already exist and the prevention could be described as 'secondary'. The physiotherapist's professional role in preventative work emanates from special knowledge about physiology and biomechanics of the musculoskeletal system and the ability to foresee the consequences of loading that system. Together with the engineers, physiotherapists can provide technical solutions to ergonomic problems and fulfil the criteria for the ergonomic design of workplaces. Such proposals are presented to the management of the workplace and it is their responsibility to implement them (SAF, LO, PTK, 1979).

Despite earlier evaluations, the proposals for the workplace may be subjected to further modifications after consultation with the users and the management. This involvement of a total team, including the user, is essential to ensure the development of a good working environment. When the modified workplace is accepted by the workers, the contribution of the ergonomist is complete.

OBSERVED PROBLEMS

A great part of total sick leave in Sweden is claimed to be due to the loading of the musculoskeletal system during work, either solely or in combination with ageing.

Today, heavy physical load at work is decreasing due to mechanization and automation. Nevertheless, the percentage of workers in the Labour Workers Union (LO) who regard physical strain during work as a problem has increased. For example, in 1970, 51% of the workers considered physical strain as the greatest problem in the work environment, whereas in 1980, this figure had risen to 71% (Arbetarskyddsfonden 1982).

In earlier years, work-related musculoskeletal disorders were observed to occur most frequently in association with the lumbar spine. However, the modern industrial design has changed this picture. Today, the neck and shoulders appear to be the most critical regions for injury or discomfort (Maeda 1977).

Nowadays much of the work done in industry and in offices is very specialized. That is to say, most of the workers perform the same movements and assume the same posture at their machine, visual display unit (VDU) or desk for the whole of the working day. Most of the work is carried out in the seated position, and very often as a monotonous and repetitive task. As most of those tasks need good vision, the posture of the head is often fixed in a forward flexed position to enable the worker to see the fixture, screen or writing material. Such postures cause strain both in the joints and muscles of the neck and in the thoracic and lumbar back regions. Furthermore there is almost always a compromise between the view distance and the optimal arm level for working with the hands and fingers. This often means that the arms must be held elevated and/or abducted during the working cycles, so causing strain on the muscles and tendons of the shoulder. If the demand for such positions is combined with repetitive movements, the strain is increased.

Continuous strain may lead to symptoms of disorder. The

symptoms observed in these groups of workers are muscular tenderness and tension and fibromyositis in the shoulder and neck region and tendinitis in the upper extremities (Bjelle et al 1979, 1981, Luopajärvi et al 1979; Kvarnström 1983; Larsson et al 1987). These symptoms are sometimes referred to as Occupational Cervico-brachial Disorders (OCD) (Maeda 1977), or Occupational Overuse Syndrome (OOS) (National Occupational Health and Safety Commission, Australia 1986).

DESIGN FOR PREVENTION

The details of a number of projects in which the authors have participated are presented in this chapter. They provide examples of secondary prevention and are presented to illustrate the different approaches and methods which may be used in the ergonomic design of workplaces.

When contributing to the resolution of ergonomic problems in industry, the physiotherapist follows a number of major steps, as follows:

Identification of the problem. One factor alone or several in combination may influence the work-load. These could include the workplace layout, the design of implements, the task or assignment, the working technique, the work organization or the approach to salary payment.

Analysis and investigation of the problem. When the problem has been identified and the causal factors analysed, a suitable method for studying the details of the problem should be chosen. Depending on the character of those causal factors, study methods could make use of questionnaires and interviews, medical examinations, analyses of movements and posture and/or a mock-up of the working situation.

Proposals for solution of the problem. Results of the detailed analyses provide the basis for proposed solutions. Recommendations may, for example, relate to a change in workplace layout or in work organization.

Implementation of the proposals. A crucial factor in ensuring the implementation of recommendations for introducing preventative practices in the work environment is to supply knowledge of ergonomic principles to the executives. They carry a major responsibility for introducing improvements to the work environment and they are ultimately responsible for maintaining good working conditions.

During this 'implementation' stage of the project, the ergonomist should provide basic knowledge of ergonomics to both the employers and the employees. This is one method of facilitating the introduction of new work organization and work methods (Ahlstrand et al 1986).

Evaluation of the results. Whenever proposals for improvement are implemented, the improvement should be evaluated to determine whether or not they have been successful in reducing the problems previously perceived. Evaluation may be effected through use, for example, of questionnaires and interviews, or analyses of movements and posture.

INVESTIGATIONS

Descriptions of some ergonomic problems resolved by the physiotherapist as a consultant member of an ergonomics team help to demonstrate the contribution which might be made by a physiotherapist in industry.

Cutting operation at canning bench

Work at a canning bench in the fish-preserving industry was investigated (from Jaderberg et al 1984).

The fishing industry on the west coast of Sweden has a long tradition and traditional sex roles are deeply rooted. Men deliver and transport the fish and products. Women clean, trim, slice and put the treated fish into cans while sitting at a special table, known as a canning bench.

The natural changes in work which were previously available through less specialized work tasks do not exist any more. Today, work at the canning bench has become much more monotonous and provides no opportunity for breaks. Furthermore, salary by piecework agreement is a natural incentive to increase the pace of work. Pauses are regulated by contract, but most workers accumulate pauses to gain longer but fewer breaks and this tends to increase the monotony of the job.

Examination of work-injury statistics revealed that the canning bench workers were significantly more exposed to carving injuries and physical stress illnesses than the average active worker in Sweden. The neck, shoulders, arms, and hands appeared to be especially exposed during work.

Identifying the problems

Through studying the job, both directly and on video, it was possible to determine and analyse the position and movements of body segments of the workers during their activities.

Workplace layout. The fixed measurements of the workplace layout created difficulties for the workers in adapting their working posture to cater for individual variations in body sizes.

Design of implements. The design of the work implements (knives as well as chopping-board) forced the hands into inappropriate movement patterns and work positions.

The task or assignment. The nature of the assignments offered few opportunities for variation in activity. The operations involved were physically similar, giving rise to lengthy static muscular strain as well as involving repetitive movement patterns. The work at the canning bench demanded clear eyesight and considerable precision, both of which contribute to tense and fixed working postures.

Working technique varied considerably from one person to another. The canning bench workers' insufficient knowledge and maybe even motivation for adoption of appropriate working techniques could influence their physical strain negatively.

Working hours. The weekly working hours were distributed over only 4 and a half days, so that each full day was longer than the usual working hours under a 5 day per week work scheme. The prolonged working hours could lead to an increased physical load on the person, with accumulated fatigue.

Approach to salary payment. The worker's payment was by 'piecework' agreement. This arrangement can contribute to too high a working speed, which in turn involves an increased risk for prolonged physical load. The piecework arrangement results in less willingness on the part of the worker to take short breaks or to vary working postures.

Analysis of work problems and formulation of recommendations

Upon analysing the working postures and movement patterns, it became obvious that in order to reduce the physical strain on the canning bench workers, the project had to be divided into two parts.

In the the first part, consideration had to be given to designing flexible workplaces and to providing information to the workers about the importance of pauses, relaxation and variations in work methods.

In the second part, consideration had to be given to the design of implements which would match both the demands of the task and the different sizes of the hands.

Mock-up. To faciliate the re-design process, a workplace mock-up was constructed with the co-operation of technicians. Appropriate ergonomic criteria for the design of this workplace were formulated. These included the following:

— It should be possible to maintain standing as well as sitting positions at the cutting table
— The cutting table should be at right angles to the production line
— The size of the table should be adapted to the task–and the chair should provide an appropriate working relationship to the table and the task
— The chopping board should be individually adjustable.

As a result of the tests in the experimental mock-up, recommendations could be made which satisfied the stated ergonomic criteria. Additionally, ergonomic information was given to the employers by means of a videotape which featured their own working environment. A special folder was made to supplement the videotape. It also included a training programme and a relaxation programme.

Evaluation of results

Experiments were undertaken to develop a new design for bench and chair, to modify the chopping-board design and to improve working technique instructions. After evaluation by the workers, modifications were made. The results showed an improvement in comfort when working at the new canning bench.

The second part of the project involved an investigation of the role of the knives in producing work-load for the hands and arms. The aim was to develop a better knife design, the use of which would reduce the risks of producing the typical physical stress complaints related to this work.

Methods

The study concentrated on estimating the strain on the hand and arm and on how the design of the knives could influence such strain. Work tasks, work positions, movement patterns and grasps were monitored and registered. The position and the movements of the loaded hand during work were analysed.

Work tasks. The most common preserved fish products in this canning industry are sliced herring, herring pieces, Matje herring pieces and anchovy fillets. In order to produce these items, the work at the canning bench consists principally of four separate cutting operations: trimming, piecing, slicing and cleaning.

Knives. Four different knives were used by workers at the canning bench (Fig. 7.1). All knives were of the conventional type, with handles of wood and blades of stainless steel. No variations in knife size to match the various hand sizes were available and all workers used the same size of knife.

The length and width of the blades changed by grinding. Some of the workers preferred thinner and shorter blades and ground them to their preferred size when the knife was new. Other knives changed over time with the sharpening after use.

Injuries and complaints. An examination of the forearms and hands of 118 canning bench workers was made to determine the type, localization and frequency of injuries and complaints. The workers were interviewed at their work-site by an industrial nurse who also inspected their hands and registered any signs of damage.

The outline of each worker's outspread hand was drawn in pencil on paper. The sites of injury were marked on the hand profile, together with the site of any subjective complaints, such as pain, aching, numbness and pricking sensations. Only four of the 118 canning bench workers examined were found to be completely free of complaints and injuries. A combination of several different problems were shown to be common among the workers.

Analyses revealed that the wrists were most exposed to musculoskeletal rheumatic disorders as expressed in stiffness, swelling and

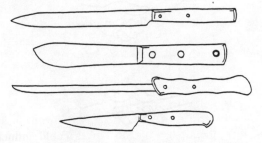

Fig. 7.1   Knives used for trimming, piecing, slicing and cleaning.

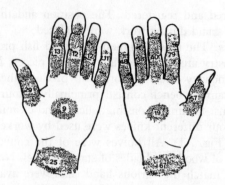

Fig. 7.2 Diagrammatic representation of incidence of musculoskeletal disorders in the hands. The numbers marked on the diagram show the distribution of musculoskeletal rheumatic disorders in the left and right hands.

pain. Thumbs and forefingers were the second site of frequent disorder. The hand using the knife, most frequently the right hand, was much more exposed than the other hand as Figure 7.2 reveals.

From the results of this study it was concluded that working at the canning bench gives rise to lengthy static muscular strain, forces the hands into inappropriate movement patterns and work positions, gives rise to neurological symptoms such as numbness and pricking sensations and gives rise to callus, blisters, rub injuries and carving sores.

Connection between knives and complaints. When the hand grasps around the handle and at the same time adapts the movement direction of the blade to the chopping board, the wrist is forced to the side of the little finger. Such a hand position is unnatural (Fig. 7.3).

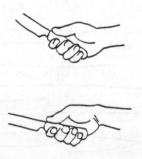

Fig. 7.3 (a) The natural hand position gives no cutting position.
(b) The cutting position gives an unnatural hand position.

When the hand is forced into an unnatural position, the muscles in the hand, arm and shoulder are more involved. Also, in order to gain free space for the hand movement, the shoulder needs to be raised. As a result, there is:

— increased work-load for the small muscles in the hand and the muscles which bend the fingers and stabilize the wrist
— harmful load for the tendons and joints in hand and wrist: risk of nerve compression
— increased static muscular strain in the muscles to compensate for the distorted work position.

The data relating to injuries and complaints suggested that many disorders in the hand and wrist as well as in the shoulder, neck and back were caused by the shape, surface structure and other qualities of the knives.

A painful hand loses a great deal of its precision and the risk for carving injuries increases.

Development of new knives

The starting point for the design of new cutting knives was consideration of the physical working positions which are natural and feel comfortable. The goal was to identify movement patterns and grasps which could ensure effective generation of power and power transmission, at the same time as providing sufficient precision. For this purpose, the hands of 167 canning bench workers were measured and the length and the width of their hands registered. Through mapping and analysing physical stress complaints related to work movement and hand positions, it was possible to express ergonomic criteria for new knife designs.

The shape and surface structure of the handles, the shape, form and sharpness of the blades and the weight and balance of the knives proved to be of great significance in allowing the work to be carried out comfortably, so that unnecessary muscle exertion, badly distributed pressure on the skin and nerves etc., could be avoided.

Experimental trials. Evaluation by means of practical tests consisted of successive ergonomic experiments where prototype knives were tested in as realistic a situation as possible. Registration of the whole work situation was made by means of photography and video film before and after modification of the prototypes.

Subjects and test occasions. The following criteria were used

for selecting the persons for inclusion in the test.
The subjects should:

— not be extremely young or old workers
— be professional workers
— belong to the group of quick and medium quick workers
— represent varying hand sizes
— represent workers both with and without disorders in the
  neck, shoulder, arm and hand
— represent all factories in the project involved
— be aware of the aim of the project and have a positive
  attitude to test situations.

Between 12 and 38 subjects participated in each of nine
scheduled test situations. In addition, many other workers tried
using the prototypes since the knives were available in their factory
and they willingly offered spontaneous comments.

Laboratory tests were undertaken as well as 1 to 2 days testing
at the ordinary workplaces within the factories. The project team
used structured interviews by checklists to record all relevant
details about the prototypes. Three tests were continued for 2 to 3
weeks, and in these cases, personnel within the factories took
responsibility for making the recordings, using the checklists as a
guide.

Results

Prototype designs. As a result of this study, four types of knives
were developed and manufactured as prototype designs for the four
different cutting operations. While they were designed for special
tasks within the preserved fish industry, tests have shown that they
can also be used effectively in other areas such as cold buffet
preparation and the household.

For trimming. The new knife has been designed using the same
principle and grip as for the conventional knife. The biggest improvement is the handle shape, weight and balance of the knife.

For pieces. The knife has been designed using a completely new
principle: the handle has a downward angle and therefore permits
work with a straight wrist and hand in a powerful grip; at the same
time the shoulder can retain its normally lowered position. The new
handle has also given the knife better balance than the conventional
one.

For slices. Two alternatives of this knife have been developed with regard to two separate handling methods. One knife has a conical (thicker backwards) handle which allows an improved rotation of the knife with the help of ring and little finger. The other knife has a handle of even thickness for those who perform the rotary movement principally with forefinger–thumb. There has been an improvement in the weight, balance and handle shape of both the knives.

For cleaning. The new anchovy knife is handled with the same grip and movement patterns as the conventional knife, but is lighter, has a thinner and more effective blade and an improved handle.

Evaluation

With the help of the practical tests and a series of test knives which were developed in stages, in co-operation with the personnel, a final product was created.

While it is too early to answer the question of how the physical stress complaints have been influenced by application of the new design features, those canning bench workers who have tried the knives for a longer period of time report that the amount of hard skin has been reduced as well as the degree of fatigue in the hand and arm.

Long-term testing has shown that the majority of test subjects preferred the new knives to their previously used implements.

Engine drivers — anthropometrics versus dimensions of the driver's cab

The report of a comprehensive study of Swedish engine drivers illustrates other features of the physiotherapist's contribution to ergonomics.

One part of the study, reported here, covers 'Ergonomic aspects of the railway engine as a workplace'. This presentation is based on the reports by Hedberg et al (1978a,b,c, 1979, 1981a,b) and Hedberg (1987). The study was initiated by Statens Jarnvagar (the Swedish Railway Company) as a result of a previous study which had shown that the driver's cab probably was designed for the dimensions of men taller than the average Swedish man. At the time of the study, the drivers in Sweden were sometimes forced to sit driving for up to 5 consecutive hours. This was done in a fixed body position. The drivers had to manipulate hand controls with both hands at the same time as they were pressing a safety foot pedal with one or both feet. Therefore it was very important to develop a workplace which was as comfortable as possible.

At the time of the study, many of the active drivers were relatively old and all of them were men. The main purpose of the investigation was to provide a basis for designing the cab of a common Swedish engine (the Rc4 engine) to suit the dimensions of both the present and the future population of men and women drivers.

In order to investigate if there had been any discrepancy between the body size of the present drivers and the cabin and if this had caused any physical problems among the drivers, a study was designed to achieve the following objectives: to collect a representative sample of the anthropometric measurements of the engine drivers; to investigate the dimensions of the cab and correlate them with the anthropometric measurements of the drivers; and to investigate the prevalence of musculoskeletal disorders among the engine drivers.

The findings of the inquiries on musculoskeletal disorders could then be correlated with the anthropometric measurements in relation to the dimensions of the engine cab.

Procedure

Material and methods. 150 male engine drivers and 91 male driver trainees were randomly selected and agreed to be subjects for the study. The trainees were chosen as representatives of the future drivers, but as there was only one female trainee she was excluded from the study.

Anthropometric measurements were taken on each of the subjects. The dimensions were chosen to match the specific purpose of the study. Measurements were made with a standard GPM anthropometer. An adjustable chair with a flat horizontal seat was used to obtain a well-defined sitting posture. The subjects were barefooted and dressed in underwear. Standard anthropometric techniques were used as presented by Lewin (1969). Six of the anthropometric measurements taken were in the standing and 16 in the sitting position (Fig. 7.4).

Sketches of the cab were studied and supplemented with measurements taken in the actual Rc4 cab (Fig. 7.5), and the dimensions of the cab were correlated with the relevant anthropometric measurements of the drivers.

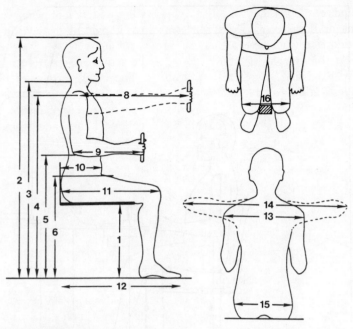

Fig. 7.4 Anthropometric measurements of sitting posture. (Reproduced by permission of Butterworth Scientific Ltd.)

A questionnaire containing questions about the prevalence of musculoskeletal disorders was presented to the subjects. They answered this questionnaire in the presence of a physiotherapist who also asked questions about their complaints in the musculoskeletal system (e.g. aching, pain, discomfort) during the previous 12 months and earlier in their life. Subjects were also asked to point out what kind of factors in the working environment (e.g. indoor climate, working posture, vibrations, etc.) they considered might have influenced their health.

Results

Anthropometrics. Collation and analysis of the results indicated that the trainees were an average of 25 mm taller than the present population of drivers. Comparisons of dimensions of the subjects in this study and other male Swedish groups of the same ages indicated that there were no notable differences. Younger generations in developed countries could be expected to be taller than their parental generation. As an example of the wide variation in the

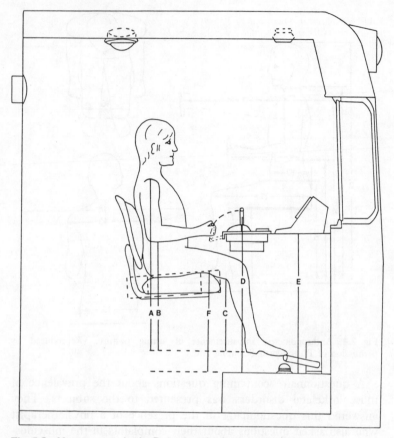

Fig. 7.5 Measurements in the Rc4 cab and relevant anthropometric
measurements of the driver representing the 5th percentile value in stature.
(Reproduced by permission of Butterworth Scientific Ltd.)

body size within the total group examined, the values for stature,
elbow height in sitting and acromion-handgrip are presented for the
fifth percentile of the drivers (I) and the 95th percentile of the
trainees (II) (See Table 7.1).

Drivers' body size and cab dimensions. The anthropometric
measurements of the present drivers differed markedly from the
dimensions of the cab of the Rc4 engine. The cab seemed to be
suited to very tall drivers, and those drivers who were at and below
the mean value for body size had difficulties in achieving a comfortable ergonomically good posture when driving. A good and
comfortable working posture should allow the drivers to sit with the

Table 7.1 Anthropometric measurements: I. 5th percentile values of engine
drivers; II. 95th percentile values of trainees

Dimension	Percentile measurements (cm)	
	I	II
Stature	164.9	184.5
Sitting acromion height	94.3	109.0
Acromion-handgrip	61.5	70.0

feet resting at the foot stool and the elbows kept near the angle of
90 degrees, i.e. the controls should be at the elbow level. However,
in the cab, one of the main controls was located 240 mm above the
mean value for elbow height when sitting. This control was
operated 39% of the working time. Other discrepancies forced the
drivers to work in a forward bent position beyond their normal
reach distance. The safety control consisted of a foot pedal placed
on the footstool under the control table. It had to be depressed for
the total driving time with one or both feet. The placement of such
important controls in relation to the chair was very important,
therefore. Although the chair was adjustable in seat height, rake
and depth and in rake of the back support, this was not sufficient
to satisfy the variations in body sizes of the users.

Musculoskeletal disorders. The frequency of musculoskeletal
disorders among the 150 drivers was highest in the lower back, the
neck and the shoulders, as is illustrated in Figure 7.6 (modified
from Hedberg 1987). The frequency increased with advancing age.

Identifying the problems

The incidence of rheumatic complaints, the anthropometric measurements and the dimensions of the cab were correlated to
determine whether the discrepancy between body size and cab
dimensions had any influence on the prevalence of musculoskeletal disorders. Drivers with and without disorders were compared.
Drivers with disorders were divided into five groups according to
the location of the symptoms: the neck and/or the shoulders, the
arms and/or the hands, the lower back, the hips and/or knees, the
legs and/or feet. Each subject in each group was compared with a
pain-free subject of the same age, with regard to the following
dimensions: stature, sitting height, acromial height when sitting,
elbow height when sitting and thigh height. Acromion-handgrip,
elbow-handgrip and buttock-patella values were also compared.

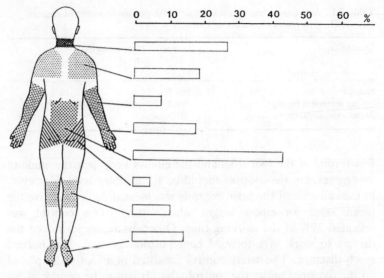

Fig. 7.6 Body chart demonstrating the percentage of engine drivers who had had musculoskeletal complaints in different parts of the body at any time during the preceding 12 months (modified from Hedberg G 1987 in Arbete Och Halsa 1987: 9 edited by the Swedish Board of Occupational Health and Safety).

The results of the comparison of the matched pairs of drivers showed that:

— The relevant dimensions of drivers with pain in neck and shoulders were significantly smaller than in the 'controls' for all measurements except elbow height.
— Drivers with pain in arms and hands did not show any significant differences in anthropometric dimensions compared with the control group.
— Drivers with low back pain were significantly shorter than the controls in sitting height, thigh height, acromion-handgrip and buttock-patella length.
— Drivers with pain in hips and knees and with pains in legs and feet were significantly shorter than the controls in sitting height, acromial height and thigh height. Those with pain in the hips and knees were also shorter in stature.

It can be seen from these results that the stature is inadequate as a single anthropometric measurement in an analysis of musculoskeletal disorders and a sitting working posture.

Proposals for improvement of the Rc4 engine cabin

The recommendations given were based on the following facts:

— Both men and women should be able to work in the engines in the future.
— The drivers should be able to drive in both the sitting and the standing positions. The main safety regulator should be a foot pedal and there should be a control table in front of the driver.

To ensure a design which would meet the requirements of all future drivers, the 95th percentile value of the Swedish engine drivers and the 5th percentile values of a group of Swedish women (Berglund et al) were used as anthropometric guidelines. In this way, all drivers were supposed to be able to maintain an ergonomically sound working posture.

The most important proposals for improvement were:

— The fixed control table should be of a height of 900 mm (lowered 80 mm).
— The thickness of the table should be 40 mm at the most (lowered 4 cm).
— The table edge should be smooth to avoid pressure on the arm.
— The seat and the footrest should be adjustable. To accommodate for the inter-individual differences between the elbow height and the seat height the seat should be adjustable by 110 mm in height and the footrest 170 mm to provide 570–740 mm below the table surface.
— The seat should be adjustable by at least 150 mm in the forward direction. To be positioned out of the way for the standing driver, it should also be movable back or sideways.
— There should be some support for the arms.

Recommendations regarding the placement of some of the regulators and instruments were also given.

Proposals implemented

To a great extent, the proposals were followed when the Rc5 engine was constructed. This was true both for height adjustments and for the flexibility and location of the regulators. Some of the differences in measurements implemented in the new design were the following:

— table height 965 versus 900 mm
— table thickness 47 versus 40 mm
— footrest adjustability 580–740 versus 570–740 mm, and seat adjustment in forward direction 180 versus 150 mm.

Evaluation of the improvements

The new cab was evaluated by experienced drivers. This was done in a separate study by Hedberg (1987) as an inquiry among a random sample of 50 drivers who had been working in the new cabin of the Rc5 engine for at least 3 months. The questionnaire contained questions concerning the background of the drivers, their age, stature and weight.

The drivers had to state their attitude to the design of the cab on a scale with five alternatives: very good, good, neither good nor bad, bad and very bad. There was also an alternative 'no opinion'.
  Regarding certain specified aspects of the cab, the drivers were asked in the questionnaire to make comparisons between the designs of the cab in Rc4 and that in Rc5. They were asked if they thought that the design of Rc5 was better, there was no difference, or it was worse than that of Rc4. There was also an alternative 'no opinion'. On every question the driver also had the opportunity of expressing his own views about the part of the cab in the question.

By drawings of the Rc5 cab and measurements in the Rc5 cab, the cab design was studied with respect to size, position and possible adjustments of the different parts of the interior.

The calculations of the dimensions of the cab, together with the earlier mentioned anthropometric measurements of the engine drivers, were the basis for an ergonomic analysis of the cab. A comparison between recommended and actual measurements in the Rc5 cab was made.

The suggested improvements were generally appreciated by the drivers interviewed. The results also showed that most of the drivers considered the design of the cab to be better in Rc5 than in Rc4. They especially appreciated the adjustable footrest as it allowed an individually adjusted position for driving.

This study illustrates the importance of using anthropometric measurements as a basis for ergonomics and design of a workplace, as emphasized in Chapter 2.

Medical secretaries: musculo-skeletal health status and design of equipment

One of the major tasks for medical secretaries is the typing of case sheets as dictated by the doctors.

In one of the university hospitals in Sweden, the medical secretaries made frequent visits to the ergonomist describing complaints of the musculoskeletal system. Therefore it was considered important to study the problem by means of a structured investigation and this was done by Björkstén & Jonsson (1987).

To identify the problems among the secretaries, an inquiry study was initiated and undertaken at two hospitals. One purpose of the study was to investigate the localization, severity of discomfort or disorders and the nature of the complaints of the musculoskeletal system. Another purpose was to seek the subjective opinion of the secretaries about the quality of their working environment. The possible correlation between complaints and environment was also studied. In a separate but simultaneously performed study by Björkstén et al (1985), the muscular load on the shoulder muscles during typewriting was analysed by means of electromyography (EMG).

The following questions were addressed:

1. How many of the medical secretaries had experienced complaints of the muscular system at any time during the previous 12 months?
2. How many of them had reported complaints during the last 7 days?
3. How many had been prevented from doing their work at any time during the previous 12 months due to the complaints?
4. Was there any correlation between complaints of the musculoskeletal system and:
   — age?
   — the length of time in the profession?
   — the amount of typewriting from dictate?
5. Was there any correlation between the prevalence of complaints from the neck or shoulders and any special work environmental factor?
6. What was the degree of severity of complaints in the neck and shoulder region?

Subjects

The subjects in the inquiry investigation were 381 female medical secretaries from two different university hospitals, who volunteered to participate. They had all been employed in the profession for at least 12 months and had not been absent from work for more than 3 months during that time. In the EMG study, 10 healthy medical secretaries aged 21–41 years participated. They were all experienced typists.

Methods

Three forms were used for the inquiry. These questionnaires were formulated in a Nordic co-operative project. The advantage of using such a common questionnaire form, an example of which is illustrated in Chapter 3, is that it allows a comparison of the prevalence of musculoskeletal disorders between different occupational groups in several countries (Kuorinka et al 1987).

Through these questionnaires the following background facts were noted: sex, age, time in profession, work-time per week, body weight, stature, right- or left-handedness. Questions about present work tasks and equipment were also asked. In the first comprehensive questionnaire, information about prevalence of musculoskeletal disorders in the whole body was sought. To gain more details concerning the complaints from neck and shoulders, and the grade of severity of those disorders, special forms for each of those body regions were used.

Procedure

Explanations as to how the forms should be filled out were given to groups of about 15 secretaries at a time. Although each person answered their questionnaire separately, the instructor was present throughout to clarify any problem. Participants were also helped by the instructions and body maps contained within the forms. Several opportunities were provided for the secretaries to participate in the study. Analysis of the responses was carried out statistically using frequency analysis, correlations and multiple regression analysis.

The experimental procedure for the EMG study was the following: the subjects were interviewed and examined by a physician, one or two days before the experiment, if possible. On this occasion, the maximal voluntary force of contraction (MVC) was measured for shoulder elevation and forward flexion in the shoulder joint. With bipolar surface electrodes placed on the upper portion of the right trapezius muscle, the secretaries first made a series of test contractions. This allowed the myoelectric results of monitoring static muscle work to be expressed in terms of the relative force of contraction. Subjects were then given three different 5-minute typing tasks, two of which were laid out as in a professional setting, one a dictation and the other a typescript.

Results

Analysis revealed that the highest frequency of disorders occurred in the neck, shoulders and low-back regions. Results showed that during the previous 12 months, 53% of the secretaries had experienced pain in the neck, 47% in the shoulders and 42% in the low back. A correlation between the incidence of disorders in the neck and shoulders during the previous 12 months and advancing age was significant at the 0.05 level.

A small but not significant correlation with time spent in the secretarial profession was shown when the secretaries had been working for more than 8 years. No correlation was found between the incidence of disorders and the task of typing from dictation. The results relating to the organization and pace of work showed that the secretaries were rather satisfied with their working environment except for the indoor climate. Two thirds of them found their job responsible and stimulating, while in only one fifth could the organization or planning of their work be considered to be a detrimental influence.

The results from the EMG study indicated that the static muscular load was at a level of about 4% MVC during the 5-minute period of analysis.

A separate study designed to develop better technical equipment for medical secretaries was carried out at this time by Karlqvist & Osterman (1984). This study was initiated by an inquiry study among other groups of medical secretaries and it showed the same pattern of musculoskeletal disorders as did the study described here. It also showed that the incidence of musculoskeletal disorders among medical secretaries was related to their work with dictaphone equipment.

As mentioned earlier, work with a dictaphone is a very common assignment for medical secretaries today. Because accurate medical documentation is so vital, this is one of the most important aspects of the secretary's responsibilities. As the work is exacting and requires concentration, it could easily lead to tight working postures, particularly during long continuous duty without pauses. The dictaphone may be directed by either hand or foot controls and the operator keeps both the hand and foot in readiness to read quickly. As the secretary usually tries to have the shortest possible distance to the controls, their position may influence hand or foot work negatively.

Because of the implications of the results of the inquiry study, a further investigation was carried out.

The purpose of this study was threefold:

— To collect basic data for the design of foot-controlled dictaphones with respect to size, form, resistance and method of application, in order to ensure both good sitting posture and low physical strain in the foot and leg during use.
— To evaluate different hand-controlled dictaphones from a physical strain point of view and any effects that may be produced while learning to use them.
— To collect basic data for designing hand-controlled dictaphones.

Methods

An introductory inventory provided knowledge about types of equipment in use and working technique. During follow-up workplace visits, medical secretaries were studied and filmed during duty. Analyses provided the basis for further study. Alternative foot or hand movements were assessed in relation to normal movements in foot or hand and the logic in control functions. The best of the alternatives were tested as mock-ups and the experiences were collated for formulation of the specific demands to be applied in test equipment. These mock-ups were evaluated by medical secretaries during their ordinary work and their assessments formed the basis for the ergonomic design criteria later formulated.

Ergonomic criteria

As an example, the ergonomic criteria developed for design of hand-controlled dictaphones will be discussed. Criteria for function, design and movement were formulated.

Function: Criteria relating to function included the following:

— The instrument shall direct 'forward', 'stop' and 'reverse'.

— The instrument shall have two keys, one for 'forward' and 'stop' and one for 'reverse'.

The keys shall be placed in such a way that their depression is logical in relation to the movements of the hand, and indicating 'forward/stop' to the right and 'reverse' to the left.

— Activity of the dictaphone shall be achieved without delay.
— 'Forward/stop' shall be activated with a light depression of the key.
— 'Reverse' shall be activated with the key pushed down and maintained in that position for as long as required.

Design: Criteria relating to hand-controlled dictaphone design included the following:

— The keys shall either replace or be placed close over the left part of the space-bar.
— The key for 'forward/stop' shall not be longer than the depth of depression required for the thumb in order to avoid activating the adjoining key.
— The 'reverse' key can be of the same length or fill up the remainder of the space-bar.
— The width of the keys shall be such as to cover the space-bar or to correspond with it.

Movement:

— The length of the depression movement shall be short or correspond to that of the space-bar, and the feedback of the depression motion shall be pronounced.
— The direction of the key depression shall be vertical or correspond to that of the space-bar.
— If a detached control is used it shall be stable.

Other criteria specified that:
— The control shall be easy to handle, easy to deposit, simple to clean, easy to maintain and stand normal handling.
— The appearance shall be in accordance with up-to-date typewriters.

Discussion

The muscular load on the trapezius muscle during typewriting was found to be at a level which might be too strenuous to maintain throughout the whole working day. This could explain why even among the younger secretaries there were complaints of musculoskeletal problems. While the static muscular load for the upper trapezius in the EMG study was found to be 4% MVC, it has been suggested by Jonsson (1982) that a static muscular load should not exceed 2% MVC if maintained during the entire working day.

The secretaries questioned in the inquiry study stated that they were satisfied with their equipment which consisted of typewriters and furniture. However, the prevalence of disorders, especially in the neck and shoulders, must be considered as being too high.

The findings of these studies prompted a solution in which an alternative method of work organization was proposed, with the possibility of arranging the job to suit individual requirements and the opportunity to vary activity by alternating with other tasks.

The result of the evaluative study in which alternative designs were assessed showed that it is possible to achieve great improvements in the degree of strain experienced in muscles and joints when working with dictaphones, by improving the design of the controls.

In many dictaphones, hand controls demand movements, especially in the thumb, which do not correspond with normal patterns of motion. While the study described here was too limited to be able to assert that such design features would lead to musculoskeletal disorders among medical secretaries, the risk cannot be ignored.

The use of hand controls in a dictaphone has a negative effect on the typewriting itself, especially on the operator's fingering and rhythm. The negative effect is most marked when use of the hand controls for a dictaphone are introduced before sufficient skill in typing has been achieved.

The hand control developed as a result of the observational study and subsequently tested, can be managed with normal movements of the thumb and with the application of low force. The control does not influence the fingering since it requires use of only the left thumb which normally takes very little or no part in typing. The hands do not have to leave their working area over the keys, so that the typing rhythm may be more easily maintained. The introduction of these controls during typing training offers much less risk than the existing control design. Interestingly, this study showed the difficulty for the workers themselves in identifying the cause of their musculoskeletal problems.

Ergonomics and work organization when redesigning a sorting section

At certain cutting and sorting departments within the wood industry, sickness absence is common. This is due to different types of injuries caused by excessive body wear, despite the fact that companies have designed the work stations according to recommended ergonomic guidelines.

Production within the wood industry is dominated by three assignments—sorting, transport and working up of materials. These assignments are repeated many times during the process between the sawed wood product and the finished product. Only in very special cases can classifying of timber be done by technical aids, for example image analysis. The manual sorting work and timber assessment are done by specially educated sorters.

In this project, cutting and sorting work was studied both from the ergonomic and work organization points of view (Karlqvist et al 1984). The studies were concentrated on the type of work classified as 'sorting of light wood details', in this case parquet blocks.

In sorting processes, timber and materials are classified depending on appearance, colour, different defects and for the kind of final product for which they are aimed.

Identify the problem

The problems revealed in this industry were identified through interviews, work studies, analyses from videotapes and photographs.

At an early stage it was quite clear that sorting of timber material demanded considerable effort from the workers. Sorting work is strenuous both physically and mentally. From a timber flow that continuously passes in front of the sorter, the quality of the timber must be estimated. It is important that a correct classification be made since that has a determining influence on the final product and on the economy of the company. A good quality visual environment is essential.

Work tasks. Work as a sorter consists of three different assignments or tasks: sorting, inspection/removal and carrying/shifting. The sorters rotate between these stations every 30 minutes.

In order to develop a priority basis for avoiding musculoskeletal disorders founded on ergonomic criteria, three stages were used for the assessment of physical loads.

Methods

In stage 1, a questionnaire was used to map out complaints in specific muscles and joints. Comparisons with other groups could then be made. Stage 2 involved a detailed analysis of physical load in different body regions. Stage 3 consisted of an ergonomic assessment lasting for one whole work cycle where physical loads were classified separately. Body wear points for different body regions were given for each work station.

Results

Questionnaire (stage 1). The complaints of the 72 sorters were distributed over body regions as follows: 61% showed complaints in the wrist/hands, 58% in shoulders and 46% in the neck. This high percentage of sorters showing musculoskeletal disorders confirms the assertion that 'monotonous sitting, highly repetitive work with light details', as occurs in sorting, are likely to lead to musculoskeletal problems. The questionnaire also revealed that complaints in the elbows/hands occurred frequently in young age groups and with only a few years' experience in the occupation.

Detailed analysis of physical load (stage 2).

Sorting stations. Observation of the activities carried out by the sorters revealed that the workers were required to lift heavy bundles of wood from awkward positions. Heavy rotation of the back when placing parquet block bundles in the outer areas of the workplace as shown in Figure 7.7 could lead to considerable stresses being imposed on all regions of the back. To see well at 'high-level sitting', the sorter had to work with a bent neck and a rounded back which easily leads to fatigue and spinal pain.

It was obvious that stresses were also imposed on the hands during sorting (See Fig. 7.8). For example, when several blocks were collected in the hand, the extent of the grip was often at its maximum and the effort great. Maximum finger extension and large grip force overload the joints of both the hand and the small finger muscles. The movement pattern in the wrist during block removal was characterized by extreme positions in the wrist (including ulnar deviation) and in the elbow joint, due to the high frequency of lifting in combination with frequent turnings.

Inspection/removal station. Analysis of the physical load at the inspection and removal station showed that the inspectors turned the parquet block bundles and, to ensure that the pieces of wood stayed together, the inspector applied pressure inwards with the hands

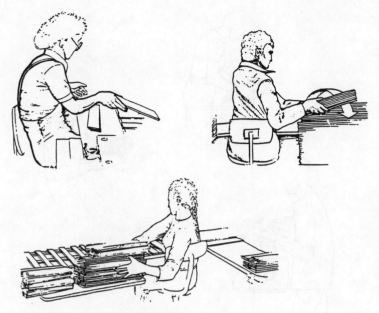

Fig. 7.7 Trunk movements at the sorting station.

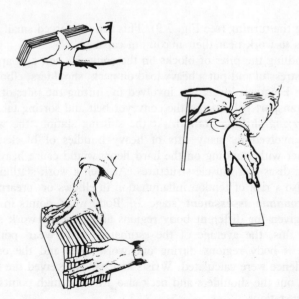

Fig. 7.8 Examples of common grips used when removing individual parquet blocks and bundles.

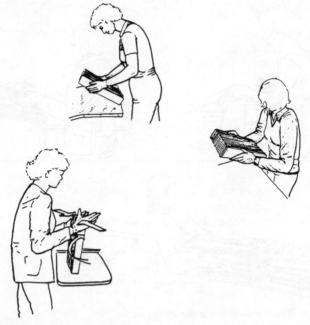

Fig. 7.9 Inspectors turning block bundles.

during the turning (see Fig. 7.9). This activity forced small muscle groups to work near their maximum capacity.

Handling the piles of blocks on the conveyor belt also appeared to be stressful and put a heavy load on neck, shoulders, elbows and hands. Frequent lifting was involved in shifting the piles of blocks to a transport pallet from the conveyor belt and sorting tables.

Carrying/shifting station. At the shifting station, the workers were involved in many lifts of heavy bundles of blocks. This, together with standing on the hard floor, would cause heavy wear on the discs and muscle structures. At such a work station, there was also a risk of tendon inflammation in elbows or forearms.

Ergonomic assessment (stage 3). 'Body wear' points in sorters were given for different body regions and for each work station. From this, the average of the estimated 'body wear' points for different body regions during one work cycle and the order of precedence were calculated. Wrists and hands received the highest score, but the shoulders and neck also attracted high points in the sorting stations.

Summary

In the group of 72 sorters studied, 81% proved to have injuries in the upper extremities due to body wear. During the first year as a sorter, 60% of the workers experienced shoulder, arm and wrist complaints.

Although the places of work had been built according to ergonomic guidelines, the way in which the transport flow influenced the sorters' ability to work according to the theoretic plan had not been taken into consideration. The sorters' positive attitude towards the work situation in spite of the problems is important. The worker attitude stresses how important are the community group attitudes and the co-operative spirit for worker satisfaction and their desire to continue work.

Specific conclusions drawn from this study included the following points:

— The real work level is not determined by the reciprocal heights of chairs and tables, but rather by the piles of work material in front of and beside the sorter.
— The real work area is not determined by the hinged chairs or, for instance, by the U-shape of the place of work, but rather by the need to attend to the transport flow which requires that the sorter sits facing in a certain direction.
— The work of the hands is not determined by the properties of individual wood blocks, but by the number of blocks that can be handled in one grip and by the movement pattern of the hands.
— Job rotation only partly satisfies the need for variation, as certain stresses reappear at all work stations.
— Scheduled breaks do not satisfy the individual's need for pauses when fatigue occurs.

Proposals

In order to solve the problems, different aspects of redesigning a whole sorting section were discussed by management, workers, technicians, social workers and ergonomists.

The principal recommendation was to drastically lower the physical load for the sorters while productivity and work content/satisfaction were maintained and possibly increased.

In order to be able to sort timber satisfactorily, working space must be designed to allow the personnel to stand or sit close to the timber. Light must be adapted to visual distance and to the size of the details being viewed, and it must allow a good perception of colour. Work environment must not be allowed to be boisterous. Since sorting work is mentally strenuous, working periods must be short and physical work varied.

Proposals implemented

An alternative sorting section was recommended, which incorporated ergonomic criteria as well as criteria for effective work organization. The new proposals were accepted and a modified sorting section constructed.

As Figure 7.10 illustrates, in the new sorting station, selected parquet blocks are moved towards the sorter on the conveyor belt. Selected blocks are fed out laterally on a belt perpendicular to the main flow. These two blocks as well as blocks that are moved to the extra conveyor belts in front of the sorters go to pilers. The machines sort bundles that have been inspected and transfer them to the transport pallets.

Evaluations

The descriptions of working positions and their consequences on muscles and joints are based on observations of the individual

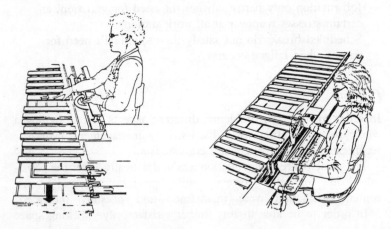

Fig. 7.10 The modified sorting station.

places of work and take into account the movements which occur commonly when working with small detailed components or parts.

The results of this project stress the importance of analysing the place of work when the technical system and the work organization are first designed. The suggested measures for improvement indicate that the traditional technical solutions can be used to improve the work situation and to reduce complaints. In-depth analyses are, however, necessary to determine how the work organization can be improved without losing the positive values that the sorters now find in their job.

In this project, compromises were made from the ergonomic requirements initially stated. This demonstrates that such requirements alone cannot direct the design. Work organization measures can, however, help to neutralize the negative effects of the compromises.

Conclusions

The projects described in this chapter are examples of the different methods of approach and the different proposals which might be recommended in order to offer ergonomic solutions to problems in some workplaces. That is, they provide examples of secondary prevention.

The ideal situation would be to install industrial physiotherapists as members of design teams, along with architects and designers, at an early stage of a project (Kilbom 1987).

It is essential that the importance of an ergonomically correct design is pointed out by a specialist at the drawing board stage, as it is both cheaper and easier to alter ideas at that stage of the process. While it is helpful for the physiotherapist to be educated not only in ergonomics but also in the art of architecture and design work, it is also important to note that the role of the physiotherapist is to advise and support other professionals in their work and to make them understand the need to consider biomechanical and physiological factors in the design of workplaces (Kilbom 1987).

The ultimate goal of this interdisciplinary work between engineers, architects, designers and industrial physiotherapists is the comfort and maintained physical fitness of the workers.

Spilling et al (1987) have shown that an ergonomically well-designed workplace reduces sick-leave. They have also performed a cost-benefit analysis of the improvement and found that it is a good investment.

While many of the present workplaces are of a good ergonomic design, the monotonous and repetitive work over a too long period of time causes musculoskeletal disorders. A wish for the future is that physiotherapists concerned with prevention will be able to influence the organization of work.

REFERENCES

Ahlstrand H, Lidehäll P, Svanberg K 1986 Statens institut för byggnadsforskning. Forskningsrapport SB: 2. In Swedish only
Arbetarskyddsfonden 1982 Nack-och skulderbesvär i arbetslivet. Forskning och forskningsbehov. (Occupational neck and shoulder problems. Research and need for research. Rapport 1982: 1. In Swedish only)
Arbetarskyddsfonden 1982 Arbetsrelaterade besvär i halsrygg och skuldra. En kunskapsöversikt. (Work related problems from cervical spine and shoulder. A survey.) Rapport 1982: 2 sid. 75. In Swedish only
Arbetarskyddsstyrelsen 1986 Research activities at the Swedish Board of Occupational Safety and Health. ADI 335
Bengtsson A 1986 Primary fibromyalgia, a clinical and laboratory study. Linköping University Medical Dissertations no 224
Berglund L, Lewin T, Aldman B Year unknown. Kroppsmått i sittande hos vuxna. Rapport baserad på undersökningar av kvinnor i åldrarna 15–70 år. Del1. Band 2. Deskription av variationer i sittmått hos kvinnor. Göteborg: Anatomiska institutionen, Göteborgs Universitet och Institutionen för trafiksäkerhet, Chalners tekniska högskola
Bjelle A, Hagberg M, Michaelsson G 1979 Clinical and ergonomic factors in prolonged shoulder pain among industrial workers. Scandinavian Journal of Work, Environment & Health 5: 205–210
Bjelle A, Hagberg M, Michaelson C 1981 Occupational and individual factors in acute shoulder-neck disorders among industrial workers. British Journal of Industrial Medicine 38: 356–363
Björkstén M G, Jonsson B 1987 Besvär från rörelse organen bland lakarsekreterare Arbete och hàlsa 1987: 34
Björkstén M G, Itani T, Jonsson B, Yoshizawa M 1985 Evaluation of muscular load in shoulder and forearm muscles among medical secretaries during occupational typing and some non-occupational activities. Biomechanics X-A. In: Jonsson B (ed) Proceeding of the 10th International Congress on Biomechanics
Hedberg G 1987 Evaluation of the driver's cab in the Rc5 engine. Applied Ergonomics 18.1: 35–42
Hedberg G 1987 Epidemiological and ergonomic studies of professional drivers. Arbete och hälsa 1987: 9
Hedberg G, Björkstén M, Ouchterlony-Jonsson E, Jonsson B 1978a Undersökningsrapport 1978: 14. Lokförarnas kroppsmått och förekomst av besvär från leder och muskler i relation till förarplatsens utformning Delrapport 1: Lokförarnas kroppsmått och muskelstyrka
Hedberg G, Bjödrkstén M, Ouchterlony-Jonsson E, Jonsson B 1978b Undersökningsrapport 1978: 14. Lokförarnas kroppsmått och förekomst av besvär från leder och muskler i relation till förarplatsens utformning Delrapport 2: Lokförarnas hälsotillstånd och dess samband med förarplatsens dimensioner i Rc-loket
Hedberg G, Björkstén M, Ouchterlony-Jonsson E, Brundin L, Björksten M 1978c Undersökningsrapport 1978: 39. Lokförarnas kroppsmätt och förekomst av besvär från leder och muskler i relation till förarolatsens utformning.

Delrapport 3: Frekvens och tidsstudie över användning av vissa reglage i Rc-lok
Hedberg G, Björkstén M, Ouchterlony-Jonsson E 1979 Undersöknings-rapport 1979: 6. Lokförarnas kroppsmått och förekomst av besvär från leder och muskler i relation till förarplatsens utformning. Delrapport 4: Analys av och förslag till utformning av förarplatsen i Rc-lok
Hedberg G, Björkstén M, Ouchterlony-Jonsson E, Jonsson B 1981a Anthropometric study of Swedish engine drivers. Ergonomics 24: 257–264
Hedberg G, Björkstén M, Ouchterlony-Jonsson E, Jonsson, B 1981b Rheumatic complaints among Swedish engine drivers in relation to the dimension of the driver's cab in the Rc engine. Applied Ergonomics 12: 93–97
Jonsson B 1982 Measurement and evaluation of local muscular strain in the shoulder during constrained work. Journal of Human Ergology 11: 73–88
Jäderberg E, Karlqvist L, Juhlin S-E 1984 Skärarbete vid läggbord (Cutting operation at canning bench) ASF 81 -0264, 82 -0672
Karlqvist L, Söderqvist A, Osterman, M-A 1984 Ergonomics and work organization when redesigning a sorting section. Wood Technology Report Nr 61
Karlqvist L, Österman M-A 1984 Hand och fotreglage för diktafoner. (Hand and foot controls for dictophones) ASF 82 -0667. In Swedish only
Kilbom Å 1987 Current aspects of the prevention of repetitive trauma disorders in Sweden. Abstract of The Volvo/IFSSH-conference on the prevention of brachial injuries and repetitive trauma disorders
Kuorinka I, Jonsson B, Kilbom Å, Vinterberg H, Biering-Sorensen F, Andersson G, Jorgensen K 1987 Standardized Nordic questionnaires for the analysis of musculoskeletal symptoms. Applied Ergonomics 18.2: 233–237
Kvarnström S 1983 Occurrence of musculoskeletal disorders in a manufacturing industry, with special attention to occupational shoulder disorders. Scandinavian Journal of Rehabilitation Medicine (suppl 8)
Larsson L, Bengtsson A, Bodegaård L, Henriksson K G, Larsson J 1987 Light microscopial and biochemical muscle changes in work-related myalgia
Lewin T 1969 Anthropometrical studies on Swedish industrial workers when standing and sitting. Ergonomics 12: 883–902
Luopajärvi T, Kuorinka I, Virolainen M, Holmberg 1979 Prevalence of tenosynovitis and other injuries of the upper extremities in repetitive work. Scandinavian Journal of Work, Environment & Health 5 (suppl 3): 48–55
Maeda K 1977 Occupational cervicobrachial disorder and its causative factors. Journal of Human Ergology 6: 193–202
National Occupational Health and Safety Commission, Australia 1986 The prevention and management of occupational overuse syndrome.
SAF (The Swedish Employers Confederation), LO (The Swedish Confederation of Trade Unions) and PTK (The Swedish Federation of Salaried Employees in Industry and Service) 1979 Working environment agreement
Spilling S, Aarås A, and Eitrheim J 1987 Kostnadsanalyse av arbeidsmiljöinvesteringer ved STK:s telefonfabrik på Kongsvinger (STK-K). Engelsk översättning: In Norwegian only

8. Lifting and ergonomics

S. Kumar

INTRODUCTION

Lifting, in a generic sense, may be performed by all higher order primates. However, the contemporary occupational lifting is uniquely human. This uniqueness emerges from the adoption of upright bipedalism by the *Homo sapiens*. Upright posture, though disadvantageous in some ways, by emancipating the forelimbs from locomotor activities has permitted the evolution of highly dextrous hands and arms capable of versatile manipulative skills. In adaptation to this situation, the original quadrupedal trunk mechanics are entirely altered. The body, ultimately supported on two feet, rests on a raised and firm platform—the pelvic girdle, which provides an anchorage for the spine—the prime mobile skeleton of the trunk; thus, in all bipedal activities the axial skeleton is required to transmit all forces acting from the trunk to the pelvis without forelimb support. In the lumbar region, the vertebrae are the sole skeletal elements available for force transmission. The lumbar vertebral segment is highly mobile. For the reasons stated, the lumbar region is subjected to large compressive, shearing and rotational forces in a variety of activities, the activity of lifting being one of the most stressful, as well as a frequently performed task.

The initial activities of survival of the stone age man involving lifting, e.g. carrying food, seeking shelters, etc., have given way to more complex vocational and industrial processes and leisure pursuits. Each one of these is contrived to maximize either productivity or performance. It is the level of achievement which is associated with the sense of satisfaction of accomplishment. In the process, then, the vulnerable human structure is compromised, precipitating low-back pain—one of the most common afflictions of the modern industrial society. In fact, Kelsey & White (1980) have estimated that up to 80% of the population will have low-back pain some

183

time during their working life. In the United States, this affliction has been estimated to cost 15.85 billion dollars (Holbrook et al 1984). Kumar et al (1987) estimated that the total transaction cost of low-back pain in the province of Alberta, Canada alone cost $114 and $99 million dollars for the years 1983 and 1984 respectively. They also reported that back injuries constituted 22.7% of all compensatable injuries in Alberta.

Lifting has been shown to be associated with low-back pain by many authors. In an epidemiologic case-control study, Kelsey et al (1984) showed that persons with jobs which required lifting objects in excess of 25 lb (11.4 kg) on an average of more than 25 times per day had over three times the risk for acute prolapsed lumbar intervertebral disc as people whose job did not involve lifting such heavy objects as frequently. Any superimposed axial rotation during lifting was associated with elevated risk. These activities are common in warehousing, agriculture, construction, manufacturing and other industries. Service industries like policing, fire fighting, catering, laundering and the like also require a significant degree of lifting and materials handling. Exposure to such risks is no where so pronounced as in some sectors of the health care industry. Physical therapists are constantly lifting and handling their patients. Similarly, nursing aides are involved in long shifts of patient lifting and handling. Kumar (1988a), in studying nine randomly selected group homes in the Edmonton area which collectively employed 173 nursing aides, found 62% prevalence of low-back pain in these personnel.

NATURE OF LIFTING

Kinanthropometry of lifting

The nature of the stresses sustained by the human back during lifting are multiple, including vertical compression, horizontal shear, rotary torque and a variety of combinations of these. They are determined by the initial, final and intermediate postures, the velocity of movement, and the load carried by the subject during the task performed. During such an activity, every structural element of the human trunk, i.e. the vertebrae, the spinal ligaments and the spinal muscles, will take part and endure the stress. Due to the degree of freedom of movement and its magnitude, different structural elements are stressed differently in different phases of any given lift. The type of motion is controlled by the form of the apophyseal joints, but its magnitude is regulated by the thickness of the intervertebral disc.

There are six possible types of movement at any given intervertebral joint, these being rotation about and translation along each of the sagittal, vertical and coronal axes. The degree to which such movements can occur is limited by the complex interaction of the vertebral articulations, the spinal ligaments, the intervertebral discs and the spinal musculature. The largest movement is normally rotation about the coronal axis, that is flexion and extension. Rotation about the sagittal axis, namely lateral flexion, can also be extensive but usually is less than sagittal movement. Axial rotation about the vertical axis appears to be highly limited at most vertebral levels. Translation along the sagittal axis causing antero-posterior displacement of vertebrae upon each other is small. Translation along the coronal axis, meaning lateral displacement of the vertebrae, is also very small. Translation along the vertical axis representing vertical displacement (compression and distraction) is extremely limited. Since lifting involves raising a load from point A to point B, it is their relative positions with respect to the worker and his postural constraints which will determine the types and extent of motion necessary for the activity. An idealized simple lift in the sagittal plane may involve only rotation about the coronal axis and translation along the sagittal axis. However, even with a slight asymmetry of the motion, rotation about and translation along the sagittal and vertical axes could be evoked, specially due to the coupling of lateral flexion and axial rotation. A variable task demand, therefore, may stress different spinal structural elements to a different level of their respective tolerance limit. Further, it is impossible to determine these levels due to individual variability in the structural and mobility characteristics, previous stress history and the level of kinanthropometric stress in relation to the tolerance characteristics. Such a limitation obscures the information which may permit a better control of low-back pain/injury incidents.

Biomechanics of lifting

Lifting follows Newtonian mechanics. However, the intricacy of the mechanics of a segmented rod (like the spine), with multiple curvatures and variable intersegmental control, working as a cantilever while moving the segments and stabilizing them at a position of optimum mechanical advantage, is self-evident. The act of stoop lifting which a man performs so frequently in everyday life is one of the physically most stressful and mechanically complex operations. In this movement, the spinal mechanism may be compared to the jib of a crane. The safe working load of a mobile cantilever crane varies with the degree of the verticality of the jib, being the least in the horizontal and the most in the vertical position. Bradford & Spurling (1945) calculated that a person holding a weight of 100 lb (45 kg) in his arms, 75 cm in front of the fulcrum formed by the lumbo-sacral disc, will require a tension of 1500 lb (682 kg) in his erectores spinae which act on a short lever arm of approximately 5 cm. They considered that the total pressure generated in the intervertebral disc will be a sum of these two figures, namely 1600 lb (727 kg). This neglects the weight of the trunk above the fulcrum level. Although the assumption of the length of the lever arm on which the weight acts is unrealistic, the idea is sound. Morris et al (1961) calculated that when a person is lifting a weight of 200 lb (91 kg) from the ground with a 40° flexion of the spine on the pelvis, the weight acts at a distance of 14 in (35.6 cm) and the mass of the head, neck and forelimbs acts at a distance of 18 in (45.7 cm) in front of the fifth lumbar disc, the compressive force within the disc will amount to 2071 lbs (941 kg). Following actual compression experiments, Brown et al (1957) described the lumbar discs as capable of withstanding an axial compression of 1000–1300 lb (455–490 kg). The vertebral end-plates have been found to be most susceptible to failure under compression. Eie (1966) found in autopsy specimens that failure of vertebral components occurred in spines subjected to axial loading beyond 650 kg. If one looks at the figures observed to be the failure strengths of the spinal elements and the calculated figures of the stresses developed and successfully tolerated, without any injurious effect, one cannot but be struck by an obvious discrepancy.

Weightlifting generates large compressive forces acting in the long axis of the spine. The magnitude of such forces depends at any given moment on the amount of the weight being lifted, its acceleration and the posture of the trunk. The interaction of these entities determines the strength of muscular contraction required for the accomplishment of the task. To begin with, in the standing posture the centre of gravity of the trunk lies in or anterior to the first lumbar vertebra. Floyd & Silver (1955) have shown that there is virtually no muscular activity when the body is in a balanced upright position. Thus it seems that when erect, the weight of the body above a given vertebral segment acts as a direct compressive force upon that segment. As one stoops, the trunk approaches a horizontal position and so the mechanical analysis becomes more complicated. Here one has to consider musculo-skeletal mechanisms as well as other facors. As far as the spine and its muscles are concerned, a trunk in forward inclination is held in position by two equal and opposite forces forming a mechanical couple. One of these forces is produced by contraction of the erector spinae group of muscles; the other is the compressive force acting longitudinally through the vertebral bodies and their discs. The perpendicular distance between these two vector forces is the length of the lever arm acting to extend the spine against flexion forces induced by gravity. At the lumbosacral intervertebral disc, when the trunk is fully stooped, the length of this lever arm is only one-sixth of the lever arm on which the weight acts (distance between the lumbosacral disc and the centre of gravity of the upper portion of the body). Therefore, the spinal extensor couple is at a 6:1 disadvantage in relation to weight, implying a six times greater magnitude of the extensor forces needed to hold the trunk in the flexed position than when standing upright (Fig. 8.1a). For positions between horizontal and vertical, the compression at the lumbosacral disc will be in part due to the mechanical couple and in part due to

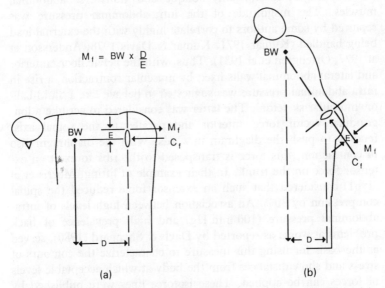

Fig. 8.1   Forces generated by extensor muscles in a stooped posture (Fig. 8.1a) and in a partially inclined trunk (Fig.8.1b). (Mf—extensor muscle force; E—moment arm of the extensor force; BW—body weight; D—moment arm of the body weight; Cf—lumbosacral compressive force.)

direct compression of the vertebral bodies by the body weight. Both these quantities vary with the angle of inclination of the trunk and, in addition, the length of the lever arm on which the weight acts also depends upon this factor. Thus, as the trunk moves from the horizontal to the vertical position, the magnitude of the mechanical couple continuously decreases and the magnitude of direct compression of the body weight progressively increases (Fig. 8.1b). The overall effect is that of stress reduction due to rapid reduction in the leverage of the weight.

Intra-abdominal pressure

The discrepancy mentioned above between the compressive forces tolerated by the spinal structures in vivo and in vitro was explained by earlier workers in terms of raised intra-abdominal pressure. An invariable significant rise in the intra-abdominal pressure during lifting activity, as reported by Bartelink (1957), Davis (1959), Morris et al (1961), Kumar (1971), Andersson et al (1977) and others, was explained to have a mechanical relieving effect on the spinal structures. It was stated to have been caused by co-contraction of the diaphragm, levator ani, oblique and transverse abdominal muscles. The magnitude of the intra-abdominal pressure was reported by some authors to correlate highly with the external load being handled (Kumar 1971, Kumar & Davis 1978, Andersson et al 1977, Ortengren et al 1981). Thus, with the pelvic floor, anterior and lateral abdominal walls fixed by muscular contraction, a rise in intra-abdominal pressure was suggested to behave like a 'fluid-ball' or 'muscular skeleton'. The latter was considered to act like a longitudinal vector force anterior and parallel to the spinal axis, tending to push the diaghram upwards. With the diaphragm also in contraction, this force is transposed to the ribs to exert an extensor force on the trunk. In their example of lifting, Morris et al (1961) considered that such an extensor force reduced the spinal compression by 30%. An association between high levels of intra-abdominal pressure (100 mm Hg) and high prevalence of back problems at work, as reported by Davis & Sheppard (1980), served as the basis for using this measure to characterize the contours of stress and show distances from the body at which acceptable levels of forces can be applied. These isoforce lines were published by Davis & Stubbs (1977a, 1977b, 1978).

Such a role of intra-abdominal pressure was widely accepted during the 60s and 70s. Currently, however, the opinion is divided.

Opponents of this theory argue that if the intra-abdominal pressure alleviates the spinal stress, an increase in the former must be reflected in a decreased intra-discal pressure as well as reduced magnitude of the erector spinae muscle activity. Nachemson et al (1986) showed that increasing intra-abdominal pressure, by performing the Valsalva manoeuvre, increased intra-discal pressure in an upright posture. This observation does not support the previously accepted cantilever mechanism of the spine. On the basis of the intra-abdominal pressure support theory, it became even more difficult to explain their observation that in a forward inclined posture (30° flexion), the same procedure reduced the intra-discal pressure. Moreover, Krag et al (1987) noted that an increased intra-abdominal pressure due to a Valsava manoeuvre in a lifting activity also increased the magnitude of the electromyographic activity of the spinal muscles. Since such a muscle response will add to the spinal load, they concluded that the intra-abdominal pressure could not be supporting the spine. Grew's (1980) observation of the generation of significant intra-abdominal pressure on the application of extensor forces to the trunk also defies the theory of the intra-abdominal pressure support mechanism. Kumar (1980) reported that in a lifting study, the peak intra-abdominal pressure was synchronous with the peak electromyographic activity of erector spinae and external obliques. If the rise in intra-abdominal pressure adds to the spinal stress, as the recent authors seem to be suggesting, the reason for its occurrence seems to be based on shaky ground. Nature has been an efficient system in weeding out the redundant and optimizing the necessary. Clearly, therefore, we do not understand this intriguing phenomenon adequately.

Muscular activity during lifting

All physical activities performed and forces exerted require muscular effort. It is through this effort that the loads are lifted. In this process, the contracting spinal muscles subject the spinal structures to considerable mechanical stress. Therefore, the spinal muscles can tell its extent. It is for this reason that considerable effort has been expended by numerous workers into studying the activity of spinal muscles. However, a lack of ability to discriminate and account for active and passive tensions of the muscles, the length of the muscle in different phases of contraction, the number and location of muscle fibres firing, and the constant relating of the EMG to tension, have frustrated efforts to derive a means to establish a reliable and predictable quantitative relationship between EMG and tension.

Electromyography, though, furnishes useful information on the temporal and qualitative aspects of muscle activity during lifting. In a balanced upright posture the spinal muscles are silent, and during flexion the erector spinae muscles contract eccentrically to control the activity (Floyd & Silver 1955). On acquisition of a fully stooped posture, a flexion relaxation of the erector spinae occurs (Floyd & Silver 1955, Schultz et al 1985). During this relaxation, the load of the spine as well as its stability is thought to be maintained by the spinal ligaments and dorso-lumbar fascia. Through the initial phases of lifting, the erector spinae remain silent, which is followed by vigorous activity (Floyd & Silver 1955). During this phase, the spine does not extend and the apparent extension occurs at the hip joint, as shown by Davis et al (1965) and Kumar (1971, 1974). When the load reaches this critical height, further extension of the spine is accompanied by vigorous activity. The magnitude of this activity has been reported by Kumar (1971), Kumar & Davis (1978) and Andersson et al (1977) to be strongly correlated to the magnitude of the load being handled. During dynamic conditions, the magnitude of the EMG recorded from erector spinae was shown by Kumar & Davis (1983) to be twice as much as of a static hold of the same load. Strong activity of the external oblique muscle synchronous with the event of weightlifting, with a pattern and magnitude coinciding and declining with that of the erector spinae, clearly demonstrates their contribution in this stressful activity (Kumar 1971). The activity of external oblique was also reported by Kumar (1971) to be strongly correlated with the magnitude of the load lifted (r=0.9, p<0.01).

Energy cost of lifting

To be of industrial significance, lifting activities have to be repetitive. At times, they have to be paced and the objects handled have to be of a given size and weight. In fact, Asfahl (1984) states that, on average, 50 tons of materials have to be moved to produce one ton of marketable product in some industries. In others, however, 180 tons of materials are moved to produce one ton of product. It is this repetitive nature of the task which places a demand on metabolic cost, which then becomes an important factor not only to ensure health and safety of the worker, but also to optimize productivity. The metabolic cost can be expressed in terms of calories spent or oxygen consumed. For most purposes, one litre of oxygen consumed equals 5.0 Kcal. Thus, by measuring oxygen uptake, the caloric cost can be determined.

Two physiological parameters characterize the ability of any worker to sustain a given rate of a task without suffering physiological fatigue, namely maximal aerobic capacity (VO_2 max), and physiological fatigue limit (Asfour et al 1988). In addition to these parameters, another concept of anaerobic threshold level of oxygen uptake which, when exceeded, will lead to lactic acidosis, was introduced by Wasserman et al (1973). However, in lifting task design, the maximum aerobic capacity has been most frequently taken as the golden standard to which things have been related. Earlier workers (Astrand 1960, Brouha 1967) advocated a 50% of VO_2 max to be an appropriate level of oxygen consumption to be used in designs for manual lifting activities. Bink (1962) and Chaffin (1972), however, recommended 33% of maximum aerobic capacity as a design criterion for lifting activities. Indeed, it is this standard which has been adopted by NIOSH (1981) in its 'Work Practices Guide for Manual Lifting'. Based on the maximum aerobic capacity of 15 Kcal (Bink 1962) and 16 Kcal of North American industrial males, a third of maximum aerobic capacity has been generally accepted at a level of 5.2 Kcal.

Objections have been raised to the application of the VO_2 max value for the design of lifting tasks. These have been based on the fact that all VO_2 max values reported were obtained during dynamic exercises, such as bicycling, treadmill running or step test. Lifting, on the other hand, has a varying degree of static component. In fact, the VO_2 max for lifting has been demonstrated to be significantly lower than those reported for other activities (Petrofsky & Lind 1978, Khalil et al 1985). It was also found to be dependent upon lifting task variables. The recommendations based on the VO_2 max for bicycle ergometry range between 33% and 50%. When the level was adjusted to the VO_2 max for lifting and lowering tasks, it represented 18.5% to 29% of VO_2 max as determined by the bicycle ergometer (Petrofsky & Lind 1978, Mital 1983a, Mital & Shell 1984, Genaidy et al 1985).

The physiological cost of lifting activity has been shown to rise with the magnitude of the load lifted, as shown by Lind & Petrofsky (1978), Garg & Saxena (1979), and Kumar (1988b). An increase in the metabolic cost of lifting with an increase in frequency of lifting is also well established (Jorgensen & Poulsen 1974, Garg & Saxena 1979). Lifting frequency and the magnitude of the lift for a given level of oxygen uptake for all three common lifting techniques (stoop, squat and free-style) were shown to have a curvilinear relationship by the aforementioned authors. The squat method (bent knee) has been shown to be most demanding (Brown 1972, Garg & Saxena 1979, Kumar 1984). The increase in the height of the lift also results in increased physiological cost (Kumar 1988b). He reported that the metabolic cost of lifting and lowering tasks increased with the reach at which the lift was performed, the height to which the load was raised, and the magnitude of load (p <0.001). The percentage increase in energy consumption over standing resting value increased from 28% to 100% when the load was raised from 2.5 kg to 10 kg, depending on the task characteristics. He found that the physiological cost increased between 11% to 41% of resting standing value when the reach of the lifting task was increased from half to full reach. However, Kumar (1984, 1988b) reported that the asymmetry of the lift (30° and 60° lateral) did not affect the physiological cost of lifting activity. In spite of the above, the asymmetric activities were concluded by Kumar to be less desirable because such loading may result in higher local and asymmetric stress (Kumar 1980), causing greater potential for injury precipitation.

Strength capability

Strength is an important parameter for ergonomics. Knowledge of it is essential for task design as well as for matching people to predetermined jobs. Chaffin et al (1978) demonstrated that the incidence rate of back injuries sustained at work increased when the job strength requirements exceeded the isometric strength of the workers. Keyserling et al (1980) found that the incidence rate among employees who were selected using isometric strength tests was approximately one-third that of employees selected using traditional medical criteria. As a result of these types of studies, isometric strength measures have often been used in industry. One of the important reasons presented by NIOSH (1981) in favour of static strength was its simplicity. Static strength testing has been performed, generally based on the 'Ergonomics Guide for the Assessment of Human Static Strength' (Chaffin 1975). Using this methodology, Chaffin et al (1978) reported static strength for arm lift, leg lift and torso lift from 443 male and 108 female workers employed in four different industries. Keyserling et al (1978) reported the isometric strength of 1239 workers in rubber, aluminium,

Table 8.1   Static lifting strength in Newtons

	Chaffin et al (1978) Male	Female	Keyserling et al (1978) Male	Female
Arm lift	382	200	382	215
Leg lift	942	416	892	392
Torso lift	545	266	441	235
High far lift	—	—	225	127
Floor lift	—	—	892	549
High near lift	—	—	539	284

steel and electronic component industries. They investigated high far lift, floor lift and high near lift in addition to arm, leg and torso lifts as reported by Chaffin et al (1978). The strength reported by these authors is given in Table 8.1.

These static strength values have been frequently used as design criteria in industry. However, it is common knowledge that most industrial tasks are dynamic in nature. Further, moving with load may affect the maximal strength performance characteristics of workers. Due to these considerations, Kroemer (1983) proposed an isoinertial method of determining maximal lifting capacity for individuals. This technique required the repeated testing of subjects with increasing weights until the maximum acceptable load could be moved through a prescribed lift distance. This type of performance test, though, could not provide a means of determining the strength capability of different stages along the trajectory of the lifting motion. This information is important since strength is likely to be altered by the changing postures used during the motion.

The first systematic comparative investigation of static and isokinetic lifting strengths at three different speeds was reported by Kumar & Chaffin (1985) and Kumar et al (1988). Significant differences between static and dynamic strengths ($p < 0.01$) in back and arm lifts ($p < 0.01$) were reported among men and women. They also reported a decrement in strength with an increment in lift speed. A lower strength capability of females compared to males was described, similar to what had been found for static mode by other authors. Findings similar to these have been reported by Kishino et al (1985). Kumar et al (1988) have reported a significant regression between static and dynamic back-lifting strength. These regressions were found to be speed specific. The strength obtained by them is shown in Figure 8.2.

The biomechanical set-up employed by different authors for

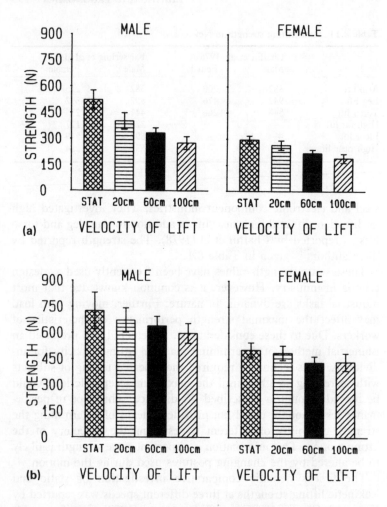

Fig. 8.2 Isometric and isokinetic strength recorded during arm lift (Fig.8.2a) and back lift (Fig. 8.2b) (from Kumar et al 1988). (Stat—isometric strength, 20 cm, 60 cm and 100 cm per second isokinetic lift strength.)

strength measurement have been different from each other, disallowing any direct comparison. To overcome this difficulty, Kumar (1987 a, b) studied the static and isokinetic strength at 60 cm per second displacement velocity at half, three-quarters and full reach in the sagittal plane. His findings are summarized in Table 8.2.

The peak strengths of the experimental sample in different categories normalized against the strength recorded in standard pos-

Table 8.2 Peak arm strength (mean and standard deviations) in N

Sex	Stat	Standard posture str.	Insometric strength			Isokinetic strength		
			Half reach	$\frac{3}{4}$ reach	Full reach	Half reach	$\frac{3}{4}$ reach	Full reach
Male	Mean	310	513	265	162	289	210	143
	SD	91	149	76	28	95	52	23
Female	Mean	158	249	169	104	169	134	99
	SD	50	91	77	39	43	40	29

Table 8.3 Peak arm strength normalized against the standard posture (SP), peak isometric strength (PIMS), and peak isokinetic strength at full reach (PIKS)

Parameter	Sex	Standard posture	Isometric strength			Isokinetic strength		
			Half reach	$\frac{3}{4}$ reach	Full reach	Half reach	$\frac{3}{4}$ reach	Full reach
Normalized against SP	Male	100	164	85	52	93	67	46
	Female	100	157	107	66	107	85	69
Normalized against PIMS	Male	60	100	52	32	56	41	28
	Female	63	100	68	42	68	54	40
Normalized against PIKS	Male	216	358	185	113	202	147	100
	Female	159	251	170	105	170	135	100

Table 8.4 Peak arm strength of females expressed as percentage of corresponding peak arm strength of males

Standard posture	Isometric strength			Isokinetic strength		
	Half reach	$\frac{3}{4}$ reach	Full reach	Half reach	$\frac{3}{4}$ reach	Full reach
50.9	48.5	63	64	58.5	63.8	69.2

ture, half-reach isometric and full-reach isokinetic conditions are shown in Table 8.3. The peak strength recorded in each category for females was significantly lower than that recorded for males, ranging between 48.5% to 69.2% of male strength values (Table 8.4). The strength capability among males as well as females was found to be inversely related to the reach distance of the task.

Psychophysics of lifting

Lifting is physiologically taxing, requiring exertion of forces, demanding on the tissue tolerance characteristics, and challenging mobility and stability all at the same time. Based on the body's ability to subconsciously integrate all the relevant stimuli and judge for their acceptability while ensuring continued wellness, a psychophysical approach has been employed. Stevens (1957) stated that magnitudes of stimuli and sensation have a quantitative relationship. He expressed this relationship as follows: $Y = K.S^n$ where Y and S are the magnitudes of the sensation and stimulus, K is a constant and n is a power to which the stimulus must be raised. Experimental work has demonstrated that for different work, different power functions apply. Further, physical and environmental factors which affect the comfort also affect the power function in the direction of their change. Thus, with fatigue, the given load feels heavier; with thermal stress the same task feels harder. Thus, an individual subjectively rates all stresses, assigning them appropriate weights, and integrates these weighted variables to come up with the magnitude of the sensation. By adjusting the magnitude of the stimulus in a given working condition, an acceptable magnitude of sensation can be derived.

Using the above premise, a number of workers have determined psychophysically acceptable magnitudes of load-lifting for different tasks. The methodology involves fixing all variables of the task, except one. For instance, the height of the lift, distance at which the lift was to be performed, frequency of lifting, size of the box, the temperature and humidity of the environment were fixed, and the subjects were given total control over the magnitude of the load to be adjusted. The subjects performed this activity for a prescribed period of time, e.g. 8 hours. During the work shift, the subjects were allowed to freely alter the load according to their perception of exertion. Most frequently, lead shots or pellets in an industrial tote box with a false bottom were used for weight. Any visual cue on the magnitude of the load was obscured by prefilling the false bottom of the box with randomly varied amounts of lead pellets. For industrial relevance, the subjects were instructed to perform on an incentive basis. This was achieved by paying the subjects according to the total amount lifted at the end of the shift—however, warning them in advance not to hurt themselves. They were also advised not to become unusually tired, weakened, overheated or out of breath as they were on the job for a long time.

Psychophysical assessment of lifting capacity has been pioneered by Snook and his colleagues. Snook (1978), in his Ergonomics Society lecture, summarized several studies carried out at Liberty Mutual Insurance Co. He presented a comprehensive set of tables for lifting and lowering loads from floor to knuckle height, knuckle height to shoulder height, and shoulder height to overhead reach. These were determined for males as well as females representing 10th, 25th, 50th, 75th and 90th percentile for lifting frequencies of 12, 6, 4, 1, 0.2 lifts per minute and one lift per 8 hour shift. Results similar to these were also reported by Ayoub et al (1978a) in their study of 73 male and 73 female subjects. Data bases from these two sources were combined to develop the 'Action Limit' load for 75th percentile females and 25th percentile males (NIOSH 1981). Ayoub et al (1983) reported lifting capacity norms for 5th, 25th, 50th, 75th and 95th percentile industrial males and females.

MODELLING OF LIFTING ACTIVITIES

Due to the complexity of lifting and its socio-economic impact, it is a widely modelled activity. The thrust of all models is to reduce hazards by predicting demands of different sorts on the human body. Modelling has been done in biomechanical, metabolic and psychophysical areas. Each one of these will be briefly and selectively reviewed.

Biomechanical modelling

Though a direct measurement of the compressive load on the spine would be the best criterion of biomechanic stress of any lifting activity, clearly it is not possible due to its invasive nature. As such, biomechanical models which estimate the compressive and shear loads at the joint of interest serve a useful purpose. Results of many studies, most notably those of Evans & Lissner (1959) and Sonoda (1962), have contributed towards a consensus of mean ultimate compressive strength of 6700 N for lumbar spinal units of people under 40 years of age and 3400 N for similar structures of people over 60 years of age. These values have been adopted by NIOSH (1981) in their 'Work Practices Guide for Manual Lifting'. In principle, modelling of lifting is based on mechanical laws of levers and Newton's laws of motion. However, anatomical and physiological complexities in kinanthropometric situations obscure the values and complicate the application of these laws. The number of unknowns frequently exceeds the number of equations available to solve the problem. This leads to an indeterminate situation, necessitating assumption and simplification of models. However, the accuracy of any model depends on the accuracy of assumptions.

Morris et al (1961) proposed a simple static model of lifting where the back extensor muscles and intra-abdominal pressure acted to balance the load held in the hand. Since then, several static and dynamic planar and three dimensional models have been proposed. Of the two-dimensional determinate static models, the one described by Chaffin & Andersson (1984) is most widely accepted. They calculate the back muscle force in the following way:

$$F_M = \frac{b(mg_{bw}) + h(mg_{load}) - D(F_A)}{E}$$

where

F_M is the erector spinae muscle force necessary to stabilize the spine

b is the moment arm of the torso at the lumbosacral disc

mg_{bw} is the weight of the body segment above the lumbosacral disc

h is the moment arm of the external load on the lumbosacral disc

mg_{load} is the weight of the load in the hands

D is the moment arm of the intra-abdominal pressure

F_A is the effective force of the intra-abdominal pressure acting at the centre of the diaphragm

E is the moment arm of the erector spinae muscles

To determine the back compressive forces employing the equilibrium equation, they state:

$$\Sigma F_{comp} = 0$$

where F_{comp} are forces acting parallel to the disc compression force. This can be elaborated as follows:

$$\sin \alpha \, mg_{bw} + \sin \alpha \, mg_{load} - F_A + F_M - F_C = 0$$

Since all values in the above equation are known except the reactive force of the compression F_C, the equation can be solved for this unknown. Similarly, the reactive shear force in a static posture across the lumbosacral disc can be solved by the following equilibrium equation:

$$\Sigma F_{SH} = 0$$

where F_{SH} is the shear force. Elaborating all forces contributing to this equation we get the following:

$$\cos \alpha \; mg_{bw} + \cos \alpha \; mg_{load} - F_S = 0$$

The only unknown quantity, the shear force, can be calculated from the above.

Due to the determinate nature of this model, its simplicity, and the ease with which all variables can be measured, this model has found wide acceptance and application. Chaffin's model has assumed a moment arm of 5 cm for the erector spinae. However, recent work (Kumar 1988c) has provided a moment arm of 6 cm for these muscles. This will make a difference of up to 20% in the results.

Schultz & Andersson (1981) reported a three-dimensional model to estimate the intersegmental resultants of the lumbar region. Their model took into consideration muscle contractions of five different muscle groups constituting 10 elements. These muscle forces, along with abdominal pressure and disc reaction forces, together made up the joint intersegmental resultants at the lumbosacral level of the trunk. Thus, they had 10 unknown muscle forces and three unknown disc forces, and only six equilibrium equations, rendering the problem indeterminate. However, they solved the problem by minimizing the disc compressive force using a linear programme subject to constraints defined by moment equilibrium equations with upper limits of the muscle stress. In 1985, McGill & Norman reported an iterated procedure which determined regression equations to predict the internal spinal joint force distributions. This model also needs many geometric values and material properties to achieve the force prediction. Kromodihardjo & Mital (1986) developed a 10 link model which computes the intersegmental resultant forces and moments at the lumbosacral disc. Cheng & Kumar (1988) presented a three-dimensional model of the human back for lifting activities. They approached the problem somewhat differently, employing two different procedures in their model calculation. First, they calculated the intersegmental resultant joint forces and moments using body weight, external loads and joint co-ordinates of 26 joints (see Fig. 8.3). In the second pro-

X-Y Plane   Z-Y Plane

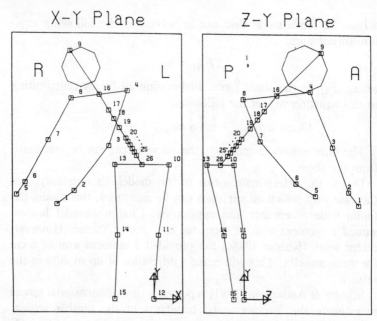

Fig. 8.3 The nodal points used in 3D back model by Cheng & Kumar (1988).

cedure, the internal musculoskeletal force distribution was determined using outputs of the first procedures as the inputs. This internal model included joint intersegmental resultants, six muscle forces, and three force components at six intervertebral disc joints (Fig. 8.4). In formulation, six muscle forces and three moment equilibrium equations at one disc joint with muscle stress (muscle force divided by physiological cross-sectional area) upper limits were used. The disc compressive force was minimized as the cost function. These solutions of muscle forces were further substituted into all six joint levels' force equilibrium equations to solve for the disc forces at all six spinal joint levels.

Metabolic model

A thorough and extensive model for predicting metabolic cost during lifting activities was presented by Garg et al (1978). They divided the complex lifting task into all its constituent activity elements. Each of these activity elements was then studied for its metabolic cost and a separate regression equation developed for each. By dividing the job into task elements and assigning a meta-

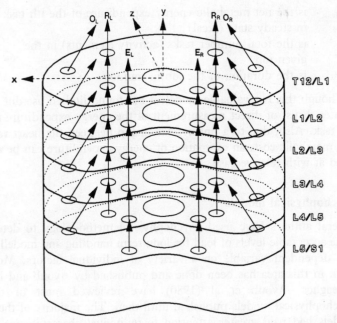

Fig. 8.4 The segmental force representation of the internal 3D model of the human back (Cheng & Kumar 1988).

bolic cost to each task based on measurable factors of force, distance, frequency, posture, technique, gender, body weight and time within each task, an energy requirement to perform that task was determined. They stated that the average metabolic cost was equal to the sum of the energy demands of the task, and the maintenance of body posture. They expressed this relation as follows:

$$\bar{E}_{job} = \frac{\sum\limits_{i\,=\,1}^{n_j} \dot{E}_{pos} \times t_i + \sum\limits_{i\,=\,1}^{n} \Delta E_{task\ i}}{T}$$

where

$\bar{E}_{job}$ is average metabolic rate of the job in (Kcal. min^{-1})

$\dot{E}_{pos}$ is rate of energy expenditure due to the maintenance of the ith posture (Kcal. min^{-1})

t_i is the duration of the ith posture

n_j is the total number of body postures employed in the job

ΔE_{task} is the net metabolic energy expenditure of the ith task in steady state (Kcal)

n is the total number tasks (activity elements) in the given job

T is the duration of the job in minutes.

Though this is a valuable model, it has found limited use due to greater thrust of direct measurement of the energy expenditure on the task. Also, due to a linear relationship between the heart rate and metabolic cost, an estimation of energy expenditure can be arrived at with relative ease.

Psychophysical models

Several authors have used psychophysical methodology to determine acceptable levels of load for long-term handling and modelled this dependent variable on a variety of individual factors. Most work in this area has been done and published by Ayoub and his colleagues. Ayoub et al (1980) have reviewed most of the psychophysical models published until then. The majority of these models had paid greater attention to individual characteristics of the operator, especially strength and endurance, to predict the lifting capacity. In later studies, independent variables pertaining to lifting tasks were also included. Mital (1983b) presented a generalized model structure which he developed using data already published in the literature for determining work rates for the upper 90% of men and women in industry. Based on task duration, the model could evaluate a material-handling job or design a needed job. In his equation, Mital (1983b) included the gender of the subject and several task variables, such as box length, vertical distance, frequency, the height level and several combinations of these. Mital (1983c) also produced some interesting results in a verification study of the psychophysical approach. He found that the industrial males, over an 8 hour work shift, lifted only 65% of what they psychophysically determined they could in a 25 minute assessment period. Over a 12 hour shift, this value was further decreased to 60%. A similar reduction to 84% and 77% was recorded for females for similar periods. The psychophysical models have to take such realities (based on a larger data base) into account and adjust accordingly.

PREVENTATIVE RESEARCH—RATIONALE AND STRATEGY

The old maxim 'prevention is better than cure' never lost its relevance but it is becoming more meaningful than ever with respect to back injuries. With a progressive change in life-style in general towards more mechanization, automation and efficiency, newer hazards are being created. In addition, the occupational hazards to the human back still remain due to the prevalence of manual material-handling in industry, amounting to approximately 50 to 180 times the weight of the items produced (Asfahl 1984). The increasing costs of medical treatment, compensation and lost production, coupled with the steadily declining value of the dollar, leave little choice other than to concentrate on research which may help control and reduce the magnitude of low-back pain problems. The human back is a dynamic system with significant and measurable diurnal changes superimposed upon the general level of ageing, degeneration and predisposition to injury or lack of it. When a predisposed person is exposed to occupational hazard, the sequence of events is quite simple (Fig. 8.5). Depending on the severity of the problem, the case may become part of the health care delivery cycle to a varying extent. A first level of such involvement is shown in Figure 8.6. However, if appropriate information about preventative procedures based on sound scien-

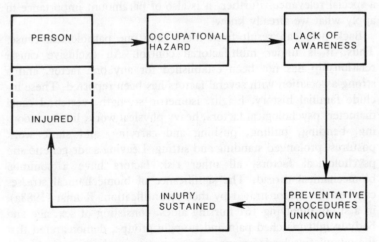

Fig. 8.5 A model of occupational accident (Kumar 1988d).

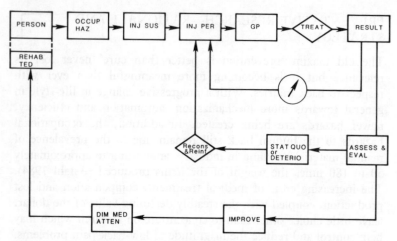

Fig. 8.6 The remediation in occupational injury—Stage I (Kumar 1988d).
(OCCUP HAZ—occupational hazard; INJ SUS—injury sustained; INJ
PER—injured person; GP—general physician; ASSES & EVAL—assessment and
evaluation; STAT QUO OR DETERIO—status quo or deterioration; RECONS
& REINF—reconsideration and reinforcement; DIM MED ATTEN—diminished
medical attention.)

tific grounds is known and available, many such injuries can be
prevented (Fig. 8.7). For a more complete description and discussion, the reader is referred to Kumar (1988d). Under these circumstances, preventative research into the low-back pain area has
a special relevance. Further, it is also of paramount importance to
apply what we already know.

Back pain can result from more than one pathological cause.
Thus, it is under multifactorial control. An exclusive causal
relationship has not been established for any one factor, and a
strong association with several factors has been reported. These include familial history, height, isometric strength, vertebral canal
diameter, psychological factors, heavy physical work, lifting, stooping, bending, pulling, pushing and carrying, and static work
postures, prolonged standing and sitting. Leaving aside genetic and
psychological factors, all other risk factors have a common
biomechanical thread. The significance of biomechanical stresses
can best be demonstrated by their quantification. Kumar (1988a),
in a study involving 161 nursing aides, consisting of sex, age and
body-weight matched pain and no-pain groups, demonstrated that
the cumulative loads among pain groups were significantly higher
($p<0.01$). Thus, the reduction of the mechanical stress on workers

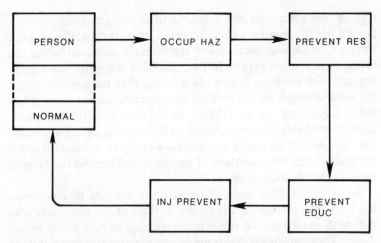

Fig. 8.7 A model for occupational injury prevention (Kumar 1988d). (OCCUP HAZ—occupational hazard; PREVENT EDUC—preventative education; PREVENT RES—preventative research, INJ PREVEN—injury prevented.)

becomes of paramount importance. Snook et al (1978) had considered three strategies for controlling the back pain problem in industry, namely (a) employment pre-selection, (b) training and (c) ergonomic job design.

Employment pre-selection, at times, may infringe on human rights. Therefore it is a sensitive issue, and no clear-cut position has been universally accepted. Snook et al (1978) investigated the effectiveness of the following pre-employment selection techniques in reducing industrial back problems:

a. medical histories;
b. medical examinations (including medical histories)
c. low-back x-ray (including medical history and medical examination), and
d. none of the above.

They found that just as many injuries were experienced by employers who used medical histories, examinations and x-rays, as by employers who used no selection criteria. The authors, however, were not certain if the findings of medical examinations were actually used in the selection process.

Chaffin et al (1978) investigated the effectiveness of isometric strength testing as a pre-employment selection criterion. In this prospective study, they studied 551 employees in six plants at the time of job placement and followed their medical history over a period of 18 months. They reported that the likelihood of a worker's sustaining back injury significantly increased when the lifting requirement approached or exceeded the employee's static strength. On the basis of this observation, they recommended that the static strength should be used as a criterion for employee selection. Keyserling et al (1980), in a tire and rubber plant, implemented this recommendation on 20 different jobs. They found that the medical incidence rate among employees screened through strength testing was one-third of the group selected on the basis of medical examination alone.

Snook et al (1978) analysed the effect of training by comparing the back pain incidences among the workers of the employers who did, with those who did not provide training on safe lifting procedures. They concluded that training was not effective in controlling low-back pain. However, they made no attempt to evaluate the quality of the training programmes. Troup & Edwards (1985) state, 'The effect of training in preventing accidents, injury or back pain has never been adequately studied over the long term, under controlled conditions. Similarly, comparisons of techniques have seldom been either comprehensive or consistent'.

Ergonomic design of the manual materials-handling tasks involving lifting, perhaps, has the most promise. Snook et al (1978) reported from their extensive survey that the tasks which less than 75% of the working population could perform without over-exertion had significantly higher back injury incidences compared to the tasks which could be performed by more than 75% of the working population without over-exertion. Based on this finding, they suggested that this is the only effective method. When one adds to this the information gleaned by the investigations of Ayoub et al (1983b), Chaffin et al (1978), Keyserling et al (1980), Bink (1962), Evans & Lissner (1959), Sonoda (1962), NIOSH (1981), and many other authors cited in other sections of this chapter, there is considerable argument in favour of ergonomic task design of lifting tasks. Kumar (1988a) has further demonstrated a statistically highly significant difference in the cumulative mechanical stress between age, sex, body-weight matched samples in the same profession with pain and no pain. It therefore lends another strategy which can be used in conjunction with other criteria for designing tasks based on psychophysical, physiological and biomechanics criteria as promulgated by NIOSH (1981). If the cumulative stress of an ergonomically designed task is to exceed the threshold range over the working life of an individual, the task may have to be adjusted. The above strategy has not been prospectively studied and validated, but deserves a chance. In the ergonomic design of a lifting task, it is important to design for the total task including coupling, work surfaces, environment and other factors which may influence the worker in his performance.

RELEVANCE TO PHYSICAL THERAPY

The ergonomics of lifting is of considerable significance to the physical therapy profession, both to the therapist and the client. A large proportion of a physiotherapist's work is physical in nature. This involves a significant force application either in treatment procedures or in lifting and transferring patients. An understanding of the application of the kinanthropometric, biomechanical, tissue tolerance, physiological and psychophysical principles to the human trunk will allow physiotherapists to better manage physical stresses. This understanding will allow therapists to make judgements on the trade-offs involved between the multiple stress factors which are important. For instance, biomechanically it is advisable to lift lighter loads more frequently. Physiologically, however, to conserve energy, the frequency must be reduced, even if the magnitude of the load must be increased. An informed therapist will try and reduce both, while optimizing the work output. It is here that kinanthropometric limits, psychophysical constraints and tissue strain recovery will also be worked into the ergonomic strategy of the management of backs.

SUMMARY, CONCLUSIONS AND FUTURE DIRECTION

Despite the fact that lifting is one of the most common activities performed during our daily activities, its impact on the human back and low-back pain profile has been profound. The complexity of the interaction between the human back and lifting activity has not yet been fully explored. To prevent human suffering and economic loss, application of ergonomic principles is recommended. Some aspects of the behaviour of human structure, such as the long-term tissue tolerance, and management of the industrial activities, such as pre-employment selection and the effects of training, need to be thoroughly investigated and incorporated in management strategy to secure a better control of the back pain problem.

REFERENCES

Andersson G B J, Ortengren R, Nachemson A 1977 Intradiscal pressure, intra-abdominal pressure and myoelectric back muscle activity related to posture and loading. Clinical Orthopaedics 129: 156–164

Asfahl C R 1984 Industrial safety and health management. Prentice-Hall, Englewood Cliffs, NJ

Asfour S S, Genaidy A M, Mital A 1988 Physiological guidelines for the design of manual lifting and lowering tasks: the state of the art. American Industrial Hygiene Association Journal 49(4): 150–160

Astrand I 1960 Aerobic work capacity in men and women with special reference to age. Acta Physiologica Scandinavica, Supplement No 169

Ayoub M M, Bethea N J, Deivanayagam S et al 1978 Determination and modelling of lifting capacity. Final Report HEW (NIOSH) GRANT No 5RO1 OH–00545–02

Ayoub M M, Mital A, Asfour S S, Bethea N J 1980 Review, evaluation and comparison of models for predicting lifting capacity. Human Factors 22: 257–269

Ayoub M M, Selan J L, Karwowski W, Rao H P R 1983a Lifting capacity determination. In: Back injuries: US Bureau of Mines IC 8948: 54–73

Ayoub M M, Selan J L, Liles D H 1983b An ergonomics approach for the design of manual material-handling tasks. Human Factors 25(5): 507–515

Bartelink D L 1957 The role of abdominal pressure in relieving the pressure on the lumbar intervertebral discs. Journal of Bone and Joint Surgery 39B: 718–725

Bink B 1962 The physical working capacity in relation to working time and age. Ergonomics 5: 25–38

Bradford F K, Spurling R G 1945 The intervertebral disc. Thomas, Illinois

Brown J R 1972 Manual lifting and related fields: an annotated bibliography. Ontario Ministry of Labour, Labour Safety Council

Brown T, Hansen R J, Yorra A J 1957 Some mechanical tests on the lumbosacral spine with particular reference to the intervertebral discs: a preliminary report. Journal of Bone and Joint Surgery 39A: 1135–1164

Brouha L 1967 Physiology in industry, 2nd edn. Pergamon Press, Oxford

Chaffin D B 1972 Some effects of physical exertion. Dept of Engineering, University of Michigan

Chaffin D B 1975 Ergonomics guide for the assessment of human static strength. American Industrial Hygiene Association Journal 36: 505–510

Chaffin D B, Herrin G D, Keyserling W M 1978 Pre-employment strength testing—an updated position. Journal of Occupational Medicine 20: 403–408

Chaffin D B, Andersson G B J 1984 Occupational biomechanics. Wiley, New York

Cheng C K, Kumar S 1988 A three dimensional biomechanical model for the human back. Manuscript

Davis P R 1959 Posture of the trunk during the lifting of weights. British Medical Journal 1: 87–89

Davis P R, Sheppard N J 1980 The pattern of accident distribution in the telecommunications industry. British Journal of Industrial Medicine 37: 175–179

Davis P R, Stubbs D A 1977a Safe levels of manual forces for young males, part I. Applied Ergonomics 8: 141–150

Davis P R, Stubbs D A 1977b Safe levels of manual forces for young males, part II. Applied Ergonomics 8: 219–228

Davis P R, Stubbs D A 1978 Safe levels of manual forces for young males, part III. Applied Ergonomics 9: 33–37

Davis P R, Troup J D G , Burnard J H 1965 Movements of the thoracic and lumbar spine when lifting: a chronocyclophotographic study. Journal of Anatomy 99: 13–26

Eie N 1966 Load capacity of the low back. Journal of Oslo City Hospitals 16: 73–98

Evans F G, Lissner H R 1959 Biomechanical studies on the lumbar spine and pelvis. Journal of Bone and Joint Surgery 41A: 218–290

Floyd W F, Silver P H S 1955 The function of erectores spinae in certain movements in man. Journal of Physiology 129: 184–203

Garg A, Chaffin D B, Herrin G D 1978 Prediction of metabolic rates for manual materials-handling jobs. American Industrial Hygiene Association Journal 39: 661–674

Garg A, Saxena U 1979 Effects of lifting frequency and techniques on physical fatigue with special reference to psychophysical methodology and metabolic rate. American Industrial Hygiene Association Journal 40: 894–903

Genaidy A M, Asfour S S, Khaill T M, Waly S M 1985 Physiological issues in manual material handling. In: Eberts R, Eberts C G (eds) Trends in ergonomics/human factors II. Elsevier, Amsterdam

Grew N D 1980 Intra-abdominal pressure response to loads applied to the torso in normal subjects. Spine 5: 149–154

Holbrook T L, Grazier K, Kelsey J L, Staufer R N 1984 The frequency of occurrence, impact and cost of selected musculoskeletal conditions in the United States. American Academy of Orthopaedic Surgeons 444

Jorgensen K, Poulsen E 1974 Physiological problems in repetitive lifting with special reference to tolerance limits to maximum lifting frequency. Ergonomics 17: 31–39

Kelsey J L, White A A (III) 1980 Epidemiology and impact of low-back pain. Spine 5(2): 133–142

Kelsey J L, Githens P B, White A A et al 1984 An epidemiologic study of lifting and twisting on the job and risk for acute prolapsed lumbar intervertebral disc. Journal of Orthopaedic Research 2(1): 61–66

Keyserling W M, Herrin G D, Chaffin D B 1978 An analysis of selected work muscle strength. In: Proceedings of the Human Factors Society: 2nd annual Meeting, Detoit

Keyserling W M, Herrin G D, Chaffin D B 1980 Isometric strength testing as a means of controlling medical incidents on strenuous jobs. Journal of Occupational Medicine 22: 332–336

Khalil T M, Genaidy S S, Vinciguerra T 1985 Physiological limits in lifting. American Industrial Hygiene Association Journal 46: 220–224

Kishino N D, Mayer T G, Gatchel R J et al 1985 Quantification of lumbar function. Part 4: Isometric and isokinetic lifting simulation in normal subjects and low-back dysfunction patients. Spine 10(10): 921–927

Krag M H, Byrne K B, Miller L, Haugh L, Pope M N 1987 Failure of intra-abdominal pressure to reduce spinal loads without and with lumbar orthoses. Proceedings of the 33rd Annual Meeting of ORS, January 19–22, San Francisco

Kroemer K H E 1983 An isoinertial technique to assess individual lifting capability. Human Factors 25(5): 493–506

Kromodihardjo S, Mital A 1986 Kinetic analysis of manual lifting activities: Part 1—Development of a three-dimensional computer model. International Journal of Industrial Ergonomics 1: 77–90

Kumar S 1971 Studies of the trunk mechanics during physical activity. PhD thesis. University of Surrey

Kumar S 1974 The study of spinal motion during weight-lifting. Irish Journal of Medical Science 143(2): 86–96

Kumar S 1980 Physiological response to weight lifting in different planes. Ergonomics 23(10): 987–993

Kumar S 1984 The physiological cost of three different methods of lifting in sagittal and lateral planes. Ergonomics 27(4): 425–433

Kumar S 1987a Arm-lift strength variation due to task parameters. In: Buckle P (Ed) Musculoskeletal disorders at work. Taylor & Francis, London, pp 37–42

Kumar S 1987b Arm lift strength at different reach distances. In: Asfour S S (ed) Trends in ergonomics/human factors IV. Elsevier, Amsterdam, pp 623–630

Kumar S 1988a Cumulative load as a risk factor for back pain. XVth Annual Meeting of the International Society for the Study of Lumbar Spine, April 13–17, Miami, Florida

Kumar S 1988b The effects of the reach and level of lifting/lowering tasks on metabolic cost in symmetric and asymmetric planes. International Journal of Industrial Ergonomics 2: 273–284

Kumar S 1988c Moment arms of spinal musculature determined from CT scans. Clinical Biomechanics 3: 137–144

Kumar S 1988d Preventative research—an effective therapy. In: Mital A, Karwowski W (eds) Ergonomics in Rehabilitation. Taylor & Francis, London

Kumar S, Davis P R 1978 Inter-relationship of physiological and biomechanical parameters during weight-lifting. In: Landry F, Orban W (eds) Anthropometry and Biomechanics of Sports Symposia Specialists Inc., Miami, pp 181–191

Kumar S, Davis P R 1983 Spinal loading in static and dynamic postures: EMG and intra-abdominal pressure study. Ergonomics 26(9): 913–922

Kumar S, Chaffin D B 1985 Static and dynamic lifting strengths of young adults. Xth Congress of International Society of Biomechanics, Umea, Sweden

Kumar S, Cheng C K, Magee D J 1987 Comparison of two rake handles. In: Asfour S S (ed) Trends in ergonomics/human factors IV. Elsevier, Amsterdam

Kumar S, Chaffin D B, Redfern M 1988 Isometric and isokinetic back and arm lifting strengths: device and measurement. Journal of Biomechanics 21(1): 35–44

Lind A R, Petrofsky J S 1978 Cardiovascular and respiratory limitations during muscular fatigue during lifting tasks. In: Drury C G (ed) Safety in manual materials handling. Publisher DHEW (NIOSH), Washington DC, pp 57–62

McGill S M, Norman R W 1985 Dynamically and statically determined low-back moments during lifting. Journal of Biomechanics 18: 877–885

Mital A 1983a Maximum frequencies acceptable to males for one-handed horizontal lifting in the sagittal plane. Human Factors 25(5): 563–571

Mital A 1983b Generalized model structure for evaluating/designing manual material-handling jobs. International Journal of Production Research 21(3): 401–412

Mital A 1983c The psychophysical approach in manual lifting—a verification study. Human Factors 25(5): 485–491

Mital A, Shell R L 1984 A comprehensive metabolic energy model for determining rest allowances for physical tasks. Journal of Methods—Time Measurements XI: 2–8

Morris J M, Lucas D B, Bresler B 1961 Role of the trunk in stability of the spine. Journal of Bone and Joint Surgery 43A: 327–351

Nachemson A L, Andersson G B J, Schultz A B 1986 Valsalva manoeuver biomechanics: effects on lumbar trunk loads of elevated intra-abdominal pressures. Spine 11: 476–479

NIOSH (National Institute for Occupational Safety and Health) 1981 Work practices guide for manual lifting. NIOSH Technical Report, publication no 81–122 US Department of Health and Human Services

Ortengren R, Andersson G B J, Nachemson A 1981 Studies of relationships between lumbar disc pressure, myoelectric back muscle activity and intra-abdominal (intragastric) pressure. Spine 6: 98–103

Petrofsky J S, Lind A R 1978 Comparison of metabolic and ventilatory responses of men to various lifting tasks and bicycle ergometry. Journal of Applied Physiology 45: 60–63

Schultz A B, Andersson G B J 1981 Analysis of loads on lumbar spine. Spine 6: 76–82

Schultz A B, Haderspeck-Grib K, Sinkora G, Warwick D N 1985 Quantitative studies of the flexion–relaxation phenomenon in the back muscles. Journal of Orthopaedic Research 3(2): 189–197

Snook S H 1978 The design of manual handling tasks. Ergonomics 21: 963–985

Snook S H, Campanelli R A, Hart J W 1978 A study of three preventive approaches to low back injury. Journal of Occupational Medicine 20: 478–481

Sonoda T 1962 Studies on the compression, tension and torsion strength of the human vertebral column. Journal of Kyoto Prefect Medical University 71: 659–702

Stevens S S 1957 On the psychophysical law. Psychological Review 64: 153–181

Troup J D G, Edwards F C 1985 Manual handling—a review paper. Health and Safety Executive, pp 1–70

Wasserman K 1986 The anaerobic threshold: definition, physiological significance and identification. Advanced Cardiology 35: 1–23

Wasserman K, Whipp B J, Koyal S N, Beaver W L 1973 Anaerobic threshold and respiratory gas exchange during exercise. Journal of Applied Physiology, 35: 236–243

9. Ergonomics—an educational challenge. A Norwegian model in ergonomic and industrial physiotherapy

R. Rustad

INTRODUCTION

Ergonomics in Norway is going through a conceptual change. Whereas it has traditionally been considered a technical and biomechanical science, over the last 15 years the concept has been widened to include psychological and educational aspects also.

In 1977, Norway adopted a new Work Environment Act. This Act was based on the older Act from 1956, but differed on two vital points. Firstly, the new law brought forth a new realization of the psychosocial aspects of the work environment by including a section in the law dealing with these kinds of problems. Secondly, the new law emphasized the importance of worker participation in solving problems in the work environment.

This second point has consequently changed the role of the various experts involved in environmental problem-solving work, from being those who analysed, defined and suggested solutions for the different problems in the work environment, to being experts using their knowledge to educate, advise and initiate action among those who have the problem or problems. Because of this, ergonomics has increasingly become an educational challenge for the professional groups interested and involved in it. Two examples of this new concept are described. The first is a report of a project carried out within a hospital in Oslo which concerned the nursing staff and the approach taken to prevent the development of low-back pain as a result of the manual lifting and handling of patients. The second example comes from the meat-processing industry and describes how the environmental work was organized there in order to secure participation from all parties concerned.

It is important to note that the changing role of the industrial physiotherapist/ergonomist leads to an increased need for a wider

213

knowledge of the educational and psychosocial factors in meeting the new demands made by the clients or user groups.

ERGONOMICS AND INDUSTRIAL PHYSIOTHERAPY IN NORWAY

In all countries, research and practice of ergonomics are closely related to the technological, social and economic development of those countries. They are also closely related to the importance that is placed upon ergonomics in the individual country, and to the way in which ergonomics as a science is defined.

Along with the rest of Scandinavia, Norway is a highly developed industrial country. Despite this, ergonomics has never really been considered as an important science in itself. Ergonomic considerations concerning work procedures or work equipment have been solved as the need has arisen. This has led to ergonomic problems being regarded as technical problems needing technical solutions only, and the feeling that there was little or no need either for long-term planning of ergonomic solutions or for evaluation of the complexity of the different problems that might arise.

Consequently, ergonomics as such has been subject to a very limited definition. Production procedures and equipment have traditionally been the responsibility of production engineers, and have been considered by them to be a field outside the competence of the ergonomist.

In Norway, organizational work, such as work procedures, shift work and work patterns, has been the domain of economists and management staff and has been considered a field outside the ergonomist's interest. Work psychology and the effects of sensory inputs on man has been the exclusive domain of psychologists, just as consideration of chemical hazards has been the exclusive domain of chemists, noise-control of engineers and hygiene of occupational health nurses.

In short, ergonomics, as known in many countries as man-machine and/or man-work relations, has in Norway, and partly also in the other Scandinavian countries, been split into a number of specific areas and sciences and has lacked educated ergonomic personnel to co-ordinate and combine the group specialities into what can be called the science of ergonomics.

Even though limited by definition, ergonomics in Norway has chiefly centred its interest on man and on the effects on man's health of certain features arising from the work environment. There are many reasons for this. As has already been mentioned, the lack of co-ordination between the many environmentally-related problem groups has resulted in the individual professions being left with a monopoly on 'their' problem. Another major reason is that ergonomics in Norway is, and has been, a field dominated by the industrial physiotherapist.

Physiotherapists were first recruited in large numbers into industrial work in Norway in the late 1950s and early '60s. In the beginning, the reasons for this were simple. Workers who developed work-related musculoskeletal injuries often required physical therapy treatment. Norwegian law entitled them to leave for treatment without loss of pay and this was costly to the employer. Consequently, physiotherapists were employed to give treatment at the workplace while at the same time analysing the cause of work-related disabilities and suggesting improvements to prevent or reduce their occurrence. This was considered a far less costly alternative for the employer.

Over the years, increasing numbers of physiotherapists were recruited into work as industrial physiotherapists and ergonomists. Today, approximately 500 physiotherapists are engaged within this field of work in Norway.

For physiotherapists, industrial work proved to be a field where preventive health care was obviously needed and this, combined with an equally obvious need for expert personnel, is the principal reason why such a large number of physiotherapists are now working in this field.

During the last 10 years, new technological developments, such as the introduction of the computerized office, have also created a boost in the demand for physiotherapists in the occupational health services. This is largely due to the problems of working with Visual Display Terminals (VDTs).

That physiotherapists became the group to 'conquer' the field of ergonomics as a profession in Norway has not only created the role of the industrial physiotherapist, but has also formed ergonomics in Norway as such.

There are few differences in Scandinavia in this field. In Sweden, however, more engineers and medical practitioners are involved in ergonomics than there are in Norway. In Denmark, ergonomics has become a field for which both physiotherapists and occupational therapists are responsible. In Finland and Iceland, ergonomics is chiefly the domain of the physiotherapists.

THE NORWEGIAN CONCEPT OF ERGONOMICS

In Norway there has been a desire to develop ergonomics as a science in its own right. The field has been dominated by physiotherapists and other health personnel, rather than by engineers and technicians. One of the results of this has been that the traditional attitude towards ergonomics has become synonymous with work physiology and work-station analysis. Because physiotherapists were the only professional group in Norway using the word 'ergonomics', the concepts of physiotherapy and ergonomics tended to become blurred by people in the community. This sometimes meant that the word 'ergonomics' was often confused with the physiotherapist's clinical work and the development of musculoskeletal pain and injuries. Figure 9.1 illustrates the traditional view of ergonomics in Norway. While the total work environment has been included within the circle, this has not traditionally been defined as part of the ergonomic sciences in Norway.

Consistent with the historic development in this field, recent trends among Norwegian physiotherapists/ergonomists have been to aim towards broadening and correcting the traditional misconception of ergonomics in the community at large. Moreover, since ergonomics is a science based upon a number of specialist fields, it has been necessary to build up a range of interdisciplinary knowledge.

The current aim is to broaden the concept of ergonomics from being one of concern for lifting or sitting 'correctly' to one of understanding ergonomics as a science which involves all parts of the environmental circle (Fig. 9.1).

Fortunately, other professional groups in Norway are also turning towards ergonomics as a field of interest.

The Working Environment Act of 1977—a conceptual change

According to the traditional concept of education within specialized fields, the ergonomist in Norway has been regarded as an expert in the field, even though this has been defined rather narrowly. Expert knowledge is necessary in all sciences and this of course also applies to ergonomics. The development of such expert knowledge is often connected to one or more professions, or to the establishment of new professional groups. The reasons for this are mainly to secure the further development of professional interest and to monopolize the field of knowledge within the group of professionals working within it.

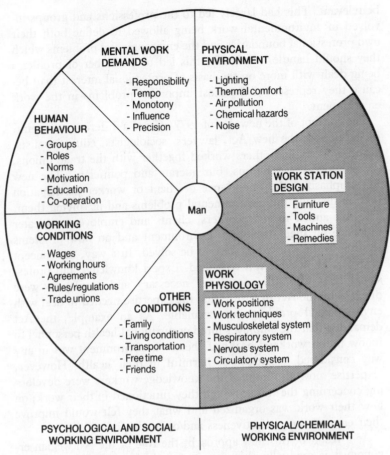

MENTAL WORK DEMANDS
- Responsibility
- Tempo
- Monotony
- Influence
- Precision

PHYSICAL ENVIRONMENT
- Lighting
- Thermal comfort
- Air pollution
- Chemical hazards
- Noise

HUMAN BEHAVIOUR
- Groups
- Roles
- Norms
- Motivation
- Education
- Co-operation

WORK STATION DESIGN
- Furniture
- Tools
- Machines
- Remedies

WORKING CONDITIONS
- Wages
- Working hours
- Agreements
- Rules/regulations
- Trade unions

Man

OTHER CONDITIONS
- Family
- Living conditions
- Transportation
- Free time
- Friends

WORK PHYSIOLOGY
- Work positions
- Work techniques
- Musculoskeletal system
- Respiratory system
- Nervous system
- Circulatory system

PSYCHOLOGICAL AND SOCIAL WORKING ENVIRONMENT

PHYSICAL/CHEMICAL WORKING ENVIRONMENT

Fig. 9.1 The traditional view of ergonomics in Norway (marked by shading).

These mechanisms in the development of professions are well documented in the social sciences (Torgersen 1972). Documentation shows that expert knowledge can be a hindrance to public knowledge, often making people reluctant to rely upon their own ability to solve a specific problem, a situation alluded to in Chapter 3.

When the Norwegian Working Environment Act was revised in 1977, these mechanisms were discussed at length. The former Act (of 1956) had stated the necessity of using expert knowledge in environmental work, but had not in any way discussed how this expertise was meant to be used or the type of expertise that would be relevant. This had largely led to the professions and groups involved in environmental work being allowed to define both their own professional boundaries and the environmental problems which they should handle. Naturally, this led to a number of problems being dealt with more on the basis of professional interest than because they represented the most important problems in the work environment.

The concept of the new Act of 1977 offered a different viewpoint. In developing the new Act, lawyers, sociologists, educationalists, health workers and others worked together with the trade unions, the employers' federations, bureaucrats and politicians. The new Act emphasized the importance of client or worker participation both in defining the environmental problems and in solving them. The Act aimed to give workers, clients and employees a greater influence on their own work environment and on how problems relating to the workplace were to be solved. In a way, the concept of expert knowledge was redefined. Expert knowledge and professional help was still considered necessary and employers were directed by the Act to ensure that the expertise needed to deal with environmental problems was available. As an example, the Act demanded that the employer hired occupational health personnel to follow up on workers' health if the work environment was in any way considered hazardous or harmful to their health. However, 'expertise' now also implied the knowledge workers were developing concerning the way in which they functioned in their work, on how their work was organized and what they felt would improve their environment, effectiveness and/or productivity.

As a result of this new approach, the role of the Norwegian ergonomist is gradually changing from being 'an expert', trying to solve problems for other people, to becoming an educator, initiating environmental work and using ergonomic expertise to guide people through a problem-solving process.

The following are descriptions of examples where this approach has been taken. The examples and the conclusions that are drawn are not scientifically tested and represent, therefore, only indications of a trend.

DESCRIBING AN ERGONOMIC PROBLEM 1

Musculoskeletal injuries and low-back pain among nursing staff

In Norway, as in most other countries with extensive health-care systems, nursing staff (nurses, nursing aides) are frequently subject to a variety of musculoskeletal injuries, the most common resulting in low-back pain. This is generally considered to be due to the fact that manual lifting is extensive, to the manual-lifting techniques used and to the handling of patients requiring special care such as on surgical, accident or orthopaedic units, geriatric patients or those admitted with mental or physical handicaps.

In Norway, musculoskeletal injuries and low-back pain are two of the most frequent causes of sick-leave and early retirement for nurses and nursing aides. This kind of problem now affects approximately 15% of all females working as nurses or nursing aides in Norway (Ebeltoft 1986).

Throughout the world, a considerable amount of research and clinical experimentation has been done concerning these problems. The most common solutions in many of the industrialized countries have been to handle the problem in one or more of three different ways. In the first, nursing staff have been taught and given advice on physical training. This has been done on the theoretical basis that a stronger individual will be less subject to physical injuries as it is scientifically proven that well-trained individuals endure physical stress better than poorly trained individuals. A number of different studies have shown this (Carlsöö 1972, Basmaijan 1978, Astrand & Rodahl 1985). In the second approach, nursing staff have been taught and instructed on how to lift and move correctly. This has been based on the assumption that although manual lifting is hazardous, it can be done in a safe way if performed in accordance with biomechanical principles. By this is meant lifting while keeping the natural curvature of the spine, holding the weight close to the body and keeping stress and tension on the spinal structures to a minimum. Thirdly, various lifting aids or mechanical devices which could be of help in different patient-care situations, have been constructed.

In spite of all efforts to improve the working conditions for nursing staff, the problem of acute low-back pain and other musculoskeletal injuries have increased in Norway, as in other countries, over the past years. It has become clear that despite these efforts, results show that they are not sufficiently substantial to prevent injuries and problems to any great degree.

Why is this so?

At Aker Hospital in Oslo, the occupational health services had been working for several years with these problems using a traditional approach. However, this did not seem to reduce the incidence of musculoskeletal injuries and low-back pain to any degree. In 1981, therefore, it was decided to try an alternative way of working with the problem, which would be more 'in the spirit' of the Working Environment Act of 1977 and more in agreement with the pedagogic principles in that same Act.

The hospital commenced by defining their problem as being something more than a mechanical, anatomical or physiological problem. The problems facing the nursing staff were often the result of a multitude of factors of which the individual's physical condition played only a small part.

This re-definition of the nursing staff's problems led to the realization by all parties that because of the complexity of possible work-related factors, a problem or an injury must be dealt with individually and analysed as such. It also led to the realization that no problems could be satisfactorily analysed or concluded by expert advisors with little or no inside experience, either of the job or of the individual's mental and physical reactions to working conditions. With these considerations in mind, it was decided to start an educational programme for the nursing staff. This programme was to be administered by the occupational health service through the industrial physiotherapist.

Aker Hospital employs approximately 2500 people and more than 1000 of these are nursing staff. A further 2–3000 part-time workers are also connected with the hospital. It seemed an impossible task for one physiotherapist, acting as an ergonomics advisor, to run courses for all employees as this would have taken years of continuous courses. It was decided, therefore, to establish a model where selected personnel were given training as 'back-instructors'. These personnel would then be expected to work with their colleagues among the nursing staff and act as educators, initiators and advisors within their own departments or wards at the hospital. Figure 9.2 illustrates diagrammatically the model which was established.

The educational programme was designed in such away as to relate to the participants' practical work. No specific classes in anatomy or work-physiology were included, as is the case in most other similar educational programmes. This does not mean that in this programme knowledge of these subjects was totally missing. However, such information was only given when participants asked questions which demanded such knowledge or when they discussed practical problems or needed to obtain further information in order to fully understand why they were experiencing a specific problem.

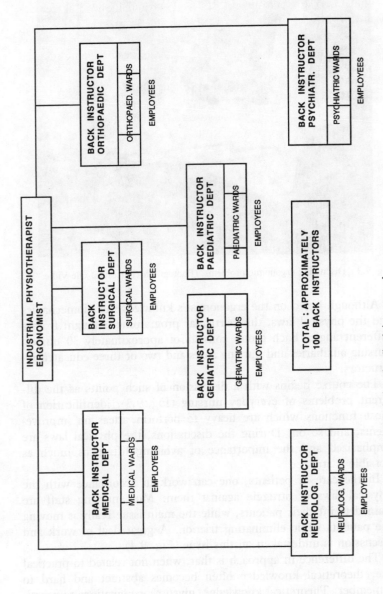

Fig. 9.2 Schematic diagram on the model of educating 'back instructors'.

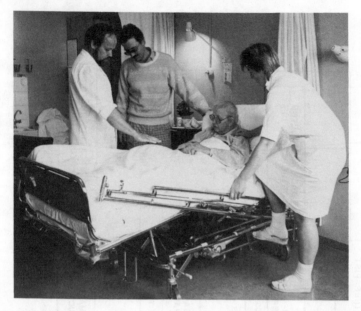

Fig. 9.3 Discussing ergonomic problems. (Photograph courtesy of Ole Vidje.)

Although based on the ergonomist's knowledge of biomechanics and the physical laws, this particular programme is taught from a different angle. Each group consists of approximately 30 nurses, nursing auxiliaries and nursing aides and two or three educated instructors.

The course begins with a discussion of such points as the different problems of everyday nursing (Fig. 9.3), identification of those functions which are heavy to perform, ideas on improvements, and so on. During the discussions, the physical laws are emphasized and the importance of avoiding lifting as much as possible is stressed.

In the care of patients, one can work in accordance with the physical laws or struggle against them. Most nursing staff are trained to lift their patients, while the main issue really is moving the patients while eliminating friction. A great deal of work and discussion is undertaken on this issue (Fig. 9.4).

The difference in approach is that, when not related to practical use, theoretical knowledge often becomes abstract and hard to remember. Theoretical knowledge, given as explanations to practical problems at hand, is, in a totally different way, accepted and retained by the participants.

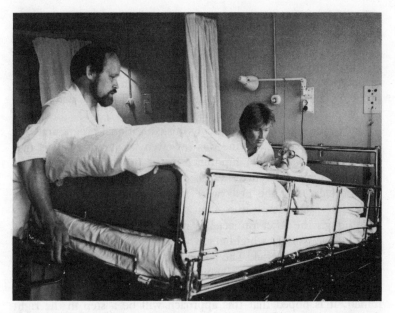

Fig. 9.4 Utilizing ergonomic knowledge in patient care. (Photograph courtesy of Ole Vidje.)

It could be said that these two different approaches represent two ways of perceiving the world. The first way considers theoretical knowledge as components or bricks to be selected and utilized as the need arises. Knowledge has its own value and is considered to be independent of our actions. Alternatively, it may be said that knowledge will always be a part of and also influenced by our actions. This is also true when doing research or in accumulating knowledge in other ways. For example, theoretical researchers will always extend their knowledge by carrying out experiments or accumulating other research results.

The educational programme at Aker was built on these beliefs: that commencing with the nursing staff's everyday problems and building on theoretical knowledge where this was relevant, was better than starting out with theoretical knowledge (such as anatomy) and then trying to fit in the practical problems being experienced by the participants. In accordance with the belief that nursing staff are the most knowledgeable people when it comes to their own work environment and that the ergonomic advisory personnel are more knowledgeable in their area, classes are conducted in dialogue, addressing such questions as: What are the specific problems? What are the different solutions, if any? Where can they be applied?

The essence of this approach is that it is impossible to teach anyone to lift 'correctly' or work 'correctly' as long as they do not realize that they have a problem. People often have to experience problems and understand that the problems do exist, before they can accept any behavioural changes.

One of the effects of introducing this educational programme was that the bed-making routine was reviewed, as it was obvious that this represented a major hindrance in the further development of the programme. The method of bed-making was revised because it became clear that the beds were made in a way that gave more priority to aesthetic pleasure than practical value.

Although the Aker project has not been finally evaluated, it is felt that the work has highlighted valuable points among the nursing staff at the hospital. The pedagogic idea is also an effect of the conceptual change brought about by the revision of the Work Environment Act of 1977. While the results have yet to be determined, it is hoped that this approach will be a step in the right direction.

DESCRIBING AN ERGONOMIC PROBLEM II

Musculoskeletal injuries in workers in the meat processing industry

The production of meat for consumption is really an extensive process. It starts with the breeding of the animals, continues on through the slaughterhouse and then the processing area (cutting, handling and packing), before the product is shipped out to the consumer as a neatly packed piece of steak or pork. Throughout the production line, workers develop musculoskeletal injuries due to manual lifting, handling heavy weights and adopting awkward working positions while processing the meat.

The meat processing industry is a male-dominated workplace, since it requires a great deal of muscular power. There are, however, quite a few women at work in those parts of the industry which handle the end products such as sausages, cooked meats and sandwich spreads.

The parting of carcasses into fillets, steaks, ribs or roasts is done by lifting, handling and cutting the carcasses of approximately 70–140 kg to the normal consumer-friendly weight. This work requires

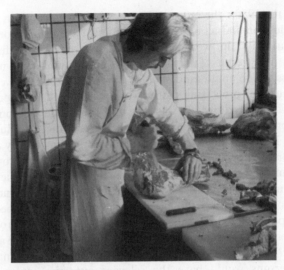

Fig. 9.5 Cutting beef by traditional methods.

a strong back and a strong arm. In this work there are, so far, only men.

For reasons of hygiene and health, all meat is kept frozen while stored. During processing, the temperature in the meat is not allowed to rise above 10°C, as this would allow the unwanted growth of bacteria. Because of these requirements, meat processing takes place in cooled rooms (10°–12°C).

This industry is traditionally very conservative and changes have taken place very slowly. Many of the work procedures used today are similar to those used 10, 20 or even 30 years ago (Fig. 9.5).

There are three major occupational health problems in the meat-processing industry:

1. Cut wounds due to handling and cutting carcasses and meats. It is well documented that musculoskeletal injuries are more common in cold environments, and since these men are working in low temperatures, there is a high incidence of cut wounds (Burton & Edholm 1955, Hassi 1982, Wiles & Edwards 1982). This is principally because the knives often slip out of the meat due to the cold temperatures.
2. Hearing deficiencies, due to the high noise level during processing.
3. Musculosketetal injuries and low-back pain, due to extensive handling of weights in the production process.

Since the 1950s, the industry has mostly concentrated on increasing production and all other considerations have been secondary to this. Naturally, the work environment in a number of firms has suffered as a result of this and there are a number of unsolved problems which could (and should) have been dealt with earlier.

At one meat-processing plant, work was started to improve the production procedures. It was felt that this could be done while also improving the work environment. As most meat production in Norway is principally for consumption within the country and not for export, the primary interest of the factory was in improving the quality of the product rather than in increasing the production. In the beginning of this process, the management was convinced that this involved allowing the production engineers, the special advisory personnel from the suppliers of the new production equipment and the production manager, to agree on where and how to install the new production line. It was taken for granted that these persons would have the relevant expertise to be able to achieve this satisfactorily.

There was disagreement, however, about this approach. The local shop steward and the local environmental ombudsman felt that there were a lot of environmental problems that would only be solved satisfactorily if the employees were allowed to participate actively in this review.

As the Working Environment Act of 1977 specifies that the occupational health service should be heard in such matters, contact was made and the industrial physiotherapist consulted. After 6 months of discussions between the involved parties, this initiative led to the establishment of a 'task force' or what might be called an 'environmental committee', with representatives from the management, the workers and the occupational health services. This committee was given a mandate to examine, evaluate and suggest possible options for a new production line.

The production manager was appointed leader of the work committee with the leading environmental ombudsman as his close contact. The occupational health services were to be consulted on the different suggestions and to evaluate possible negative health effects. In practice, the industrial physiotherapist worked closely with the production manager and the ombudsman in a continuous discussion on the various suggestions.

There were several positive effects of this work. The new way of organizing the environmental work encouraged the involvement of the workers and vitalized their discussions. It was now considered

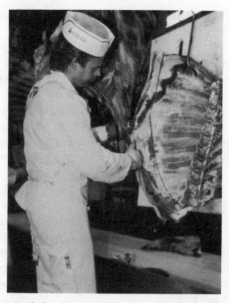

Fig. 9.6 Cutting beef after instalment of new production equipment.

that the workers' knowledge of the production processes was valuable and could be regarded as 'equally important as' the knowledge of the experts. In turn, this led to a greater degree of involvement and interest among the workers with regard to their own jobs and their own work environment and to quite a few valuable suggestions and ideas being offered for improvement (Fig. 9.6).

It was felt that as a result of this approach, the social network improved and communication and co-operation between management and workforce were more effective than previously.

Further effects of adopting this problem-solving process were seen. As interest was being shown in the workers' experiences and ideas, they offered other ideas and suggestions for improving the work environment more frequently and more freely. Noise, which had always been one of the major problems in the work environment, was reduced significantly as a result of applying suggestions from the workers.

For example, noise from the various meat saws in the factory was reduced from 94–102 dBA to about 75 dBA. For those in the surrounding work environment, noise was reduced even more to 65–70 dBA. It must be added that these suggestions did not demand a major investment, since it was possible to keep noise-control costs to a minimum.

Other improvements included less manual handling of carcasses due to new and improved production lines, where all meat is now transported mechanically; better work positions while parting meat due to new, adjustable work-tables: less strain on less. feet and low back due to improved flooring; reduced musculoskeletal strain and fewer cuts due to raising of the temperature. The latter could be achieved because the production process was handled more quickly than previously, so that there was no increase in bacterial growth in the meat. Improvements to the equipment used such as new wheels with less friction for the transport apparatus led in turn to improvements in the work environment.

The workers' influence in the process clearly led to a better work environment. Their experience in practical work was valuable when establishing the new production line. It also became quite clear that productivity increased significantly. This meant a better economic situation for the company and thus a better situation for further environmental work.

Throughout this process the occupational health services and the physiotherapist worked as educators and initiators rather than as ergonomic 'experts'. Naturally, ergonomic advice was sought and given, but only after a problem had been discussed thoroughly among those affected by it. The ergonomic advice was never offered as the final solution, but rather as suggestions meant to generate further discussions in the problem-solving process. It is important to note that all ergonomic advice was given in a manner to which the lay person could relate and in a form that did not remove the problem from those experiencing it.

However, the major effect was that a new routine was established in the environmental work. The establishment of work groups, with representatives from the management, the workers and the technical experts, was probably the most positive change that occurred. The other was the realization among all parties that problem solving was a process where everybody involved could make a valuable contribution.

ERGONOMICS—AN EDUCATIONAL CHALLENGE

These two examples from Norwegian industrial physiotherapy practice have been used to show how the work of the Norwegian industrial physiotherapist/ergonomist has changed from being solely technical with knowledge founded on anatomy, physiology and biomechanics, to being technical, psychological and educational with the need for knowledge in all these fields.

As a result, the role of the physiotherapist has changed to that of an educator and initiator of environmental work, especially when related to musculoskeletal illness and injuries. There are several reasons for this. It is mainly due to the experience gathered over recent years that it has become obvious that proper and lasting solutions can only be found if everyone involved in the problem participates in defining and solving it. This does not mean, however, that the industrial physiotherapist now only acts as an educator in problem solving or as an initiator of action. It is still necessary to have sound ergonomic expertise and to be able to give professional advice when consulted. As the field of ergonomics is growing rapidly, and reports, studies and articles are published in increasing numbers, the industrial physiotherapist must in fact accumulate an increasing amount of knowledge in order to keep abreast, and must develop a wide perspective of man–machine interaction and not just fragmentary knowledge. The need to know has not changed. What has changed is the understanding of how to communicate expert knowledge to the public and how to transform expert knowledge into user/client knowledge and, in turn, convert this knowledge into effective action.

Being an expert requires a certain amount of intelligence and a lot of study. Many people become experts, as they are very knowledgeable in their specific field. But being an expert is usually not sufficient. Clients must be able to understand the nature and meaning of the advice being given. This places demands on the expert's ability to communicate his knowledge and is one of the difficulties of being an expert advisor.

The most difficult aspect is communicating expert knowledge in such a way that it is understood by the receiver and will lead to problem-solving actions.

This is the role of the industrial physiotherapist today.

Ergonomics has become more than the understanding of technological and/or bio-mechanical problems in the work environment. Ergonomics is understanding the total interaction between man and his environment—and understanding that to be able to give adequate help in a problem-solving process the expert must, through his or her work, enable the user/clients to understand and be able to handle their own problems.

Socrates knew this, as many others after him have known it. The great Danish educator, Sören Kierkegaard (1813–1855), knew this, and his words from the mid-19th century are equally true today:

..... that, if one is to succeed in guiding someone somewhere, one must first seek to find him where he is and start there. This is the secret of the art of helping. Anyone who cannot do this, is deceiving himself into believing he can help others. For, in truth, to be able to help anyone I must understand more than him—but first of all I must understand what he understands.

If I do not understand this, my wider understanding will be of no help to him at all.

If I still, despite this lack of understanding, let my wider knowledge dominate, it must be because I am vain or proud, that I, rather than trying to help him, want to be admired by him.

But all true help begins with a humility. The helper must first humble himself before the person he wants to help, and thereby understand that helping is not the same as dominating, but serving—that helping is not the same as being the most autocratic, but the most patient—that helping is willingness to accept that one can be wrong and that one may not understand what the other person understands.

REFERENCES

Astrand P O, Rodahl K 1985 Textbook of work physiology. McGraw-Hill, New York

Basmajian J V 1978 Muscles alive. Williams & Williams, Baltimore

Burton A C, Edholm O G 1955 Man in a cold environment. Arnold, London

Carlsöö S 1972 How man moves. Heinemann, London

Ebeltoft A 1986 Fra Muskelverk til Miljöaktivitet. Universitetsforlaget, Oslo

Hassi J 1982 Working in cold conditions. Nordic council arct Med Rep (No 30)

Kierkegaard S Filosofiske smuler med avsluttende uvitenskapelige efterskrifter. Kobenhavn, 1946 English translation: 1964 Philosophical fragment of philosophy. Transl: D F Swenson/Rev: H V. Hong Kong University Press, Princeton

Torgersen U 1972 Profesjonssosiologi. Universitersforlaget, Oslo

Wiles C M, Edwards R H T 1982 The effect of temperature, ischaemia and contractile activity on the relaxation rate of human muscle. London Medical School

The Norwegian Working Environment Act of 1977, 5th edn. Oslo 1986

10. Matching work demands to functional ability

H. Watson, S. Whalley, I. McClelland

Far and away the best prize that life offers is the chance to work hard at work worth doing.

Theodore Roosevelt 1903

INTRODUCTION

First thing on a Monday morning, it is difficult to view work as a blessing. For many people, their job separates them from family, friends, hobbies, sports and other aspects of life which are valued. Yet, at the end of a day's work there is something to be said for the satisfaction which can be felt on completing any worthwhile task.

Over the years and between cultures, creeds, generations and individuals, work has been perceived as a way of life, a means to salvation, a source of exploitation, a necessary evil and, more recently, as a luxury. Indeed, it is likely that perceptions of work will continue to change as the very nature of work changes (Cornes 1984). For the present, though, work is seen by many as a central activity in their lives and even as a duty owed by each citizen to society. In turn, societies are felt to have reciprocal responsibilities towards their working-age citizens, irrespective of ability, and the 'right to work' has become a valued prize in many industrialized countries.

Disabled people of working age are no exception to the rule in wanting to work. They share a fundamental right '. . according to their capabilities, to secure and maintain employment or engage in a useful, productive and remunerative occupation. .' (UN Declaration of Rights, Article 7, 1975) and this ideal has been embodied in various laws passed over the years since the Second World War. For example, in Great Britain, the Disabled Persons (Employment)

Act 1944 set up a quota system for employing disabled people in open industry, introduced the Disablement Resettlement Officer (DRO) service, created sheltered employment facilities and encouraged the development of advisory committees and special courses of employment rehabilitation. Nonetheless, despite legislation, it has been pointed out that the degree to which disabled people can exercise their current entitlement to work depends not only on the prevailing political climate, but also on the services available and the physical, social and economic environment within which they live (DeJong 1981).

So, while in principle disabled people have the right to work, in practice they are often less successful than their non-disabled peers in realizing this right, as confirmed by the existence of legislation to protect disabled peoples' interests. For instance, Bowe (1983) found that the typical, working-age, disabled American does not work—only one in three participating in the workforce. Similarly, Croxen (1985) has suggested that disabled people in the European Community form a disproportionately high number of the unregistered unemployed. (The precise unemployment rates for all disabled people in member states is unknown due to the problem of identifying and classifying disability (Duckworth 1983) and thereby identifying a distinct population which may be counted.) Nevertheless, it has been estimated that disabled people, registered or otherwise, form a sizeable minority of working-age populations as confirmed by a social survey conducted in Great Britain (Harris et al 1971). This estimated that over 1 000 000 people of working age (and living in private households) had a physical, mental or sensory impairment which resulted in minor, appreciable, severe or very severe functional difficulty.

Undoubtedly, such estimates include people who are so severely disabled that they could never be expected to 'secure and maintain' employment in the open labour market. Yet, severely disabled individuals are unrepresentative of the vast majority of the disabled population who actually may have little in common. For ergonomists, familiar with issues of human variability, the point is obvious. However, it is widely misconceived that disabled people typically are wheelchair-bound and dependent upon others for most of their needs. The persistence of such beliefs may explain why disabled people in general are discriminated against, despite there being no reason to suppose that the majority of disabled employees are any less efficient or less capable of performing a variety of tasks than non-disabled people. In fact, Kettle (1985), for example, has provided evidence to dispel the myths that disabled employees are relatively poor attenders or any more prone to work injuries than their non-disabled colleagues.

Consider the difference between a person who is colour blind and a person who has lost a leg. Both individuals are potentially occupationally disabled. The colour-blind employee may be functionally unable to identify information coded in red/green and, consequently, would be prohibited from training for any job where colour vision was crucial. By contrast, the person with a lower limb amputation may be as functionally mobile as non-impaired people and certainly could be considered for posts requiring colour vision. From this simple example, it is clear that disability is a very individual experience which differs not only between individuals, but also relatively with the type and severity of the underlying impairment, the way in which people overcome or compensate for functional difficulties and the nature of the task in hand.

Against a backcloth of human rights, inequalities and prejudices, the role of vocational rehabilitation specialists is to expedite the return-to-work, or re-introduction into the labour market of disabled employees who might otherwise lose the opportunity to resume work. (This role is distinct from that of vocational habilitation professionals who are concerned with obtaining jobs for disabled people with no previous work experience.)

The general process of rehabilitation is initiated by physiotherapists and other members of the paramedical and medical professions in the context of treatments and services provided in hospital, the community or some occupational settings. The premise of all treatment-based regimes is that the problem lies within the individual who must be helped to regain or compensate for losses of function. So, for example, physiotherapists and occupational therapists attempt to minimize the effects of sensory, physical or mental impairment upon movement or activity, respectively. This treatment approach to rehabilitation has been strongly criticized (Dejong 1982, Stubbins 1982), since it is believed to perpetuate patient dependency and ignores the fact that attitudes and environments contribute to the experience of disability. Therefore, in a broader sense, vocational rehabilitation is concerned with what Galvin (1985) and others have termed disability management and this is as much about changing the attitudes of professionals, employers and wider society as it is about developing the abilities of disabled people.

Disability management is concerned with co-ordinating activities intended to restore an individual's working capacity by removing obstacles imposed by the environment, by making efficient use of medical and vocational rehabilitation resources, by minimizing disability-related costs and increasing the continuity between services (Galvin 1985). It is proposed that this be achieved through education and the introduction of employer-based programmes of management which emphasize positive policies towards disabled employees and adopt systematic return-to-work plans incorporating methods of job analysis, placement, modification and other related services and accommodations.

MATCHING MEN, MACHINES, WORK SPACES AND ENVIRONMENTS

Within the broad framework of disability management, the ergonomist is suitably qualified to address general systems issues and the classical ergonomic factors influencing the matching of human abilities with work demands. As a technologist 'concerned with health (in the sense of well-being) and efficiency (in the sense of optimal use of human labour)' (Singleton 1972), the ergonomist is concerned with the dual interests of employees and employers. In order to optimize health and efficiency, it is important that employees are suited to the environments within which they work. Thus, in the design of any new system this may be accomplished by the appropriate 'allocation of function' between men and machines on the basis of deciding which activities are best carried out by men and which activities are best automated. Only then is it appropriate to implement 'the classical ergonomic procedures of matching men, machines, work spaces and environments' (Singleton 1972), and there are two approaches which may be taken:

1. Either employees can be matched to jobs by careful recruitment, training or placement procedures
2. Or jobs can be matched to employees by selection, redesign, adaptations and aids to employment or other accommodations.

The first approach—fitting men to jobs—equates with the medical model of rehabilitation, the ergonomist striving to match human resources to man-made standards which may be humanly unreasonable or inequitable. Central to this method of matching is the importance placed upon people carrying out jobs as they are preordained. For example, the convention of using red for 'stop' or as a warning signal and green for 'go' is not immutable, but has been devised by colour discriminative people as a means of conveying important information. In a population where the majority of people were colour blind, symbols, auditory cues or both might be used to convey the same detail.

The second approach—fitting jobs to men—acknowledges that the cause of disability can lie outside the individual in the work environment itself. Importance is placed upon arranging work environments to suit the abilities of employees and this may be achieved by making organizational changes (as in the case of work-sharing) or material changes (such as rearranging work-station layouts).

In either event, the ergonomist (in conjunction with other rehabilitation professionals) needs to obtain detailed information about the functioning of relevant aspects of work systems and relevant abilities of disabled employees before a decision can be made about a particular person in relation to a particular job. One of the most systematic ways of obtaining such information is to employ standardized methods of assessing work demands and human abilities (Watson & Cornes 1986).

When developing a general methodology for occupational disability assessment, Singleton et al (1979) concluded that a comprehensive assessment involves four stages:

1. psychometric assessment of potential
2. psychological assessment of trainability
3. medical assessment of residual function
4. ergonomic assessment of matching to specific work, including, when necessary, the modification of the work.

The first three stages relate to obtaining information about an individual, whereas the latter stage entails assessing work from the point of view of recording work-load in relation to the abilities of an employee. This would appear a sensible recommendation as it implies that a disabled person will be considered on merit. However, many methods of medical and psychological assessment are difficult to interpret in conjunction with existing forms of ergonomic job analysis. (For a more detailed discussion of methods of psychological assessment, see Anastasi 1961).

Arguably, the most comprehensive taxonomy of disability devised by members of the medical profession is contained within the International Classification of Impairments, Disabilities and Handicaps (ICIDH) (WHO 1980). While impressive in coverage, the disability section of the ICIDH is not wholly relevant to the workplace, covering such activities as bathing, going to bed and coping with household objects. Even if used selectively, the two 10 point 'grading' systems for current ability and prognosis are difficult to interpret. For example, what does one conclude about the suitability of a person for a physically demanding job if he is coded as disabled in relation to physical strain, but not requiring aids nor assistance? Other classifications of disability severity noted by Singleton et al (1979) include the Classification of Men with Chronic Conditions by Working Capacity, the A-Z Medical Code for the Classification by Disability of Disabled Persons and the Classification by Degree of Functional Disorder. Like the ICIDH, these classifications are reported to be difficult to apply, are applicable to very specific situations or have no formal scientific basis.

Assessments commonly used by occupational therapists are oriented towards assessing activities of daily living (ADL), such as the ability to wash or dress. Examples of ADL assessments include the Barthel Index (Mahoney & Barthel 1965), the Functional Life Scale (Sarno et al 1973) and the Frenchay Activity Index (Wade et al 1985). Although highly appropriate for their original purpose, such assessments are often developed in relation to a specific patient group (e.g. the Frenchay Activity Index was devised to assess stroke patients) and are frequently only sensitive to particular tasks.

By comparison, physiotherapists employ methods of physical assessment which typically examine body systems (e.g. the locomotor, neurological or respiratory systems), or are based upon examination checklists for specific conditions (Parry 1980). or depend upon open-ended reporting (as is the case with problem-oriented medical records). It is notable that the first two of these approaches are influenced by the medical model of examination and testing which persist despite insistence that 'physiotherapy is not about pathological diagnosis—it is about disorder and about problems of function and ability' (Williams 1986). However, List (1986) has also identified a need for physiotherapists to assess, evaluate and plan treatment programmes without physician referral, a practice which has been followed in some countries, especially Australia, for many years. Physiotherapists must therefore be capable of making differential diagnoses. For this reason, it is likely that physiotherapists will continue to take a diagnostic approach to examining patients at the outset of treatment. In the future, however, they may increasingly monitor progress and evaluate the efficacy of treatment in terms of functional outcome. Certainly, there is an urgent need for the profession to develop suitable outcome measures for this purpose. Yet, it must be recognized that it is only as recently as 1978 (Coates & King 1982) that methods of assessment became part of the physiotherapy curriculum in the UK, although in some other countries they have formed part of physiotherapy education for many years. Accordingly, functional assessments currently in use either concentrate upon ADL criteria or focus upon function relating to developmental pattern of movement, e.g. ability to roll to the right, roll to the left, to 'bridge' etc.

While functional assessments employed by physiotherapists are unnecessarily detailed for work-related application and are, as yet, sketchy in their scientific development, coverage and use, functional movements (or 'elemental functions' as they are called by Jochheim et al 1984), appear to form an appropriate foundation upon which to assess the physical compatibility between men, machines, work spaces and environments. Even so, there is a pressing need to develop and refine the properties of many of these types of scale and indices. Above all there is a need to establish relationships between various assessment methods and the external criteria they seek to measure (Keith 1984), although this is clearly not a problem unique to therapeutic-type assessments.

Perhaps the most promising and certainly the most comprehensive methods for assessing human ability in relation to work demands have been devised by ergonomists, psychologists and vocational rehabilitation specialists (see Watson & Cornes 1986, for a more detailed discussion of some of these techniques). In particular, the approach taken by ergonomists is appealing in that it seeks to measure interactions occurring between employee and workplace through the structured, systematic examination of functional items relating to both. This approach necessitates the identification of criteria against which measures may be set and the use of instruments or techniques of assessment which measure differences in functional ability.

When considering the general population, a high proportion of people fall within the bounds of what is considered to be 'normal' and therefore they may be judged in relation to normative or common criteria. However, the abilities of the disabled population cannot necessarily be judged in the same way and do not necessarily conform to generally accepted patterns of ability. This being the case, it is vital that the abilities of disabled people are assessed in a systematic manner because there are no grounds for predicting what can and cannot be done.

In the context of occupational rehabilitation, the criteria employed in ergonomic-type assessment schemes are based upon functional, work-related items which are measured on a simple, ordinal scale for both the job and the person. In principle, this provides a more objective method for rating ability than is currently achieved by clinical means. It also enables a direct comparison to be made between necessary work activities and an employee's ability to perform these activities. Such techniques are still in their infancy and have many imperfections, but since so little is known about the characteristics of the disabled population at large it is virtually impossible to design instruments which are highly sensitive to important differences in functional ability. However, steps have been taken towards devising simple measurement techniques. The description which follows outlines one such scheme of assessment, called the 'Activity Matching Ability System', which was developed by ergonomists and a physiotherapist/ergonomist.

THE ACTIVITY MATCHING ABILITY SYSTEM

The Activity Matching Ability System (Whalley & Watson 1983) was developed by members of the Institute for Consumer Ergonomics under contract to the European Coal and Steel Community and in conjunction with the British Steel Corporation.

Background and aims

In 1978, the Institute for Consumer Ergonomics was asked to investigate rehabilitation procedures operating throughout the British Steel Corporation. At that time, it was common practice to provide alternative work for disabled employees, unable to perform their original work, by placing them in amenity or 'housekeeping' jobs. For example, in many cases this was achieved through informal discussion between medical officers, personnel managers, departmental managers and trade union representatives, but the nature of these informal links and the relative contribution of individuals differed dramatically from area to area. Consequently, successful placements were contingent upon the quantity and quality of information passing between different parties involved. Either incomplete knowledge about the job and/or person, or the use of ambiguous or incomprehensible terminology could result in misunderstandings which in turn could lead to inappropriate decisions being made about the future of disabled employees.

Furthermore, the potential number of jobs available to disabled employees was limited by a practice of designating specific posts to accommodate disabled people if the need arose. These posts were often menial in nature and were known as 'shelter' or 'static' jobs. Shelter jobs were so named because they were seen to protect employees from performing physically demanding work, while static jobs exempted job holders from taking otherwise obligatory promotion-line moves.

It was recognized that such resettlement provisions were quite inadequate for many employees because disabled people were so very differently affected and had such a wide variety of needs (Whittington & Stead 1980). For instance, one common 'housekeeping' activity involved sweeping. Clearly, sweeping duties under-employed the skills of experienced workers and potentially physically stressed employees with respiratory or certain locomotor disabilities.

As a result of the survey, it was recommended that a more en-lightened system of job placement should be based on a detailed means of assessing and matching disabled employees to existing production jobs. It was also recommended that these techniques should be founded upon methods of functional assessment and form part of an overall programme of rehabilitation and resettlement.

This idea was not novel in that a number of functional assessment techniques (Crewe & Athelston 1981, Jochheim 1981, Lytel & Bot-terbusch 1981, Renault 1976, Rohmert & Landau 1979, Wilcock 1982) were being developed at that time and it was believed that one of these would fulfil the requirements of the British Steel project. Thus, it was originally proposed that the aim of the new research should be:

> to select from the literature and pilot an appropriate assess-ment technique, of proven validity and reliability, which could be used to identify suitable jobs for production employees who required a job change on the grounds of disability.

During the first phase of this new project, the techniques were to be evaluated on existing job/people matches where the job in question was already being carried out by a disabled employee or a person recently returned from a period of sickness absence of longer than twelve weeks. During a second phase of the project, the predictive validity of the overall resettlement procedure was to be evaluated and, depending on the outcome of this work, the sys-tem was to be put into operation within Scunthorpe and elsewhere.

Unfortunately, soon after the initial phase of the research commenced, it became apparent that no single, existing scheme met with the project's specific requirements (Watson et al 1983). Accordingly, it was necessary to develop a new system which embodied the basic principle of assessment and matching outlined above. Thus, the purpose of the project was then to develop:

1. a job or 'activity' assessment technique which described work in terms of level of job demand for items relevant to areas of potential disability
2. a person or 'ability' assessment technique which described levels of work capacity in terms which were directly complementary to items and levels of job demand.

These two developments have been incorporated within a formal return-to-work procedure which has been called the Activity Matching Ability System (AMAS).

The development of AMAS

The first stage of the research took place between July 1982 and September 1983. The field workers were based at the Scunthorpe works of the British Steel Corporation and worked in close co-operation with members of the resident occupational health team.

Four main considerations influenced the development of the new assessment techniques:

1. The assessments had to concentrate on items relevant to tasks and activities undertaken in iron and steel production.
2. Items had to be restricted to those which could be affected by changes in ability resulting from illness or injury.
3. Job demands and functional ability had to be assessed using the same items and levels of coding to ensure that the two assessments could be directly related.
4. The new system had to be specifically designed to stand up to all the criteria originally used to evaluate existing schemes.

These criteria are presented in Figure 10.1.

A list of 100 core items (Fig. 10.2) formed the basis for each assessment and was derived from experience gained whilst piloting the Arbeitswissenschaftliches Erhebungsverfahren zur Tatigkeitsanalyse or AET (Rohmert & Landau 1979) plus Supplement (North 1980) and the Physical Demands Job Analysis or PDJA (Lytel & Botterbusch 1981). These analyses were the only ones

CRITERIA	ACTIVITY MATCHING ABILITY SYSTEM
1. Relevant to heavy industry	Specifically designed for BSC
2. Systematic	Hierarchy of sections for both job and person assessment
3. Include meaningful variables	Pertinent to the entire works and all possible disabilities returning employees may experience (WHO 1980, Whittington 1980)
4. Exclude invariables	Evaluation eliminated only two remaining invariables
5. Suitable format and access information	Activity assessment booklet with item and level description — manual redundant
6. Easy to code, update and access information	100 items, 3 point scale. Access by computer or manually by A3 charts
7. Quick to complete	Approximately 30 minutes after minimal practice
8. Require minimal training	Experts not required, designed so current BSC personnel can operate system
9. Sensitivity	Three levels of coding
10. Face validity	During evaluation job incumbents were asked for their opinion. All felt that the items were appropriate
11. Content validity	Scope and compatibility assessed on 55 steelworkers' jobs – empirical validity to be examined in phase II
12. Inter-rater agreement	As acceptable as AET and PDJA
13. Structured person assessment	Developed as a compatible unit allowing one to one matching of items and use of compatible levels
14. Computerized method of 'matching'	Potential identified and software had since been prepared for use on a micro-computer

Fig. 10.1 Criteria used to evaluate existing schemes of assessment.

under review which had been validated for use in heavy industry. Items covered by the two assessments were listed and included in or eliminated from the new system according to whether they could

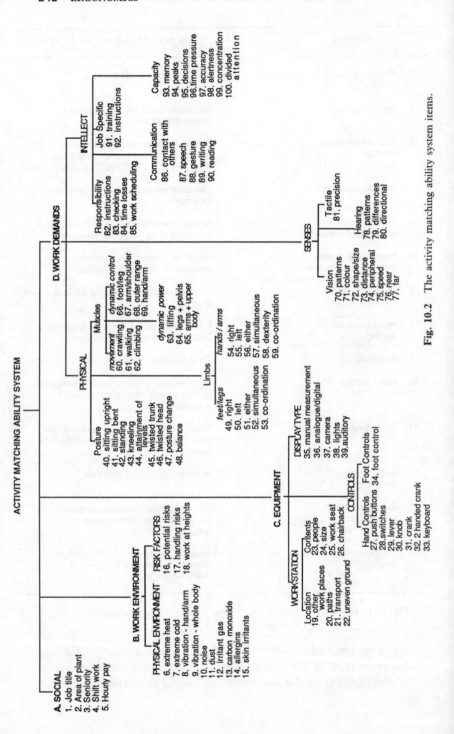

Fig. 10.2 The activity matching ability system items.

be applied to steel work jobs and whether they were relevant to topics covered in the disability section of the International Classification of Impairments, Disabilities and Handicaps (WHO 1980). Site visits and informal discussions with employees, managers, trade union representatives, safety advisors and medical staff resulted in the inclusion of other items and helped the research team establish the content and face validity of the new assessments.

Draft instruments were developed through several iterations involving pilot trials before the final versions of the activity and ability assessments were produced. The inter-rater agreement obtained when piloting the draft job assessment was similar to claims made for the AET and PDJA. In other words, approximately 85% of all items were coded alike by two independent assessors when rating 10 separate jobs.

The 'activity' assessment

The activity assessment so developed consists of a booklet of 100 items divided into four main sections as follows:

1. Section A considers social aspects of a job and covers such factors as former pay scale, status and department. Where possible, this enables a similar type of job to be identified.
2. Section B considers physical and risk factors associated with the work environment.
3. Section C examines the type of equipment in use or present at the work station, including types of control and display.
4. Section D considers physical, intellectual and sensory work demands. This is the largest section.

Items included in Section A are descriptive and uncoded, but items in all other sections are rated on an identical, three point, ordinal scale representing three levels of job demand. The wording for these three levels changes from item to item, but in essence follows the same conceptual schema of increasing demand:

1. Level 1: no demand
2. Level 2: possible demand (occasional/non-essential)
3. Level 3: major demand.

In order to facilitate the coding of job demand, items are coded in the booklet by ticking one of three annotated boxes. The sections and sub-sections in this booklet are ordered so that the social items describing job are recorded first, followed by a logical progression

(Tick the most appropriate box)

ACTIVITY MATCHING ABILITY SYSTEM
(JOB ASSESSMENT)

SECTION A: SOCIAL

1. Job title ....

2. Area of plant ....

3. Seniority ....

4. Shift work   days ☐   2 shift or ☐   3 shift ☐
                                                occ. 3   system

5. Hourly rate

SECTION B: WORK ENVIRONMENT

Physical Environment

6. EXTREME HEAT:
                    n/a ☐   occasionally: ☐   frequent job ☐
                                   not part of   requirement
                                   normal job

7. EXTREME COLD:
                    n/a ☐   in winter ☐   all year ☐
                                   only

8. VIBRATION — HAND/ARM:
                    n/a ☐   occasionally: ☐   frequent job ☐
                                   not part of   requirement
                                   normal job

9. VIBRATION — WHOLE BODY:
                    n/a ☐   occasionally: ☐   frequent job ☐
                                   not part of   requirement
                                   normal job

Fig. 10.3   Sample page of the activity assessment booklet.

through general aspects of the job to the detail of work demands.
A sample page of the job assessment booklet is shown in Figure
10.3.

The 'ability' assessment

Existing classifications and scales of functional ability were of limited help in developing the new technique. In practice, the ability assessment was outlined in conjunction with the detailed development of the activity assessment and was designed to mirror items and levels included in the latter. However, in structuring the ability assessment into a working document it became apparent that the ordering of the items should be altered and that information should be collected from a number of sources, namely the returning employee, medical personnel and department staff.

The resultant ability assessment comprises three parts (Fig. 10.4):

1. a return-to-work questionnaire for completion by the employee
2. a medical report for completion by medical or para-medic staff
3. discussion items assessed by departmental representative in the context of a round table meeting.

The main reason for including a return-to-work questionnaire, was to establish whether the employee felt ready to work. The first part of this questionnaire relates to current job detail covering job title, area of plant, seniority status, shifts and former hourly rate of pay. The second part of the form contains four questions which examine the employee's attitude towards an early return, a change of job, working at heights and working in confined spaces.

The medical report is the largest section and has been designed for completion by any member of the occupational health team. Seventy-nine items fall into this category and are sub-divided into five sections which may be completed hierarchically. The sections are as follows:

1. Section 1 consists of a standard examination covering the ability to adopt different postures, the ability to lift, seating requirements, mobility and access, susceptibility to risk factors and tolerance to environmental factors.
2. Section 2 consists of a more detailed examination of limb function which includes the ability to operate foot and hand controls.
3. Section 3 covers vision and hearing.
4. Section 4 deals with communication in terms of the ability to speak, signal, write and read.
5. Section 5 deals with mental abilities such as alertness, the ability to concentrate and to divide attention between several tasks.

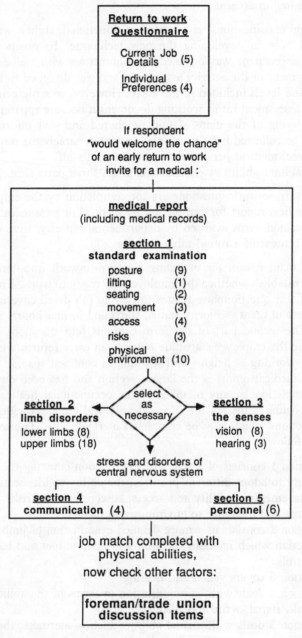

Fig. 10.4 Format of the ability assessment.

The grouping of items within the ability assessment sections does not correspond with the grouping of items within the activity assessment sections. However, within each section for both the activity and the ability assessments, each specific item is numbered to facilitate the matching procedure. Thus, the item numbered 40 in the activity assessment (Fig. 10.2) is matched directly with item number 40 in the ability assessment (Fig. 10.5).

The three levels of ability relating to each item broadly represent the following scale of diminishing ability:

1. Level 1:able
2. Level 2:has difficulty
3. Level 3:unable.

These levels coincide with corresponding levels of coding for a job. In other words, increasing demand for a particular job activity (Level 3) relates to diminishing ability to perform that activity (Level 3).

The medical report items have been arranged into a two page summary form (Fig. 10.5). An accompanying manual lists the precise levels for each item and suggests certain functional tests which could be used to establish the different levels of ability. These tests are offered as suggestions only since the time scale for the study did not allow the validation of individual tests. However, it was important that assessors should be prompted into testing for functional performance rather than relying upon their professional opinion as to the person's capacity to cope with a task. Ultimately, the selection of appropriate tests is left to the discretion of the assessor, but the purpose of introducing testing was to move towards a more objective method for examining ability with less opportunity for bias.

A third category of 14 items deals with work behaviour and organization, manual measurement and displays, and represents a Department's input to the activity assessment. These items are not rated, but form the basis of discussions between medical personnel, departmental staff and employee.

The matching procedure

For each of the 100 items, the three levels of coding for the job and person result in nine possible combinations of demand versus ability. As shown in Table 10.1, five of these pairings are ideal, the job making no demand upon the human operator or the person

SECTION 1 : STANDARD EXAMINATION

Posture					Work Station Access				
Sitting 'upright'	40	☐	☐	☐	Locomotion: other work places	19	☐	☐	☐
Sitting 'bent'	41	☐	☐	☐	Access: climbing	20	☐	☐	☐
Standing naturally	42	☐	☐	☐	Transport needs	21	☐	☐	☐
Kneeling	43	☐	☐	☐	Uneven ground	22	☐	☐	☐
Stooping, crouching	44	☐	☐	☐	**Risk Factors**				
Twisted body	45	☐	☐	☐	Shiftwork	4	☐	☐	☐
Turning head	46	☐	☐	☐	Loss of conciousness	17	☐	☐	☐
Posture changes	47	☐	☐	☐	Work with others	23	☐	☐	☐
Balance/equilibrium	48	☐	☐	☐	**Physical Environment**				
					Extreme heat tolerance	6	☐	☐	☐
Lifting	63	☐	☐	☐	Extreme cold tolerance	7	☐	☐	☐
Seating					Vibration: hand/arm	8	☐	☐	☐
Work seat	25	☐	☐	☐	Vibration: whole body	9	☐	☐	☐
Back seat	26	☐	☐	☐	Noise tolerance	10	☐	☐	☐
					Inhalants: dust	11	☐	☐	☐
Movement					Inhalants: irritant gas (SO_2)	12	☐	☐	☐
Crawling/sliding	60	☐	☐	☐	Inhalants: carbon monoxide	13	☐	☐	☐
Walking	61	☐	☐	☐	Allergens	14	☐	☐	☐
Climbing	62	☐	☐	☐	Skin irritants	15	☐	☐	☐

Fig. 10.5 Sample page of the medical report summary form.

having normal ability. Three of the combinations are less desirable, the person having difficulty in meeting a major or potential job demand or being unable to meet a possible demand. Finally, one

Table 10.1 Possible combinations of demand versus ability

Activity assessment Level of demand	Ability assessment Level of ability	Matching decision
1 Major	Able	Ideal
2 Major	Difficulty	*Possible*
3 Major	Unable	*Unsuitable*
4 Possible	Able	Ideal
5 Possible	Difficulty	*Possible*
6 Possible	Unable	*Possible*
7 None	Able	Ideal
8 None	Difficulty	Ideal
9 None	Unable	Ideal

pairing is totally unsuitable, the person being quite unable to meet a major job demand.

When carrying out a match, all 100 pairs of items must be considered for any job/person combination. In theory, a perfect match arises when a person is able to do all that is required. However, it is more likely that discrepancies will arise, in which case the number of discrepancies and the nature of these will influence the final decision about placement. For example, it may be feasible to redesign aspects of a job or provide job aids in order to overcome particular difficulties.

In the case of the British Steel project, the matching process was achieved manually by using a system of overlays based on a diagrammatic layout of items shown in Figure 10.2, but in which each item is followed by a small coding box. In this process, job assessment details are transcribed on to a paper copy of this summary form using colour coding to indicate different levels of job demand. An identical summary form, printed on a transparent overlay, is used to summarize the ability profile. Colour coding is also used to indicate different levels of ability. The coding represents the following:

1. Red indicates a major job demand (if on the activity profile) and inability to perform that demand (if on the ability profile).
2. Green indicates a possible demand and difficulty in performing that demand.
3. Black or a blank box indicates no job demand and normal ability.

Thus, red overlaying red clearly highlights a major job demand which a person is not capable of performing. Combinations of red with green or green with green indicate areas of potential difficulty, whilst any combination of colour with black indicates a perfect match.

The compatibility of the two assessments

The compatibility of the technique was evaluated by comparing activity/ability assessments completed for disabled people who were currently in a post. In order to examine compatibility in this way, several assumptions had to be made. For instance, it was assumed that disabled employees were satisfactorily placed. Contingent upon this was the further assumption that where mismatches did occur they would demonstrate inadequacies in the design of the assessments, unless other explanations could be found.

A total of 55 paired assessments were completed. Eligible individuals were identified from the work's medical records, past long-term absentee lists and by word of mouth. From this population of potentially disabled employees, a group was drawn which included people with a wide range of impairments and who were performing a variety of production jobs. Unfortunately, stratified, random-sampling techniques could not be used because the numbers of people involved were too small. Therefore, there are no statistical grounds upon which it may be claimed that this group was representative of the total population of disabled production workers. However, discussion with the medical officers suggested that the group broadly represented the types and range of impairments experienced by steelworkers at the Scunthorpe Works. Only one person declined to take part in the study.

The job information was collected by an ergonomist and physiotherapist/ergonomist. The ability assessments were completed by seven raters, comprising two medical officers, two physiotherapists and three nursing officers. A comparison of these two assessments provided a measure of their compatibility. Table 10.2 summarizes the data and demonstrates the extent and area of the discrepancies occurring over the entire sample (expressed as a percentage of the total number of possible mismatches) before and after explanations were sought. On questioning, it was found that certain inconsistencies were attributable to factors beyond the scope of the techniques. For instance, one person who was unable to walk over uneven ground, but had to do so to get to his place of work, was found to drive his moped into the work's building. Similar

Table 10.2 The type and percentage of discrepancies which were found during the evaluation of the compatibility between the two assessments

Job	Person	Before explanation	After explanation
Red 'major demand'	Red 'inability'	5.45%	0.00%
Green 'possible demand'	Red 'inability'	9.09%	5.45%
Red 'major demand'	Green 'difficulty'	45.47%	38.18%
Green 'possible demand'	Green 'difficulty'	9.09%	9.09%
Black 'no demand' and/or	Black 'able'	30.9%	47.28%

explanations were discovered for the other apparent mismatching and some of the less desirable pairings.

The high percentage of red/green combinations suggested that people were undertaking possibly difficult tasks as part of their routine duties. This finding was anticipated due to the nature of the group. Therefore, within the limitation of these summary percentages and a more detailed examination of the data between the assessors and by job/person match, it was concluded that the techniques were sufficiently compatible and sufficiently sensitive to merit further evaluation. Consequently, it was recommended that the Activity Matching Ability System should be implemented within the Scunthorpe Works in order to evaluate the empirical validity of the procedure for placing disabled people in appropriate jobs. Unfortunately, this was not possible at the time and the second phase of the work had to be planned for a later date. Part of the development for the second phase was the computerization of the matching procedure. A major consideration in the usability of the scheme is the speed with which a match can be achieved and the ease with which the data collected can be interrogated. It was always intended that the system should be computer based and that the conversion from the manual method of matching should be a major part of the implementation phase.

The return-to-work procedure

The assessment techniques described in this section are intended

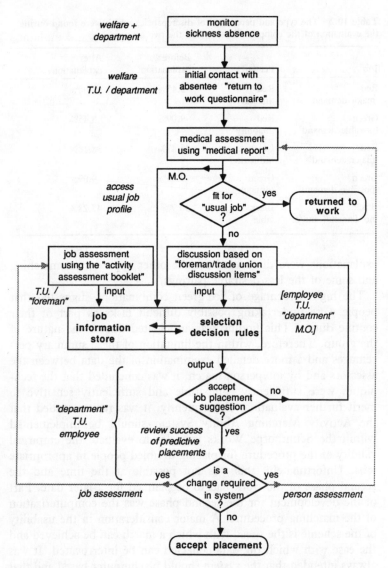

Fig. 10.6 AMAS communication flow for returning long-term sickness absentees.

for use within an overall rehabilitation and resettlement procedure (Fig. 10.6). Central to this procedure is the compilation of a job information store which is intended to provide up-to-date information about work demands associated with any one of a potential range of jobs covered by the system. The procedure is dependent upon monitoring the sickness absence of employees and initiating their timely return to work. Thus, assuming that an absentee is fit and willing to resume duty, the occupational health team will assess the person's functional capabilities and examine these in relation to their former job using the manual or computer matching facilities. It may also be desirable to scan the job information store for suitable alternatives which the person could perform by screening departments, seniority levels, vacancies or other pre-determined criteria.

The information gathered during the course of this matching exercise provides a basis for discussions between management, trade union representatives, medical staff and employee. The assessment techniques are used to effect a match based mainly upon physical aspects of job/person interactions, and, therefore, the purpose of the round table discussion is to consider extraneous variables which cannot be assessed in such a methodical manner. This discussion forum is a vital stage in the procedure and it is extremely important that the techniques are seen as tools, providing helpful information rather than pre-empting decisions about placement. In fact, the procedure incorporates a 'discussion loop' which allows a variety of alternative placements to be discussed from various viewpoints before arriving at a suitable solution.

It should be further emphasized that the system is a dynamic one requiring frequent updating of the job data and periodic re-assessment of the person to ensure that notice is taken of improvements or deteriorations in functional ability.

THE FUTURE OF MATCHING ASSESSMENT SYSTEMS

Elaborate systems of the type described in this chapter have come into being because disabled people have not been able fully to exercise the right to work according to their capabilities. It was supposed that, in the wake of industrial society, the information age would offer disabled people a more equitable basis upon which to compete for jobs. In practice, this is not necessarily true because new technology is designed to meet the needs of the majority of users who, by definition, possess normal ranges of ability. Therefore, it is likely that there will always be a need to tailor user/machine interfaces to the special requirements of certain disabled users. Having acknowledged this, it must also be noted that new technology has the potential for transforming the working lives of many people by enabling them to undertake tasks which, hitherto, they have been unable to perform. This will not obviate, but rather increase the need to describe and analyse levels of ability in the future.

One of the problems in trying to design systems and equipment for disabled people is that, unlike the concept of the average man, little is known about the average disabled person or even the characteristics of the group as a whole (Mayfield & McClelland 1985). In the main, disability statistics have concentrated upon describing the population in terms of diagnoses rather than functional capability. In consequence, disability has been associated with ill-health and general malfunction which perpetuates the idea that disability is synonymous with total debility. The reason for the development of assessment schemes of the type described here has been to demonstrate that disabled people are able to undertake jobs on an equal footing with non-disabled peers, providing that the person and the job are suitably matched. In this context 'matching' is not intended to imply a rigid approach to placement. Rather it is a means of offering evidence to support the claim that disabled people can work as efficiently as any employee. The strength of this argument has been based upon the objectivity of the techniques, and doubtless there will continue to be a need for such evidence in relation to jobs associated with new technology.

One benefit of having devised a tool capable of measuring ability, albeit in a crude sense, is that the ability assessment also offers clinicians a potential instrument for identifying functional decrements and for monitoring functional outcome and change. The applicability of the ability assessment to work-related demands means that treatments and services may be focused upon restoring or compensating for functions vital to work performance. However, it is also suggested that the concept underpinning the ability assessment could be used to develop instruments which are sufficiently sensitive to monitor patient progress during and following treatment. Such instruments would not only provide essential feedback for the therapist and patient, but would also facilitate the much needed scientific evaluation of treatment techniques.

In conclusion, it is recognized that matching assessment techniques provide rudimentary tools which require further development and refinement before they can be used more widely. Futhermore, the successful application of such tools is possible only within the context of an integrated scheme of disability management which takes proper account of clinical and psychosocial factors, family demands, financial commitments and other important variables. However, despite their current inadequacies, such techniques offer a promising and novel approach to the very complex problem of how to assess and match work demands to functional ability.

ACKNOWLEDGEMENTS

The research reported in this chapter was sponsored by the European Coal and Steel Community (research number 7247/18/047) in conjunction with the British Steel Corporation, Scunthorpe Division. Former colleagues associated with the project include Mr R. J. Feeney, Mrs M. S. Stead, Ms M. C. Whittington and Mr K. Jago.

Many people contributed to the preparation of this paper, both directly and indirectly. In particular the authors would like to acknowledge the support of the Association of British Insurers during the writing of this chapter; Mr P. Cornes and Mrs M. Smith from the Rehabilitation Studies Unit, University of Edinburgh for their editorial help and advice; and Miss E. Grieve for her assistance with the preparation of diagrams and secretarial support.

REFERENCES

Anastasi A 1961 Psychological testing. MacMillan, New York
Bowe F 1983 Demography and disability: a chartbook for rehabilitation.
    Rehabilitation Research and Training Center University of Arkansas, Arkansas
Coates H, King A 1982 The patient assessment. Churchill Livingstone,
    Edinburgh
Cornes P 1984 The future of work for people with disabilities: a view from Great
    Britain. Monograph 28 World Rehabilitation Fund, New York
Crewe N M, Athelston G T 1981 Functional assessment in vocational rehabilitation:
    a systematic approach to diagnosis and goal setting. Archives of Physical
    Medicine Rehabilitation 62: 299–305
Croxen M 1985 Employment and disability: a European perspective. In: Cornes
    P Hunter J (eds) Work disability and Rehabilitation. University Center for
    International Rehabilitation, Michigan
Dejong G 1981 Environmental accessibility and independent living outcomes:
    directions for disability policy and research. University Center for International
    Rehabilitation, Michigan
Dejong G 1982 Independent living as an analytic paradigm. Australian
    Rehabilitation Review 6(2): 45–50
Duckworth D 1983 The classification and measurement of disablement.
    HMSO, London
Galvin D E 1985 Employer-based disability management and rehabilitation
    programs. Annual Review of Rehabilitation 5
Harris A I, Cox E, Smith C R W 1971 Handicapped and impaired in Great
    Britain. Part 1 HMSO, London

Jochheim K-A 1981 Fahigkeits-und anforderungs profile fur die einglidiederung behinderter. Unpublished report from the University of Cologne Rehabilitation Centre, Cologne

Jochheim K-A, Koch M, Mittelsten-Scheid E, Schian H-M, Weinmann S 1984 Ertomis—ability and requirements profiles aid for the vocational reintegration of the disabled. 2nd edn Gemeinnutzige Stiftung ERTOMIS Bildungs-und Forderungs-GmbH, Wuppertal

Keith R A 1984 Functional assessment measures in medical rehabilitation: current status. Archives of Physical Medicine and Rehabilitation 65: 74–78

Kettle M 1985 The accidents and absence of disabled people at work. In: Cornes P, Hunter J (eds) Work, disability and Rehabilitation. University Center for International Rehabilitation, Michigan

List M 1986 Physiotherapy—a mobile Profession in health care. Physiotherapy 72(3): 122–124

Lytel R B, Botterbusch K J 1981 Physical demands job analysis: a new approach. Materials Development Center, University of Wisconsin, Wisconsin

Mahoney F I Barthel D W 1965 Functional evaluation: Barthel index. Md State Medical Journal 14: 61–65

Mayfield W, McClelland I L 1985 The value of carrying out research into aids and equipment for disabled people. Unpublished report to the Department of Health and Social Security. Institute for Consumer Ergonomics, Loughborough

North K 1980 Job analysis for the disabled, supplement of the AET. Unpublished report to the European Coal and Steel Community, ARBED, Darmstadt

Parry A 1980 Physiotherapy Assessment. Croom Helm, London

Renault 1976 Les Profils de postes, methode d'analyse des conditions de travail. Masson Sirtes, Paris

Rohmert W, Landau K 1979 Das arbeitswissenschaftliche Erhebungsverfahren zur Tatigkeitsanalyse (AET). Huber-Verlag, Bern

Rohmert W, Landau K 1983 A new technique for job analysis. English edn. Taylor and Francis, London

Sarno J E, Sarno M T, Levita E 1973 Functional life scale. Archives of Physical Medicine Rehabilitation 54: 214–220

Singleton W T 1972 Introduction to Ergonomics. World Health Organisation, Geneva

Singleton W T, Debney L M, Papworth C F 1979 Occupational disability assessment. Unpublished Applied Psychology Report 88. University of Aston, Birmingham

Stubbins J 1982 The clinical attitudes in rehabilitation a cross cultural view. Monograph 16. World Health Rehabilitation Fund. New York

United Nations 1975 Declaration of the rights of disabled Persons. United Nations 2433 Plenary Meeting

Wade D T, Legh-Smith J, Hewer R L 1985 Social activities after stroke measurement and natural history using the Frenchway Activities Index. International Rehabilitation Medicine 7(4): 176–181

Watson H J, Whalley S P, Stead M S 1983 Job and disability assessment—a selective review. Unpublished report to the British Steel Corporation and the European Coal and Steel Community. Institute for Consumer Ergonomics, Loughborough

Watson H J, Cornes P 1986 Occupational assessment of people with disabilities. In: Kettle M, Massie B (eds) Employers' guide to disabilities. Woodhead Faulkner, London

Whittington M C, Stead M S 1980 An investigation into rehabilitation in the steel industry of the United Kingdom. Unpublished report to the European Coal and Steel Community. Institute for Consumer Ergonomics, Loughborough

Whalley S P, Watson H J 1983 The rehabilitation and resettlement of occupationally disabled workers in the British Steel Corporation with siecific reference to the Scunthorpe Works, Phase 1—final report. Unpublished report to the British Steel Corporation and the European Coal and Steel Community. Institute for Consumer Ergonomics, Loughborough

Wilcock R 1982 A vocational assessment procedure. Unpublished PhD thesis. University of Leeds, Leeds

Williams J I 1986 Physiotherapy is Handling. Physiotherapy 72(2): 66–70

World Health Organization 1980 International classification of impairments, disabilities and handicaps. WHO, Geneva

11. Role of functional capacities assessment after rehabilitation

S. J. Isernhagen

THE ROLE OF FUNCTIONAL CAPACITIES ASSESSMENT (FCA)

Work injury management

Closing the 'work injury gap' is of significant importance today and will be of increasing importance tomorrow. The United States Department of Labour estimated in 1980 that workers' compensation was costing employers $22.2 billion annually. These costs had increased by 400% in 10 years and this trend towards increasing expenditure is still continuing.

On the medical side of the work injury question is the physician who has primary responsibility for taking charge of patient restoration (Isernhagen 1985). Employers and insurance companies place great dependence upon doctors who, they assume, can direct healing, release an employee to return to work, and know all the physical restrictions under which that employee can work. The employer is responsible for taking the small amount of medical information available and effecting a return to work without playing 'russian roulette' with the employee and placing him within a potentially injurious job.

In the past few years, a number of questions regarding the injured worker have been asked. For example, what can a semi-healed employee do? When can work begin? Will there be a re-injury? Employers, insurance companies and even most physicians hesitate to answer these questions. The physical therapist, however, is highly qualified to provide answers and direction for both employer and physician. The method for doing so involves accurate, comprehensive functional assessment after rehabilitation has been completed.

One of the best sources for information on ergonomic principles, which can mesh with physical principles, is the book *Occupational*

Biomechanics by Chaffin & Andersson (1984). These authors state that, 'In the discussion of mechanical trauma due to physical mismatching of a worker and the job demands it must be readily conceded that the physical capacities of a normal population can vary greatly, depending upon genetic factors, fitness, skill and many other factors. It has been a traditional role of occupational medicine to devise methods for determining a person's capacity to safely perform certain types of work.' The authors delineate methods of evaluating work-sites within a biomechanical model. This engineering background can be of particular help to the physical therapist in understanding the ergonomics approach. However, Chaffin & Andersson (1984) concentrate on designing the workplace rather than on providing methods of evaluating the worker.

To give credence to matching worker selection to workplace demands, Chaffin et al (1978) described isometric strength measurements and their application in predicting physical function on the job. These authors concluded that as job strength requirements approach or exceed demonstrated isometric strength, severity of injuries increases. They also concluded that their study confirmed the need to utilize some form of a strength-testing programme when placing people on the job.

In a study regarding chronic case resolution, Mayer et al (1985) showed definitively that quantification of functional ability through measurement of trunk musculature strength and retraining of these same muscle groups significantly increases the 'return to work' statistics.

Another viewpoint suggests that a combination of flexibility, strength and aerobic condition testing is appropriate. For example, Cady et al (1979) indicated that the level of conditioning does influence injury rates, for in their study, the most fit group of employees were injured less often and less severely than the least fit group.

Today, governmental agencies, industry and medicine are working together to provide guidelines for a safer workplace. In defining standards for the United States, the National Institute of Occupational Safety and Health has developed a *Work Practices Guide For Manual Lifting* (1983). It defines four categories that need to be studied as factors in predicting potential injury on the job.

Epidemiology: identification of the incidents, distribution and potential controls for illness and injuries in a population.

Biomechanical: musculoskeletal structure and its relationship to stresses especially when lifting.

Physiological: the human body's metabolical and circulatory responses to various loads.

Psychophysical: subjective tolerance of people to the stresses of manual materials handling.

It is submitted that a fifth category is also necessary: that of functional capacities assessment (FCA). The latter approach offers the ability to use, but go beyond, these first four principles by studying the individual movement patterns of human beings. It allows musculoskeletal and neuromuscular concepts to be assessed in functional patterns which tend to differ from individual to individual. Physiological signs are correlated with muscular activity including strength, endurance and co-ordination. Psychophysical limitations of fear or over-achievement are overcome with true functional testing. Basic functional assessments of true movement take the science of physical measurement into a more comprehensive realm.

It is obvious that scientists and medical specialists are documenting and studying abilities and disabilities relating to work. Quoted assessment methods, however, have been only of specific body components rather than of the whole person. Many of the conclusions are applicable by way of norms rather than by individual assessment.

The development of a suitable method of functional capacities evaluation has been a subject of study for a number of years. The need to provide returning employees with an exact description of their capability and the need to ensure that employees were capable of performing specific jobs was recognized. The methods described in this chapter were formulated as a result of the study of functional assessment which has taken place in the USA over the past years. Primary models were developed and studied. Clarity, objectivity and work relevance were found to be critical components. Advances in comprehensiveness and content have been noted by Isernhagen (1988).

THE DESIGN OF FUNCTIONAL CAPACITIES ASSESSMENT

Physical therapists have a wealth of abilities with which to evaluate total function. To provide correct and comprehensive information, the design of functional capacity assessments is all important. Limited tests, however technological they look, give only limited information. However, comprehensive physical therapy assessment succeeds if the following parameters are used in evaluating and establishing the assessment itself.

Parameters for evaluation

Total person

To be considered truly functional, an evaluation must test the total person so that all aspects of movement and muscle patterns can be observed. People work as a physical composite and, in attempting to retain their function despite limitations, they often develop compensatory movements. For example, a dysfunctional knee may interfere with proper body mechanics, which in turn may be the cause of subsequent injuries to the low back; a hand injury affects patterns of movements in traditionally gross motor activities such as lifting, carrying and climbing; loss of proprioception in an ankle can interfere with balance, while back problems can affect neck and shoulder functioning.

For this reason, the best functional capacity evaluators address total body functioning. In the descriptions contained herein, body segments have been evaluated in the context of total patterns of activity at work or at home.

Work-related activity

A specific effort must be made to evaluate body motions in the context of real work and daily life. For example, it is known that limited range of motion of the shoulder does not necessarily imply limited work function. On the other hand, full range of shoulder motion does not indicate that there is full work function. For this reason, the applicable work functions must be tested rather than relying on estimates of what might be limited.

To make the evaluation work related, work activities should be broken into specific musculoskeletal motions addressing strength, endurance, motion and co-ordination. The results should make reference to actual work activity. Standardized tests should be developed from relevant return-to-work forms.

Objectivity

As in any relevant testing procedure, rater bias must be eliminated.

Because the workers' compensation system is generally adversarial, it is important that work function evaluations be objective. Standardized procedures should be used and the evaluator thoroughly trained in these procedures, to reduce any chance of rater bias. In addition, the therapist raters must make their neutral position known to the patient at the initiation of the evaluation. This aids in encouraging patient compliance and also establishes that medical principles rather than subjective observations will be used.

Reproducability

The reliability of test items lies in their reproducability. It is necessary, therefore, to test the patient until consistent results show clear ability or specific limitation. Only when the therapist is assured that true work performance has been observed, may the report be written. The results often lead directly to the patient's return to work.

The most important way of assuring reliability of testing is to carry out a follow-up in the work setting. If a functional test shows that a patient is able to do x, y and z on the job, then x, y, and z should be monitored after return to work to make sure that those conclusions were correct. This establishes that proper design and evaluation techniques were used.

Function and dysfunction

Patients come to the physical therapist for functional capacities evaluation because they are not completely cured or because they may have some residual dysfunction which cannot be improved by surgery or treatment. The patient must be viewed as someone who will go forward to employment from their present functional position rather than staying behind in an attempt to reach physical perfection.

All professionals involved in the return to work process are especially interested in the patient's work capability rather than his or her disability. Each capability level established indicates potential work that the patient can do. Disability should be considered only in the context of establishing work modifications or limitations. It is the patient's ability level that should be stressed.

Use of full professional skills

By being knowledgeable about normal functional movements, the physical therapist will be able to identify physiological patterns of effort and fatigue. Accessory muscle activity should be observed when the patient is approaching the maximum level of functioning. Changes in body mechanics signal the attainment of maximum function, while physiological signs, such as sweating, pulse rates and flushing, are also noticeable. These aspects should be documented by the physical therapist for, by recording actual physical signs, credibility will be given to the conclusions reached during assessment.

Integration of motion factors

When statistics on work injuries are evaluated, it is seen that the amount of force involved in the work movement can be a factor in the injury rate. Injuries also take place when there is repetitious activity, fast pacing or a sudden change in body position. Therefore, functional capacity assessments should include reference to all of these variables.

Endurance. In many cases, the force maximum might be the same for any two given people. Yet the amount of endurance which would allow repetitious activity to take place would be considerably different. Limited endurance factors can be due to a low level of muscle capacity, joint dysfunction or lack of aerobic conditioning.

Pace. The pace at which a person can work is an individual attribute. An evaluation of speed, smoothness of motion and safety of pace allows comment on the possibility of return to work. For example, a previously injured worker may be functional if allowed to use a slow guarded pace. Work demands can be met through self-pacing on the job. On the other hand, a patient may show that fast pacing is leading to loss of safe body mechanics and may be a precursor of injury. In such a case, pacing needs to be identified as the potential cause of problems, so that it can be monitored at work.

Body mechanics. Evaluation of body mechanics is also important because of their influence on safety on the job. Consistently good, safe body mechanics are a bonus for both employer and employee. For the person who has a consistent problem with certain body mechanics, recommendations for training before return to work should be made.

Range of motion. Joint dysfunction, muscle weakness, lack of muscle endurance and decreased aerobic capacity can all affect activity through the full range of motion. Only by evaluating dynamically at all points in the range will the presence and location of a limited factor be identified.

Physiological factors and work recommendations

It is obvious that in looking at the whole person, strength testing is not sufficient. Factors such as the ability to undertake repetitive work, the pacing level, body mechanics and full motion must be evaluated to provide a thorough and comprehensive picture of the patient's abilities.

The reasons which limit the patient's maximum function are important considerations in offering recommendations. The following examples show how recommendations vary according to the cause of the limitation.

Test result: 15 kg lifting capacity, floor to work-bench height

Patient problem limiting lifting capacity	Possible work or treatment recommendation
Subject 1. Right knee dysfunction with increased symptoms and compensatory change in body mechanics at 15 kg load.	— Work-site modification needed. — Weighted objects over 15 kg should always be placed at proper height so that lifting from floor is not necessary. — Objects 15 g or less may be lifted from the floor if repetitions are limited.
Subject 2. Loss of low back stability in lifts from floor greater than 15 kg.	— If greater capacity is desired: trunk muscle exercise regime and lifting training.
Subject 3. Weak quadriceps leading to loss of stable body mechanics in loads greater than 15 kg.	— If greater capacity is desired: quadriceps and accessory muscle strength and endurance regime.
Subject 4. Wrist and finger joint symptomatic stress accompanied by loosening of grip in holds greater than 15 kg.	— Change handle size and position to allow maximum comfort and strength of grip. — If greater capacity is desired: strengthening activities for wrist and finger muscles.
Subject 5. Loss of thoracic extension position beyond 15 kg lift.	— If greater capacity is desired: back extensor exercises. — Modification of lifting position with neck extension to facilitate extensor components.

Who, when, why, where, how

In describing the details of functional capacities assessment, it is important to consider who might benefit, when is the appropriate time to make the evaluation, why it is valuable, where and how it might be carried out.

Who

A variety of patients can benefit from having a functional capacities assessment.

Musculoskeletal injuries. By far the most common work injury is musculoskeletal. If acute, it should be handled in a different manner to the chronic case. In either patient, functional assessments have been successfully and logically utilized by defining strength, endurance, motion, and other measurable musculoskeletal parameters.

Systemic disease. Those with chronic systemic diseases, such as arthritis, multiple sclerosis and diabetes, are at risk of injury and also at risk of limitations imposed by themselves or their employers. Even though these clients often have changes in their conditions over time, a good functional capacities assessment provides a baseline of their abilities and limitations. Repetition and pacing need special attention. Periodic re-evaluations are also helpful.

Neurological problems. Patients with stroke, spinal cord injury and head injury are also amenable to functional capacities assessment. In addition to testing physical functioning, such components as following directions, attention span, ability to attend to a task, co-ordination and repetitive movements must be evaluated.

Developmental disabilities. In the same vein, those with developmental delays who work in sheltered workshops are excellent candidates for functional evaluation. Judgement of their physical ability rather than their mental ability can lead to appropriate employment.

Stabilized cardiac patients. Cardiac patients are now returned to work at a greater pace than once thought possible. By combining functional evaluation with cardiac rehabilitation, both the employer and employee can be more confident of safety at work. Abilities and limitations defined by functional tests and cardiac sufficiency tests can be blended into one report.

Chronic deconditioning. Any prolonged sedentary recovery following illness leads to aerobic and musculoskeletal deconditioning.

Thorough functional testing is appropriate with this type of patient, not only to facilitate return to work but also to suggest work-hardening principles.

When/Why

There are a number of specific times when functional capacities assessment is particularly useful.

After treatment. If there is a question about a patient's return to full work activity after stabilization of the condition, functional testing will be time appropriate and cost effective. It facilitates immediate safe return to work without the necessity of 'waiting', which itself can allow chronic physical and psychological symptoms to be manifested.

After surgery. Many surgeons wait a minimum amount of time before return to work is considered following surgery. In some cases this is appropriate, but in many cases it is artificially long. Also, without the thought of return to work, the patient, during recovery, may not be doing anything to recondition his body. In such cases, the physical therapists can offer a preparatory conditioning programme. As soon as the patient's condition has stabilized, the physical therapist can perform an FCA. The job description may also be interfaced with the testing. Through being offered at the most effective time for return to work, the assessment allows the reconditioned patient to reach work ability level sooner.

After return to work. The initial functional assessment should take place just prior to return to work so that the information will help the patient to reach his full maximum work potential. A second assessment may be given after several weeks of working. This allows the work-strengthened patient to be upgraded to a higher yet safe functional level. This graduated return to work is cost effective in terms of both workers' compensation and medical costs.

Disability determinations. In many cases, work injury is permanent and does not allow full return to work. A disability determination must then be made before there is case resolution and other employment can be found. Physicians have traditionally been responsible for determining percentage of disability. They often must use limited information such as range of motion measurements and manual muscle tests. Better information could come from functional ability and limitation assessment. Physical therapists are currently seeking to identify normal values in many functional movements. When these are obtained the percentage of disability will be clearer. In the meantime, functional capacity assessment results that indicate capability and limitation add invaluable information to court proceedings. Once case resolution is accomplished, results of functional evaluation can be used as a stepping stone to find a new occupation for the patient who has just settled the case.

Where

Medical setting. The therapeutic atmosphere of a physical therapy department lends itself to professionalism and increases patient confidence. Such a setting is considered neutral and objective and this is an important attribute in the multifaceted work injury system.

Industry. In specific circumstances, medically-based functional testing needs a segment of actual work evaluation. Indeed, for complete accuracy, the work-site needs to be used or duplicated. This combines standardized medical evaluation with work specificity.

How

Duration of testing. A simple schedule for both patients and therapists is the one-day format testing, involving between 2 and 6 hours depending upon the depth of the evaluation. Two potential difficulties of this format have been noted. The first is the inability of the therapist to ensure longitudinal reliability. Many patients have good and bad days, sometimes depending on the activities of the previous day. In the one day format, the therapist is not able to gauge whether the evaluated performance is consistent from day to day.

Another deficit is the inability to assess the physical reactions to the heavy work involved in an evaluation. A good functional capacities assessment physically stresses the patient as his maximum function is determined. The high level of test activity can in itself increase or decrease symptoms in a patient. For example, a patient who is adversely affected by repetitions or high weight loads may not show the effects until the second visit, when symptoms such as decreased range of motion, joint swelling, muscle spasm and other physical signs can be evaluated. Conversely, a patient who 'self-limits' due to fear of reinjury may be encouraged by the first day of testing and show increased confidence and increased ability on the second day.

The 2 day format which evaluates similar abilities, solves these problems. In this format, weight capacities and other critical items can be retested for accuracy and reproducability.

A third format goes beyond basic testing into long-term endurance and full work days, and is often called work-tolerance screening. This format adds factors such as overall endurance, punctuality, work habits and repetitious activities. The advantages are the in-depth simulated work evaluation and also pretraining prior to return to work. Disadvantages are the costs of the assessment and the external costs such as lodging and meals.

The most reliable of these testing formats in a short period of time appears to be the 2 day format.

Equipment. The purest form of functional assessment is that which uses the minimum of restrictive equipment and a maximum of natural body motions. However, machinery and equipment have often become the means of collecting objective, quantitative data. This technology must be used with a full understanding of what *is* tested, and what is *not* tested. Currently, two types of equipment are most prevalent. The first measures total body force such as that involved in lifting, pushing and pulling. Metered force is measured through a static or fixed-range tensiometer. There are many types of measurement apparatus but individual muscle groups are not isolated in this type of testing. The forces measured are not necessarily applicable to free moving function. Individual variables within the patients must also be recognized. For example, each person moves differently due to differences in bone lengths, distribution of muscle fibres, body shapes and centre of gravity. Joint dysfunction, muscle weakness, lack of muscle endurance and decreased aerobic capacity can all affect activity through the full range of motion. The use of isometric or limited range measurements will not provide information on these aspects.

If the testing mechanism measures only peak torque, this could be misleading as the momentum may produce peaks of a higher level than the average person is capable of taking through the full range. If a person tries to move through a weak point in his range with a weight heavier than can be tolerated, then compensation or injury could occur. Since, in practice, a person can only lift the mass that he is capable of handling through his weakest point in the range, testing must apply the same principle. For this reason, machine testing of lifting capacity through full range should be used cautiously. Although data so collected would provide valuable information regarding torque, smoothness of force curve or limited range power, care must be taken in relating such information to actual work ability.

Isokinetic testing of muscle groups is growing in popularity as a form of measurement. Its advantage lies in its ability to measure torque produced by isolated muscle groups. Such information can be correlated with functional capacity assessments in which individual muscle groups have been identified as a limiting factor in a particular work activity. The specific documentation produced by isokinetic testing can be an accessory to functional capacity assessment documentation. Isokinetic testing cannot be regarded as referring to functional movement alone, however, as it does not allow for natural body movements through full range. The type of equipment used in isokinetic testing should be thoroughly evaluated to determine the comparability of movements involved with functional testing.

Psychological parameters. The study of delayed recovery is well documented by psychologists, who have found that psychological factors can provide secondary gain for physically limited patients. However, if the proper approach is taken, these need not interfere with physical testing. 'Delayed recovery' patients are a special challenge to the physical therapist carrying out FCAs as such patients may consider any symptom as a reason not to perform a task. Such a patient must be made aware that pain and loss of function are not necessarily synonymous and that many people who have consistent pain retain their function. Conversely, a patient may go beyond safe maximum limits and feel no pain until later. The patient must be made aware that he can report discomfort symptoms but that the evaluator will consider maximum function on the basis of physiological signs rather than report of pain. Diagnoses regarding psychological dysfunction belong in the realm of the licensed psychologist or psychiatrist. However, the physical therapist may indicate when functional limitations are not of a physical nature by reporting objective signs of psychological interference with physical functioning.

COMPONENTS OF FUNCTIONAL CAPACITIES ASSESSMENT

A functional capacities assessment is comprised of a number of different components, all of which have relevance to activities of daily living. Prior to carrying out an actual FCA, medical history and physical assessment information are required.

History

A medical history should be obtained from each patient. It should appraise the physical therapist of any past physical conditions which may provide insight into current physical status. Contraindications should be known before assessment begins. It is also helpful to gain a short verbal history from the patients themselves. Their own perceptions of disabilities and limitations may prove to be closer to their real functional level than a preconceived notion developed from a medical history.

Physical assessment

To provide insight into potential performance on the assessment, the basic physical parameters should be known prior to the test. It is wise to carry out a musculoskeletal evaluation to determine the existence of any gross problems in range of motion, strength and functional patterns. Vital signs should be taken. This allows for clarification of the physical limitations which would interfere with function during the testing situation.

The components necessary for an FCA have been derived from governmental and industrial 'return to work' forms used across the United States. The typical set of components included in a functional capacities assessment are tabulated below.

1. Weight capacities
lifts	— floor to work-bench
	— horizontal
	— work-bench to shelf
push/pull	— dynamically and statically
carry	— distance variables
	— surface variables
	— unilateral/bilateral factors

Hand grip strength

2. Flexibility/Positional work
overhead activity
bending at hip
trunk rotation

squat to floor, bending hips and knees
crawling
kneeling

3. Static positioning
standing
sitting

4. Ambulatory skills
walking
stairs
ladders
rough surface
balance activities

5. Co-ordination
upper extremity co-ordination

6. Aerobic/endurance activities
(evaluated in walking, stairs, lifts, carries)

Running or bicycling may be added as extra tests, as necessary.

Weight capacities

Lifts

There are several different types of lifting, and functional evaluations choose to measure these in different ways. There should at least be a differentiation between three types of lifting. Each places different stresses on muscle groups and components of the musculoskeletal system. Since the evaluation of one type of lifting capacity does not necessarily provide information on another, all lifting items should be individually tested.

Lifting from floor to waist height involves a vertical movement of the load. The recommended starting position is flexion of hips and knees while maintaining the normal lordotic curve in the low back. This lift is metabolically strenuous yet safe because the low back is maintained in a stabilized position. The primary muscle groups stressed are the quadriceps, hip extensors, back extensors, abdominals, and elbow, wrist and finger flexor muscles. In addition, stress is placed on the cardiopulmonary system and a significant increase in pulse rate can occur if the lift is done repetitively. Cardiac precautions should be noted and followed.

Transferring a weight from one work surface to another at waist height involves a horizontal movement of the load. This does not produce the same stress on the lower extremities and cardiovascular system as the previous lift. Instead, because the weight capacity is usually higher, the additional stress is relayed to the low back and upper extremities.

Lifting from table height to shelf height is also a vertical lift. The position of the upper extremities influences the task. If the lifting technique utilizes a handle grip, the wrist will be forced into a strongly flexed and ulnar-deviated position when the lift reaches its highest point. This strain on the joint and supporting musculature may in itself become the limiting factor. Alternative methods would allow initial underhand holding of the object or changing to an underhand hold at the lift's highest level. When hand–wrist components are not unduly stressed, the anti-gravity shoulder and scapular muscles (primarily deltoid and upper trapezius) perform the heaviest functions. The ability of the patient to maintain extension in the neck and lower back is also tested. Heart rate is increased during this test. Again, cardiac precautions are important.

Carrying

The task of carrying weights differs from that of lifting in that it needs sustained contraction of upper extremity muscles and strong pelvic stability while walking. The carrying task tested can be adapted for job specificity by varying the type of container and comparing unilateral and bilateral activities.

Push–pull

Push–pull ability may be tested either statically or dynamically. The static format has the advantage of evaluating the exact amount of force generated to initiate movement. A dynamic push allows observation of body mechanics and any limitation in movement. In either case it is important that the actual force of push and pull be measured rather than merely using the weight of the object as an indicator of the assessed force. Inertia, friction and changes in floor patterns affect the force required to push or pull, and for this reason, the exact force in Newtons required to produce movement is the most accurate measure of push–pull ability.

Hand and pinch grip

Standard measurements for hand and pinch grip strengths can be taken. They may be compared against the standardized normals available as a result of research studies. One of the most valuable aspects of this type of measurement in work-related activities is that a difference between right and left hands may be noted. It is also important to determine the optimum hand grip size for use in cor-relation with hand grips at work.

Flexibility–positional work

The patient's ability to cope with working for prolonged periods in various specified positions is also evaluated.

Overhead activity

Sustaining an overhead work position stresses the endurance of the deltoid muscles, scapular muscles and upper trapezius. Assessment of their tolerance during sustained overhead reach at different heights should be made. In addition, the patient's ability to tolerate sustained cervical extension should be noted during such activities. Secondary problems such as vision or eye–hand co-ordination during work at this level may be documented. Weights may be added to simulate the use of a tool.

Bending

Frequent bending can be accomplished easily by people who have no musculoskeletal problems in the low-back area. Where trunk flexion is required to carry out the work function, it should be al-ternated with extension, and the same principle should be applied during testing. Repetitious bending at the hip is best evaluated to a forward trunk angle of 45°, where the back extensor muscles remain in control. Each flexion movement should be followed by a return to the full upright position. This allows the cumulative effect of repeated bending to be evaluated rather than the problematic sustained trunk flexion.

Squatting

In squatting to floor level, the hips and knees are flexed and normal lordosis is maintained. While this activity is strenuous and stressful on the knee joints, its inclusion is considered necessary in order to identify functional safety. If the patient has any knee joint dysfunction or a significant quadriceps weakness, the squatting cannot be performed with an upright back posture. In such a case, the stress would be transmitted to the low back which would flex to compensate for the lack of knee flexion. In testing the patient's ability to squat, the movement is repeated to fatigue or tolerance level, stopping the test if upright back posture cannot be maintained. The therapist would need to identify any limitation in depth of squatting or in number of repetitions.

Trunk rotation

Trunk rotation while lifting a weight is not recommended in work activities. If lifting or carrying is necessary during work, then patients are advised that trunk rotation should be avoided. They are encouraged to pivot at foot level rather than to rotate the trunk. In the testing situation, trunk turning without a weight may be evaluated, as this requires co-ordinated body movement.

Kneeling

To evaluate kneeling, the position should be maintained statically for 5 to 10 minutes. This allows the therapist to evaluate the effect of prolonged static contractions on the low-back and hip musculature necessary to maintain this position.

Static positioning

The patient's ability to maintain the standing or the sitting position and the duration of rest required from that position are measured. It is wise to make these observations while the patient is involved in another activity such as describing his medical history, filling out forms or doing another portion of the assessment. The length of time that a static position can be maintained is monitored as well as the time needed for rest from that position. For example, if a patient is able to tolerate standing for only 20 minutes, a 5-minute rest break might allow return to the standing job. On the other hand, it may take 25 minutes before standing can again be tolerated.

If difficulty in sitting for prolonged periods is determined, suggestions should be made for the provision of suitable devices or adaptations which would rectify the problem. If a back support or a change in work height allows an increase in sitting time, this should be documented.

Ambulatory skills

A number of skills relating to ambulation need assessment.

Walking

Walking should be evaluated in a consistent manner. Generally, walking for one quarter to three quarters of a mile allows endurance, speed and gait deviations to be evaluated. Most walking tests are performed indoors to eliminate weather variables. If only outdoor work is to be performed, an additional walking test should be done outdoors.

Stairs, ladders and inclined planes

In these activities, co-ordination, endurance and the need for suitable modifications to permit carrying need to be evaluated. Stair and ladder climbing need to be repetitious so that the cardiovascular system is stressed and any limiting factors can be identified. The patient's levels of musculoskeletal flexibility and co-ordination are also evident during these activities.

Balance

Balance testing is very helpful in establishing not only the neurological balance abilities, but also the joint proprioception and stabilization capabilities. Evaluation of balance in the forward, backward and sideways directions is recommended.

Co-ordination

Upper extremity co-ordination

There are a number of standardized upper extremity tests which may be used for this functional component. Fine and gross motor co-ordination should be evaluated along with sensory abilities. Since repetitious activity, as well as a non-neutral wrist position, can contribute to cumulative trauma, the upper extremity tests should include aspects of both.

Good upper extremity co-ordination can provide a positive statement of aptitude when the patient's ability to return to heavy work is questioned. For this reason, this particular test may be included even if the injury is to a larger area such as low back, hip or knees.

Aerobic-endurance activities

Adequate aerobic capacity is very important for a person's return to work. It may be incorporated into the testing situation by allowing activities such as stair climbing or walking to be of sufficiently long duration to measure changes in pulse and blood pressure. The floor to waist height lift is another example of a test that causes stress to the cardiopulmonary system. In addition, tests may be added, such as bicycling, step testing or running, which may increase the overall information on aerobic capacity.

Additional factors

A number of other features of testing need consideration. For example, non-skid shoes and loose fitting shorts and shirts are recommended for testing. In testing the upper extremity, it is helpful if men remove their shirts and women wear a halter top, to allow the therapist to visually inspect the muscles involved in those activities. Where a mandatory type of clothing must be worn at work, it is wise for this to be used during testing. Although this changes standardized procedure, it is more effective in testing the patient, since work is more closely simulated and limiting factors can be determined that might be related to the clothing or equipment.

If a medical device is to be worn, such as an ankle–foot orthosis, low back brace or wrist splint, then it should be worn during testing. If the devices are not consistently worn by the patient, they are not necessary during assessment as long as safety is not in question.

SCORING

Functional capacity assessment does not lend itself to a pass–fail scoring method. Instead, objective determinations of ability in strength and endurance are necessary. In addition, the physical factors which limit the activity should be delineated, so that appropriate recommendations may be made regarding additional programmes or work-site modifications. Employers in industry can comply with an employee's specified work limitations when physical reasons are given.

The variations in physical limiting factors which can occur between patients can be appreciated by reference to some of the test items.

1. In lifting from floor level, using the upright back posture with normal lordosis, normal fatigue patterns will be different between patients, depending upon the physical limiting factor. For example,
   a. If fatigue occurred in the quadriceps and they began to fail, the knees would extend prematurely with a resultant forward flexed posture of the back and hips. The testing would be stopped at this point to prevent the back extensor musculature from carrying out the majority of the lifting. Quadriceps weakness would be designated as the physical limiting factor (see Fig. 11.1).
   b. If the back extensors were the weakest component (the physical limiting factor), rounding of the upper back during the lift would be identifiable (see Fig. 11.2).
   c. If lack of a strong low-back stability were the limiting factor, the lumbar area would not be held in a stabilized position during the lift. It would show movement into flexion and extension patterns as stabilization faltered.
   d. If upper extremity flexors (usually biceps) were the weaker physical component (limiting factor), the subject would begin to lift with the weight lagging and the need to 'jerk' it into a higher position to bring the weight to table height.
2. In studying static overhead work tasks, the subject may go through patterns of position change which indicate stress or fatigue. For example,
   a. If the deltoids lose their endurance, the shoulders change position in order to rest certain muscle portions. While maintaining constant hand contact on the object, one hand may be placed more forward and the other backward. Alternatively, one hand may support at a higher level than the other. These patterns often reverse as each extremity tries to rest from the pattern it has held. Toward the end of

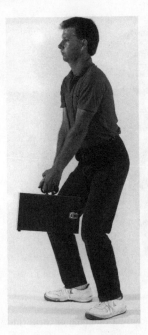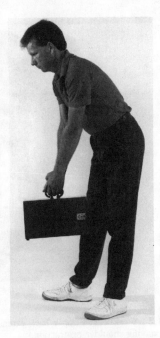

Fig. 11.1 (a) Normal lift with upright back position and normal lordosis.
(b) Quadriceps fatigue forcing knee extension before load rises—causing back
flexion.

maximum deltoid function, there is decreased shoulder joint
flexion, increased upper trapezius activity bilaterally and
increased wrist and finger extension (see Fig. 11.3a + 11.3b).
b. If the cervical extension position is a limiting factor, the
subject will place himself horizontally further from the task
and keep his neck in a neutral rather than an extended
position (see Fig. 11.3c). Because this position is more
difficult for eye–hand co-ordination, the subject without
cervical problems will not adapt this position.

The purpose of the therapist in scoring, is not only to time the
activity, count repetitions or record mass moved, but also to identify the physical limiting factor in the activity.

Recommendations made by the physical therapist are based upon
the scoring and limitation factors which were evident during functional testing. It is important that adequate documentation is
provided to accompany these recommendations, to facilitate com-

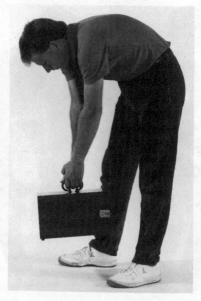

Fig. 11.2 Weakness in upper back extensors causing rounding of back with accompanying shoulder protraction.

munication and for possible future use in any potential legal aspects.

Rating scale used during a functional assessment

'Rating' in the context of functional capacities assessment means to give the patient an objective determination of functional ability level on each of the tested items. It is completed after the functional testing report has been completed. An FCA scoring report should have included listings and explanations of abilities and physical limitations, as described above. The rating, however, goes beyond this in that it compares the scores of the individual to an outside system. In making these comparisons, the outside standard used should represent the functional requirements of the task. This allows the positive factors of ability to be highlighted, and yet work restrictions to be clearly defined. At the present time, in the USA, each state has a predetermined 'rating scale' for use in the workers' compensation system. The example shown in Table 11.1 is more comprehensive than most scales, but does give the vital information

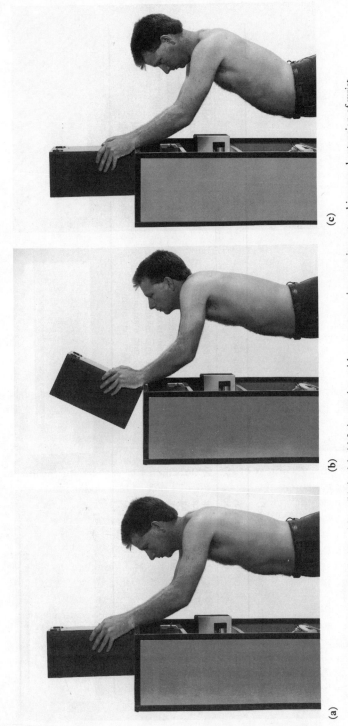

Fig. 11.3 (a) Normal overhead work position. (b) At deltoid fatigue point, with upper trapezius recruitment and increased extension of wrist and fingers. (c) Protection from cervical extension usually due to positional discomfort.

Table 11.1 Rating scale example (brief)

Function	% activity in a work day					Restrictions	Comments
	0–5%	6–25%	26–50%	50–75%	76–100%		
Lift from floor	30 kg	20 kg	5 kg	NO	NO	30 kg maximum	More rest periods should be provided as weight reaches maximum
Lift from table	50 kg	35 kg	10 kg	5 kg	5 kg	50 kg maximum	
Push	100 kg	75 kg	40 kg	15 kg	15 kg	100 kg force maximum	Cannot tolerate uneven surfaces: distance not to exceed 200 m at maximum
Pull	110 kg	80 kg	45 kg	15 kg	15 kg	110 kg force maximum	
Standing				X		40 min maximum at once	Should be allowed to change positions frequently
Sitting			X			30 min maximum at once	
Kneeling		X				15 min maximum	Provide kneeling pad
Crawling	X					100 ft maximum	Smooth surfaces only

called for in the state systems and allows for the delineation of further restrictions and explanatory comments.

At the moment, the ability of uninjured persons to perform this complement of dynamic functional activities is not fully known. Lifting has been studied in several different ways, as mentioned earlier. However, in research reported to date, the subject has been the judge of maximum function, rather than a professional physical therapist who can document the point at which safety is compromised or where physical limiting factors are identifiable. Polinsky Medical Rehabilitation Center has been studying non-injured subjects on 17 standardized work-related tasks. When performance of uninjured subjects is known, the rating scales may then go beyond an individual's capacity as determined by a physical therapist and on to a comparative analysis with normals.

OUTCOMES OF FUNCTIONAL CAPACITY ASSESSMENT

A comprehensive functional capacity assessment cannot only identify the ability of a person to do work, but can also identify any limited areas and the physical reason for those limitations. This is valuable information for the patient in his everyday life.

In relation to work, functional capacity information may lead to four possible outcomes. The use of functional capacity information in promoting case resolution for an individual patient illustrates these outcomes.

'Return to work' statements

To be used in 'return to work' statements, the functional testing must be compared to functional components in a job description. Where a functional job description is provided, the therapist can then make a statement such as the following:

> The patient's functional abilities are adequate to meet all physical aspects in the enclosed job description of a carpenter. The exception is lifting and carrying, which must be limited to 30 kg.

If no job description has been provided, the therapist's statement might be:

> Return to work can be functionally accomplished if the job requires activities listed in this report as functionally able. Special conditions in future work would indicate a limitation of 15 kg in lifting from the floor and 25 kg in lifting or carrying from table height. Kneeling should also be eliminated.

Therefore, the physical therapist can convey by report or by conference the information regarding physical abilities as they relate to the work itself. Physicians, employers, rehabilitation consultants and the patient/employee should be given this information.

Job or job-site modification

When compared to the job description, a functional assessment might indicate a physical limitation which would prevent the patient from returning to work. If a simple modification could be made to the work or work-site, return to work could be accomplished without compromising the worker's physical safety.

For example, lifting from the floor or squatting to the floor might be limited due to permanent knee joint dysfunction. During the functional evaluation, the patient may have compromised his back safety by forward bending during lifting or squatting, thus causing increased back symptoms. The return to work of this employee could be accomplished if all of his work were brought up to work-bench height by means of pallets and shelving, or by changing the placement of controls or tools to waist-height level.

An assembly line worker with carpal tunnel syndrome may be able to continue work if hand grips were changed on the tools to allow a neutral position, rather than one of flexion and ulnar deviation, which is common during the use of many tools. The lack of ability to perform repetitious activity may be alleviated by allowing the employee to vary the type of work performed. By such job rotation, symptoms which preclude work should not develop. However, overall, the employee should achieve the same amount of work in one day.

Employers have been found to be very willing to make changes to the work-site or the work itself to allow an employee to return to work where the physical reason has been documented in an FCA.

Work hardening

Physical strengths and weaknesses are well documented through the functional capacity assessment, which relates to work items. A description of functional capacity and limitations can provide the basis for future goals in further rehabilitation and training for both the patient and the physical therapist. It also establishes the basis for a physical restoration or 'work-hardening' programme, which is a medically supervised plan in which the patient's function is progressively increased in order to attain an appropriate level for a return to work. The work hardening programme defines the identified physical problems and the plan of action to be followed in order to reach the specified goals relating to work demands.

If a lifting limitation, an inability to do repetitious activity, or a decrease in aerobic capacity present major return-to-work problems, a work-hardening programme may be instituted. After the work hardening has been completed, a further evaluation would delineate specifically the 'return to work' physical parameters, as outlined earlier.

For example, the functional capacity assessment might reveal that lifting from the floor and squatting limitations were due to weak quadriceps muscles and that low endurance in the deltoids allowed only short periods of time in overhead work ability. A third problem area might be evidence of an increased pulse rate during stair climbing, lifting and other strenuous activity. The patient may have begun the functional evaluation with a relatively high resting pulse rate, indicating a deconditioning situation. A work-hardening programme could then be specifically addressed, not only to the physical body functions needing restoration, but also to the work ability which would be improved if these functions were increased An increase in quadriceps strength would allow lifting of greater masses from the floor, would increase stair climbing endurance and would increase the ability to squat to the floor and return to the upright position safely. An increase in deltoid strength would allow overhead work to be done for longer periods of time and also with heavier weights (tools). An increase in aerobic conditioning would not only make the patient more fit generally, but would also increase ability and endurance of stair climbing, walking, lifting and carrying and any other activities which generally raise the pulse rate. Therefore, several physical restoration activities can be included as part of the work hardening and they work together to increase the overall functional level.

In work hardening, exercise would not be the only appropriate factor. Work simulation is necessary to allow the patient to replicate the motions and work activities he will be required to do upon return to work. Therefore, if improvement in lifting and carrying capacity is desired, not only would strengthening activities be necessary, but also the exact shape of objects and the distance of their placements would be replicated. Overhead work could be simulated by using weights or the actual tool. The height of the overhead work would match job requirements. In aerobic activities, the extent and type of work would also be important.

Work hardening increases the functional abilities of the patient and allows positive feedback toward actual work activities which ensure safety upon return to work.

Case resolution

In many instances, litigation is a part of the worker's compensation case management. The physical therapist responsible for the functional capacities assessment may be called upon to give functional ability information relating to work. This is used by attorneys, judges, physicians and the workers' compensation systems to aid in settlement of an employee's claim. The functional assessment also provides the employee with information that can determine abilities and limitations in future work.

RESEARCH IN FUNCTIONAL CAPACITY ASSESSMENT

As in all areas of physical therapy practice, further research is needed to ensure that the most effective programmes are developed. In particular, research should continue in two areas concerned with functional assessment.

Data collected from assessments on patients need to be studied for relationships of variables influencing functional ability. Variables might include diagnosis, time off work, time post-injury, type of work, height, weight, gender, age, blood pressure, resting pulse rate, increase in blood pressure after activity and increase in pulse rate after activity. Also, study will show inter-relationships between functional items. For example, if a person can lift 10 kg safely from the floor, will this translate into an estimate of his ability to lift that amount from table height? Will that translate into an amount he can lift and carry? Other correlations could be evident between upper extremity tasks, flexibility tasks, endurance tasks, etc.

Research on normals will also be very helpful to functional capacity evaluations. Once these same variables and relationships can be studied on normals, the importance of findings on patients will be enhanced. While normal or 'average' information will never replace individual evaluation and neither should it, it does provide a basis on which to state criteria for rating the patient's functional level during assessment. The multiple variables involved in functional assessment lend themselves to an understanding of total function even beyond the work realm.

The data produced by a study carried out by Isernhagen et al (1987) for FCA Network Polinsky Medical Rehabiliation Center, Duluth, Minnesota, could provide clinicians with clearer directions for evaluation and restorative care. That study investigated the relationship of age and gender to functional performance in patients and uninjured subjects and is described below.

A study of the relationship of age and gender to functional performance

Materials and methods

Extensive testing of subjects in a consistent manner provides the opportunity for an analysis of inter-relationships between variables in the subjects themselves and their performance. For this reason, a data bank was established in 1981 by Polinsky Medical Rehabilitation Center. The initial purpose of the data bank was to determine any trends that existed in patient performance. When age and gender consistently appeared to be important variables, those tasks more affected by age and gender were selected for particular attention.

The procedures for testing and scoring for the functional capacities assessment remained consistent during the period of the study. To ensure standardization of approach, all testing therapists were educated on testing and scoring procedures during a 2-day training session. When testing subjects, these therapists followed a 5-hour (over 2 days) assessment protocol on standardized generic work-related tests.

To allow a comparison of the influence of age and gender on performance in patients following injury with that of uninjured ('normal') subjects, the FCA tests were also applied to a group of uninjured volunteers. Their performance was analysed on those tests which had appeared most affected by age and gender in the patient population. These areas were 'weight capacities', 'stair climbing' and 'balance' and tests for those were as follows:

a. Weight capacities
　　(i) Stand up lift (floor to table height): maximum mass lifted safely for 10 repetitions.
　　(ii) Level lift (table height to table height): maximum mass lifted safely for 10 repetitions

(iii) Weight carry (weight carried 30 m): maximum mass carried safely and time needed to perform the carry.
b. Stair climbing
   (i) Pace: number of stairs per minute
   (ii) Endurance: maximum time stair climbing could be tolerated, up to 4 minutes.
c. Balance
   (i) Forward walk: time needed to complete 15 m test and number of errors during performance
   (ii) Forward heel to toe: time needed to complete 15 m test and number of errors during performance
   (iii) Backward heel to toe: time needed to complete 15 m test and number of errors during performance
   (iv) Sideways walk: time needed to complete 15 m test and number of errors during performance.

A total of 1696 subjects were tested including 1643 patients following injury and 153 uninjured subjects. The data were separated into six categories, with three age groups falling into each of the male and female subgroups: young(16–34); middle (35–55); and advanced (56–75). Table 11.2 shows the numbers in each group.

Table 11.2 Distribution of age and gender in injured and uninjured subject groups

Age group	Injured n = 1643		Uninjured n = 153	
	F	M	F	M
Young	150	436	25	24
Middle	291	606	27	25
Advanced	48	112	25	27

Results

Following computer analysis, results were examined according to relative performance in each of the three tests selected for comparison purposes.

Weight capacities. From Table 11.3, it can be observed that in all age and gender categories, the masses lifted or carried were lower in the patient group than in the uninjured group. The difference in performance by males and females in each of the

Table 11.3 Comparison of mean performance in FCA test of weight capacity

| Test | | Weight capacity (lb) | | | | | |
| | | Female | | | Male | | |
		Y	M	A	Y	M	A
		n = 150	n = 291	n = 48	n = 436	n = 606	n = 112
P A T I E N T S	Stand up lift	23.78	19.97	16.36	39.33	33.39	28.96
	Level lift	34.20	30.90	21.45	48.05	43.00	37.16
	Weight carried	32.15	26.99	20.54	50.87	46.43	37.23
		n = 25	n = 27	n = 25	n = 24	n = 25	n = 27
U N I N J U R E D	Stand up lift	41.92	28.37	14.32	67.41	64.44	51.85
	Level lift	59.16	49.51	48.72	82.70	82.24	73.66
	Weight carried	1.28	51.92	52.84	84.66	84.24	77.55

Age groups:
Y = 16–34 years
M = 35–55 years
A = 56–75 years

different age categories can also be readily seen. In all three weight capacity tests, females had significantly less capacity than males.

The influence of age on weight capacity is apparent in both the uninjured and the patient population, showing a decline in ability with increasing age for both groups. In the uninjured population, there was a more marked decline in performance for females by middle age than for males.

Stair climbing. Table 11.4 reveals that patients performed less well than the uninjured group in all age and gender subgroups. Most patients were unable to complete the 4 minutes of stair climbing. Age proved to be an important factor in determining endurance level in stair climbing for both men and women, although the effect was not noticeable until 'advanced' age in the uninjured group and then was not as marked a decrease as in the patient group. Females showed less endurance than males in the patient population, but for the relatively short 4 minute test, any difference in endurance

Table 11.4 Comparison of mean performances in FCA test of stair climbing

Test		Mean performance					
		Female			Male		
		Y	M	A	Y	M	A
		n = 150	n = 291	n = 48	n = 436	n = 606	n = 112
P A T I E N T S	Endurance (min)	3.49	3.16	2.97	3.70	3.41	3.28
	Pace (No/min)	67.69	47.77	36.08	68.09	54.90	48.64
		n = 25	n = 27	n = 25	n = 24	n = 25	n = 27
U N I N J U R E D	Endurance (min)	4.00	4.00	3.86	4.00	4.00	3.95
	Pace (No/min)	98.79	80.22	73.45	100.00	92.16	78.96

Age groups:
Y = 16–34 years
M = 35–55 years
A = 56–75 years

ability between uninjured men and women was not revealed except to a slight degree at advanced age.

The pace of stair climbing was also affected by age, the pace decreasing progressively with increasing age. Both the rate of decline and its magnitude were more marked in the patient population than in the uninjured subjects. The gender difference in pace of stair climbing, in which men performed better than women, was apparent for both subject groups.

Balance. Table 11.5 compares both the time taken to complete each of the four balance tests and the number of errors made during each test. The patient group performed less well than the uninjured group in every age and gender category. Age was shown to have an important influence on time taken and errors recorded, both of these variables increasing with age, with only one exception. It appears that those with greater age took more time, which may

Table 11.5 Comparison of mean performance in FCA test of balance

Test		Mean performance					
		Female			Male		
		Y	M	A	Y	M	A
		n = 150	n = 291	n = 48	n = 436	n = 606	n = 112
P A T I E N T S	Balance (min)						
	A.	0.60	0.81	1.01	0.55	0.68	0.68
	B.	1.14	1.36	1.81	1.02	1.14	1.14
	C.	1.64	1.88	1.78	1.30	1.44	1.40
	D.	0.84	1.05	1.35	0.75	0.94	1.00
	(No. of errors)						
	A.	0.09	0.48	1.57	0.12	0.30	0.53
	B.	0.32	1.19	3.02	0.30	0.73	1.37
	C.	1.61	2.35	4.40	1.15	1.79	2.80
	D.	0.27	0.42	0.97	0.25	0.39	0.59

Test		Mean performance					
		Female			Male		
		Y	M	A	Y	M	A
		n = 25	n = 27	n = 25	n = 24	n = 25	n = 27
U N I N J U R E D	Balance						
	A.	0.3580	0.4185	0.4513	0.3715	0.3687	0.4062
	B.	0.8067	0.8883	1.09	0.7340	0.7793	0.8198
	C.	1.24	1.24	1.75	0.98	1.13	1.21
	D.	0.5367	0.5907	0.7240	0.4757	0.5307	0.5623
	No. of errors						
	A.	0.0400	0.0741	0.1600	0.0833	0.1200	0.0370
	B.	0.2000	0.2222	0.8750	0.1250	0.4800	0.5926
	C.	0.92	1.22	2.66	0.54	0.76	2.66
	D.	0.2000	0.0370	0.6000	0.2083	0.0000	0.7037

Age groups:
Y = 16–34 years
M = 35–55 years
A = 56–75 years

indicate more effort, and yet they made more errors in the balance tests.

Females in both subject groups took longer to complete the balance tests than did males in all four balance activities. Females in the patient population made more errors than males but the difference between males and females in the balance tests was less clear in the uninjured subjects.

Clinical implications

As a group, the patient population, both male and female subjects of all ages, scored lower on all test capacities evaluated. Not suprisingly, the uninjured population appeared much more functional and capable as an overall group.

In both the patient and the uninjured populations, women generally had less capacity than men in all weightlifting tests. They also appeared to have less endurance and a slower pace in stair climbing. In some balance activities they performed less ably than males.

It was obvious from this study that increasing age affects performance in the functional activities tested. With an increase in age came a decrease in the amount of weight lifted, a decrease in the pace and endurance of stair climbing and an increase in the incidence of errors and the time required to complete a balance test.

In looking at the individual effects of age and gender, it is observed that the older worker and the female worker have lesser capacities than younger or male workers, and they may therefore be at greater risk of injury either on the job or at home. The older female, by virtue of the influence of both age and gender on the capacity for certain tasks, would be at the greatest disadvantage.

The occupational medicine clinician needs to make a return-to-work recommendation or a suggestion which would facilitate the restoration of work function. Some results of this study may assist clinicians in formulating those recommendations.

1. Job risk in weighted activities, anti-gravity endurance activities (stair climbing) and tasks requiring balance may be greater for females and older workers. Work activities which combine these factors could place a worker at an even greater risk of injury.

2. Since patients who might return to work are shown to have significantly decreased abilities compared to the uninjured, patient workers may be at greater risk of further injury. Therefore, work-

hardening programmes can be of importance in increasing the functional level to that of the average worker. If a restoration programme is not possible, the low patient scores suggest that physical restrictions are an important consideration upon return to the job. The results of the comparative study also highlight the necessity for a thorough, individual functional capacities assessment to allow the individual worker to have specific functional return-to-work recommendations.

3. Job analysis is particularly important for the total workplace in identifying when physical lifts and carries, aerobic conditions and balance are needed on the job. This job analysis might then be viewed in the light of the type of workforce present at the job and it may indicate whether age and gender limitations might exist in any particular work condition.

4. Pre-employment and pre-placement screening will be helpful in identifying abilities and limitations on an individual basis.

Recommendations for future research

The three functional areas that were discussed in this presentation—lifting capacities, balance and stair climbing—would be excellent areas for further specific research. Variables other than age and gender may also be studied to clarify their full influence on functional abilities. Some of these could include diagnosis, height, weight, exercise levels and health habits. Longitudinal studies would also be helpful to determine whether there are individual variations in the changing capacities with age.

PHYSICAL THERAPISTS IN INDUSTRIAL MEDICINE

Functional capacity assessment has a natural ability to complement and strengthen other industrial medicine programmes. As physical therapists develop their professional skills in these areas and explain their value to physicians and industry, their expertise is likely to be sought in the following areas.

Pre-employment screening

The emphasis in pre-employment screening is on prevention of injury and this requires a professional determination of an employee's risk of injury. A large range of risk identifiers have been used, including the person's medical history, a general medical examination, x-ray and strength testing of isolated muscle groups. The physical therapist can add significantly to the body of knowledge available for pre-selection purposes with both musculoskeletal evaluation and selected functional capacities assessment items.

While the development of a screening process that could identify abnormalities in musculoskeletal attributes is seen as an advantage, caution needs to be taken not to over-react to their relationship to functional problems. Specific and typical measurements made by the physical therapist were evaluated for predictive value by Biering-Sorensen (1984). His extensive review of the literature raises doubts that cornerstone measurements such as hamstring length, height, weight, leg length and leg lowering ability can be correlated with risk of future injury.

Functional evaluation of physical capacities that are identified by job description remains the physical therapist's stronghold. If capabilities in such areas as lifting, bending and carrying are measured, not only will the employer's questions on work ability be answered, but also assistance will be given in matching the worker with a safe job. Evaluating the capability for lifting and carrying 36 kg (80 lb) should be regarded no differently to the routine testing of ability to type at a specified rate (e.g. 80 words per minute). Designated functional capacities can be assessed by the therapist for pre-employment ability. The difference lies in selecting only pertinent components and matching them exactly to the work demands. A method of matching work demands with functional capacity was described in Chapter 10. Follow-up studies will be needed to increase the validity of accurate prediction.

Work-site—ergonomic evaluation

To make the workplace safe in a musculoskeletal sense, work postures, motions and stresses need to be studied. Forces applied and repetitions achieved provide basic measurable information. In addition, observations regarding the person's physical functioning on a particular job can reveal those work movements which cause flexion, extension, rotation, etc. Repetitions and the degree of co-ordination possible should also be part of the job-site evaluation. The physical therapist would write a report based on medical and physical stresses. The industry would then have understandable and logical information upon which to base a modification of the work-site design and the physical therapist would have the basis of comparison for functional capacities assessments.

Education and training

The value of educating employees in body mechanics has been well documented. This need has not diminished; in fact, statistics indicate the need for continued involvement to refresh the employee's knowledge and add additional comprehensive viewpoints.

The development of specialized training that complements safety education is also valuable. For example, the physical therapist can design transfer training for nursing personnel, lifting practices for stock persons, and posture awareness for office workers. By combining this basic education with specific work tasks, there should be a decrease in injury and an increase in productivity.

Health and fitness

Concurrent with an accentuated public interest in fitness, industry has recognized its value. Many employers now encourage both on- and off-the-job participation in fitness programmes. There is more, however, that the physical therapist can add to this system. Job requirements can be analysed and matched to the available exercise programmes to increase work tolerance. Exercise breaks at the work-site can be designed. Fitness can be made specific to the job tasks in order to increase strength, endurance and flexibility, and improve relaxation.

Work hardening

As described earlier in this chapter, work hardening is a medically supervised programme of increasing patient function with the goal of returning to work at an appropriate level. The following features are important to the process.

Professional supervision

During the work-hardening process, the physical therapist should be directly involved in evaluation, programme monitoring and the final functional assessment.

Goal specificity

Work-hardening goals should be specific in identifying physical problems, the plan of action and projected functional outcome.

Job direction

A job description should be used whenever possible to aid the therapist and employee towards pertinent work goals and objectives. Actual work stations or work simulations should be used.

Programme intensity

Because workers' compensation costs have increased dramatically, due in part to prolonged recovery periods, work-hardening programmes should be intensive and time specific. A good work-hardening programme can be time effective by allowing longer treatment periods and a shortened overall programme.

Employment integration

Thorough communication with the employer, rehabilitation consultant and insurance company is necessary to ensure a successful return to work. Once an employee has reached his or her goal, the therapist should participate in defining actual return-to-work specifications. Follow-up studies after the person's return to work are also necessary and helpful in designing future programmes.

THE PHYSICAL THERAPIST'S CHALLENGE

The future of functional capacities assessment in physical therapy can be directed by some pertinent professional goals.

First, the physical therapist's assessments should be accurate on an individual basis. There will be no guesswork or 'inferential leap' involved when each individual has been give a thorough functional assessment. By transmitting this accurate information to the employee, employer and all other professionals involved, the employee should be able to work at a safe level without entering the adversarial system often found in work injury cases. Keeping accurate records on case resolution and return-to-work success is critical at this early point in the professional development of physical therapists in this area.

Research should also be carried out on data collected from functional capacities assessment items. More functional parameters promote or limit function than are currently known. Some of the areas of a functional nature that need to be studied include the relationship of motion, joint stability, posture and body mechanics to functional abilities. While strength and endurance may be correlated with individual functions, research may indicate a relationship of abilities between these items.

Additional data required relates to the correlation of function with age, gender and fitness levels. Multiple variables are involved in functional capacities assessment, and greater knowledge in this area can only enhance understanding of total physical function, even beyond the work realm.

Knowledge and integration of ideas from other professions are necessary in the development of physical therapy in this field. Not only must literature and research findings from ergonomists, engineers, industry, insurance companies and governmental agencies, and other health professions, be read and applied, but also those professional groups need to be educated in the interest and function of physical therapists. As specialists in their own field, physical therapists have a certain expertise. It is important that such expertise should not lead, however, to professional isolation.

Physical therapists belong in work injury management. The patient can be taken from the realm of treatment of injury through thorough rehabilitation; and a safe and timely return to work can be effected with functional capacities assessment. Study of the field, perfection of skills and development of follow-up research offer the physical therapist both a challenge and an opportunity of satisfaction in the functional realm of the industrial world.

REFERENCES

Biering-Sorensen F 1984 Physical measurements as risk indicators for low back trouble over a one-year period. Spine 9 (2): 106–119
Cady L D, Bischoff D P, O'Connell E, Thomas P C, Allan J H 1979 Strength and fitness and subsequent back injuries in firefighters. Journal of Occupational Medicine 21(4): 269–272
Chaffin D B, Andersson G B J 1984 Occupational biomechanics. Wiley, New York
Chaffin D B, Herrin G D, Keyserling W M 1978 Pre-employment strength testing. Journal of Occupational Medicine 20(6): 403–408
Isernhagen S 1985 The physical therapist and the injured worker: the right match. Whirlpool 8(4): 24–26
Isernhagen S 1988 Functional Capacity Evaluation. In: Isernhagen S (Ed) Work injury: management and prevention. Aspen, Rockville
Isernhagen S J, Mokros K, Miller M, Johnson L 1987 The relationship of age and gender to functional performance: patients and uninjured subjects. Research Report for FCA Network, Polinsky Medical Rehabilitation Centre, Duluth MN
Mayer T C, Gatchel R J, Kishino N et al 1985 Objective assessment of spine function following industrial injury. Spine 10(6): 482–493
National Institute of Occupational Safety and Health 1983 Work practices guide for manual lifting. American Industrial Hygiene Association, Akron, OH

SECTION TWO

Appendix

Active participation in a professional group or society concerned with the advancement of the discipline of ergonomics can not only provide a better understanding of its aims and objectives, but also offer a stimulus to closer involvement and application of ergonomic principles. Reference to journals relevant to ergonomics can also broaden knowledge and deepen the appreciation of the full scope of ergonomics and its contribution to the health of the community.

To facilitate this communication and understanding, sources of contact and reference are provided below.

Part A. Ergonomics societies

A number of ergonomics and human factors societies in various countries throughout the world are affiliated with the International Ergonomics Association (IEA). Sixteen societies are represented on the IEA Council and one (the Human Ergology Society) is an affiliated society of the IEA Council. Because the Secretariats of Societies change from time to time, full addresses have not been listed. It is presumed that reference to a current telephone listing would provide local information.

Brazilian Ergonomics Association Abergo, Brazil
Ergonomics Society, United Kingdom
Ergonomics Society of Australia, Australia
Gessellschaft fur arbeitswissenschaft. West Germany
HF Association of Canada/Ace, Canada
Human Factors Society, USA
Hungarian Society for Organization & Management Science, Hungary
Japan Ergonomics Research Society, Japan
Nederlandse Vereniging Voor Ergonomie, The Netherlands

301

Nordic Ergonomics Society, Sweden
Polish Ergonomics Society, Poland
Societa Italiana Di Ergonomia, Italy
Societe D'Ergonomie De Langue, France
The Association of Ergonomics Societies of Yugoslavia, Yugoslavia
Seaes/South-East Asian Ergonomics Society, Indonesia
Belgian Ergonomics Society, Belgium
Human Ergology Society, Japan.

Part B. Journals

Those who plan to read more widely in the area of ergonomics would benefit from reference to the journals which either focus particularly on ergonomic issues or include in their publications, articles featuring some facet of ergonomics.

1. Journals relevant to ergonomics

Applied Ergonomics, IPC Science & Technology Press, Surrey, England
Ergonomics, Taylor & Francis, London
Ergonomics Abstracts, Taylor & Francis, London
Human Factors, Human Factors Society, Santa Monica California
International Journal of Industrial Ergonomics, Elsevier Science, Amsterdam.

2. Journals which include papers on some facet of ergonomics

Australian Journal of Physiotherapy, Australian Physiotherapy Association, Melbourne, Australia
Aviation, Space and Environmental Medicine, Aerospace Medical Association, Alexandria, VA
Behaviour and Information Technology, Taylor & Francis, London
British Journal of Industrial Medicine, British Medical Association, London
Human Biology, Wayne State University Press, Detroit
Journal of Applied Psychology, American Psychological Association, Washington, DC
Journal of Applied Physiology, American Physiological Society, Bethesda, Maryland
Journal of Biomechanics, Pergamon Press, Oxford

Journal of Human Ergology, University of Tokyo Press, Tokyo
Journal of Occupational Behaviour, Wiley, NY
Journal of Occupational Psychology, British Psychological Society,
  Leicester
Journal of Occupational Medicine, American Occupational Medicine
  Association, Baltimore
Scandinavian Journal of Rehabilitative Medicine, Almqvist and
  Wiksell, Uppsala
Scandinavian Journal of Work Environment and Health, Finnish In-
  stitute of Occupational Health, Helsinki
Spine, Lippincott, Hagerstown, Md.

Annotated bibliography

This annotated bibliography provides an overview of literature in the areas explored within this volume. The annotations, prepared by the authors of the volume, are designed to give some insight into the content of each reference. While not meant to be totally comprehensive, this bibliography does offer some guidance to the reader as to the breadth of material available in those aspects of ergonomics which are particularly relevant to the physiotherapist.

A. ERGONOMICS

Astrand P, Rodahl K 1986 Textbook of work physiology. McGraw Hill, New York.
   This text provides a good overview of basic physiology. Its purpose is to bring together into one volume the various factors affecting human physical performance in a manner that is comprehensible to the physiologist, the physical educator and the clinician. Each chapter has been written as a fairly complete entity, relatively independently from the rest of the book. With this arrangement, the book may also be useful to those who wish to penetrate more deeply into a particular field or a limited area of study.

Corlett N, Wilson J, Manenica I (eds) 1986 The ergonomics of working postures: models, methods and cases. Taylor & Francis, London.
   The proceedings of the First International Occupational Ergonomics Symposium, Zadar, Yugoslavia, 1985, are collated in this book. Topics include postural risk factors and disease; methods for measuring body posture; models of posture; measures of the effects of posture; seats and sitting.

Eason K 1988 Information technology and organizational change. Taylor & Francis, London.
   The importance of considering the individual needs of the office worker is emphasized in this book. After addressing the challenge of information technology, the author describes methods of system design and organizational change and, importantly, the design of the technical system for human use.

European Journal of Applied Physiology and Occupational Physiology 1988 Occupational muscle pain and injury 57(3).
   A thorough review of the recent state of research and knowledge of work-related musculoskeletal disorders is contained in this issue of the journal. It should help the physiotherapist to understand such problems more fundamentally.

Grandjean E 1984 Ergonomics and health in modern offices. Taylor & Francis, London. Proceedings of the International Conference on Ergonomic and Health Aspects in Modern Offices. Turin, 1983.
This book comprises different studies concerning environmental factors such as indoor climate, music and noise and lighting of modern offices. Ergonomics, visual functions, cognitive aspects and evaluation and design of VDT work stations are discussed and presented in separate chapters in this serious attempt to cover the subject.

Grandjean E 1988 Fitting the task to the man. Taylor & Francis, London.
An excellent and complete survey of ergonomics today is offered by this book. Professor Etienne Grandjean has been one of the leading figures in ergonomics in Europe for over 30 years. His main research interests were the sitting posture, fatigue and working conditions in industries and, for the last decade, VDT work stations. He has published some 300 scientific papers and edited the first edition of *Fitting the task to the man* in 1963, which has since been translated into 10 different languages. As with the preceding editions, the fourth edition concentrates on basic issues of ergonomics and their occupational applications and endeavours to offer the reader as many practical hints as possible. The aim and purpose of this new edition remains the same—to impart the important elements of ergonomics in a simple and lucid form to all those who are responsible for putting into practice the principles of occupational ergonomics.

Grandjean E, Hünting W, Nishiyana K 1984 Preferred VDT work-station design, body posture and physical impairment. Applied Ergonomics 15: 99–104.
This article is one of numerous papers published by a group of researchers in Switzerland headed by Professor Etienne Grandjean. The group has also collaborated with Japanese researchers and in this way many Japanese techniques for studying neck and upper extremities disorders, including the use of body charts, have been transferred to Europe and the rest of the world. The methods and results reported in this paper are contentious for many reasons, not the least being the use of 'comfort' ratings to determine work postures. However, the methodology for determining work postures is simple and relatively reliable and has been used in other studies. These results are widely quoted, although they should be interpreted with care.

Grandjean E, Hünting W, Pidermann M 1983 VDT work station design: preferred settings and their effects. Human Factors 25: 161–175.
The preferred settings, body postures and subjective evaluations were assessed during subjects' customary working activities at a VDT work station. The operators' preferred body postures were distinctly different from those recommended in textbooks and other publications. This study of body postures revealed that most operators tend to lean backwards 97°–121°. The physical complaints in the neck–shoulder and back area diminish with the preferred settings. In this study, there was practically no correlation between preferred settings and anthropometric data of body length or eye levels above the floor.

Grune S 1985 VDT work stations—a bibliography. K G Saur-Verlag, Munchen.
This book offers an extensive bibliography of over 3000 references of international origin, dealing with various aspects of visual display terminal use. The principal section of the book contains chapters addressing basic principles of ergonomics with special emphasis on man-machine-interaction and design of furniture and the environment, and on particular features of VDT work. The remainder of the book collates details relating to standards, guidelines and rules.

International Institute for Labours Studies 1987 From research to practice—a long road. A report on co-operation between the Union of Commercial Workers in Finland and the Finnish Institute of Occupational Health. Geneva, Switzerland/Vaanta, Finland.
This report deals with how research can be carried out in order to obtain a practical application in an industry. The report shows that co-operation between the researchers and the workers is essential in order to gain optimal research results and to ensure that the research is possible to apply to the workers' practical work. The report also outlines *how* this co-operative work can be organized.

Kvålseth T O (ed) Ergonomics of work-station design. Butterworths, London.
Practical job design tools and approaches are the focus of this book, which contains some of the papers presented in Oslo in 1980 under the auspices of the International Ergonomics Association and the Nordic Ergonomics Society. Guidelines for work-station design, ergonomics methodology and an analysis of the ergonomic implementation process are included.

Nygard C-H, Luopajärvi T, Cedercreutz G, Ilmarinen J Musculoskeletal capacity of employees aged 44 to 55 years in physical, mental and mixed work. European Journal of Applied Physiology 56: 555–561.
This article is one component of a series of articles with Nygard as author. The research describes strengths and weaknesses in a currently working population in Finland. For the purposes of identifying variables, the authors divided the working groups according to gender and then according to physical type of work performed—physical, mental and mixed. The study showed a decrease in musculoskeletal capacity of middle-aged workers, greater than anticipated by previous research. These findings suggest to Nygard et al that regular health checks of employees should include an assessment of musculoskeletal capacity. There is also an indication that doing heavy work not only does not protect one from weakness, but may actually be a factor to consider.

Rohmert W, Landau K 1983 A new technique for job analysis. Taylor & Francis, London.
This book describes one ergonomic job analysis procedure, developed in Germany, which is based upon the stress/strain concept of work. The technique, known as the AET, was developed in the process of analysing 4000 shop floor and management jobs. The book is divided into two main parts: Part I explains the meaning and purpose of job analysis, in general, and describes the uses and method of evaluating the AET, in particular. Part II covers the classification of codes and provides a manual in the form of a checklist of items included in the procedure which are sub-divided into three parts: Part A, The man at work system; Part B, Task analysis; Part C, Analysis of work demands. In all, 216 job factors are covered which are said to include all features of the material or object being worked on, the equipment being used and the work environment. The book is recommended as an essential guide for work analysts, ergonomists and managers who are interested in using the AET.

Shakel B (ed) 1984 Applied ergonomics handbook. Butterworths, London.
An introduction to and guidelines for many of the fundamental concerns of ergonomics which are of particular interest to the physiotherapist are presented in this Handbook. Considerable attention is given to the design and analysis of a work station both for the able-bodied and the disabled worker.

Singleton W T 1972 Introduction to ergonomics. World Health Organization, Geneva.
This manual on ergonomics sets out the basic principles in simple language using an abundance of illustrations. Chapters cover: the provision of energy; the application of forces; problems of body size and posture; the effects of climate; limitations of the sense organs; the design of controls and displays; man/machine information exchange; work conditions; age, vigilance and accidents; individual and systems behaviour; the design of work; assessment, presentation and interpretation of evidence; and finally, comments on the past and future application of ergonomics. Each chapter concludes with a summary of general principles and notes on special cases and these are further exemplified in graphic form in a series of illustrations.

Snook S H 1978 The design of manual handling tasks. Ergonomics 21(12)R:963–985.
The author has synthesized the results of studies conducted by him and his co-workers in this paper. Psychophysical methodology was used, where subjects were asked to exercise the process of self-selection for optimizing a materials-handling task after varying certain selected variables of the task. The author studied the activities of lifting, lowering, pushing, pulling, carrying and walking. The effects of height, distance, frequency of the tasks, the size and weight of the object, the differences in worker sex, age and physique, and the heat stress were studied. The author has presented extensive tables giving the maximum weights that are acceptable to 10, 25, 50, 75 and 90% of the North American working population. The author claims to have established in an evaluative study that jobs designed using these criteria could reduce the back pain problem by one third. He claims that such a task design was significantly more effective than employment, pre-employment or worker training.

van Wely P 1970 Design and disease. Applied Ergonomics 1: 262–269.
This paper was possibly the first to discuss the link between ergonomic factors in the workplace, particularly work-loads and postures determined by poorly designed equipment, furniture and work spaces, and the development of musculoskeletal complaints. It appeared in the first edition of the journal, *Applied Ergonomics*, and alerted the ergonomics world to the predictability and preventability of these conditions, through ergonomics.

Williams T A 1988 Computers, work and health. Taylor & Francis, London.
The problems for health and safety which may exist within offices designed around computer technology are acknowledged in this book. It addresses the implications for injury and the different approaches to design which may be taken by the ergonomist in dealing with occupational health and safety problems in the office.

B. BIOMECHANICS

Chaffin D B, Andersson G 1984 Occupational biomechanics. Wiley, New York.
The book covers different aspects of biomechanics as an instrument for analysis and prediction of physical workload. It is divided into two parts. The first part provides a description of the structure and function of the musculoskeletal system and the methodological areas that define the science of occupational biomechanics. The second part presents six contemporary applications of occupational biomechanics.

Frankel V, Nordin M 1980 Basic biomechanics of the skeletal system. Lea & Febiger, Philadelphia.

This book has been written to serve as an introduction to biomechanics for those who deal with disorders of the skeletal system. The authors, an orthopaedic surgeon and a physiotherapist, have provided a well-conceived bridge between engineering concepts and clinical practice. A major determinant of effective function is the force tolerance and mobility of the skeletal system. Increases in the intensity of activity of all age groups and extended human longevity are presenting new demands on these physical qualities. To develop an appropriate clinical response, biomechanical information must be acquired and the knowledge translated into therapeutic guidelines.

Garg A, Chaffin D B, Herrin G D 1978 Prediction of metabolic rates of manual materials-handling jobs. American Industrial Hygiene Association Journal 39: 661–674.

The authors of this paper have described a systematic way of determining the metabolic cost of manual materials-handling using a mathematical model. The basic premise used is that it is possible to dissect the lifting task into its individual components. Further, by determining the metabolic cost of these components and their duration, the total cost of the task can be computed. Thus, by dividing the job into task elements and assigning a metabolic cost to each task based on measurable factors of force, distance, frequency, posture, technique, gender, body weight and time within each task, an energy requirement to perform just that task can be determined. The authors suggest that the average metabolic cost will be the sum of the costs of the task and the maintenance of body posture over time. The authors validated their model by studying 48 tasks and reported a correlation coefficient of 0.95 between the measured and predicted physiological costs.

Morris J M, Lucas D B, Bresler M S 1961 Role of the trunk in stability of the spine. Journal of Bone and Joint Surgery 43-A(3): 327–351.

This is one of the first papers which describes a biomechanical model of lifting activity. This paper also lent support to the observations made earlier by Davis (1956) and Bartelink (1957) of the mechanical support forthcoming from the pressure of the truncal cavities during lifting activities. In their study, the authors recorded the postures photographically, and the myoelectric activity of the abdominal, thoracic and back muscles. They also measured the intra-thoracic and intra-abdominal pressures. By calculating load on the spine and the relieving effect of the intra-abdominal pressure, they suggested that the latter contributes towards 30% relief.

Schüldt K 1988 On neck muscle activity and load reduction in sitting postures. An electromyographic and biomechanical study with applications in ergonomics and rehabilitation. Scandinavian Journal of Rehabilitative Medicine Supplement 19: 9–49.

In this thesis on the biomechanics and muscular function of the cervical spine, it was shown that work postures can be optimized to diminish neck muscle load and that ergonomic aids, arm support or suspension can reduce neck muscle load. It was also demonstrated that the relationship between EMG activity of the posterior neck muscles and muscular moment during neck extension is non-linear, with a greater increase in activity at high moments. The muscular activity in the posterior neck muscles is related to the position of the lower-cervical-upper-thoracic spine during maximum isometric neck extension. The effect of different isometric test contractions on the EMG activity level of the posterior neck muscles is shown.

Schultz A B, Andersson G B J 1981 Analysis of load on the lumbar spine. Spine 6(1): 76–82.

This paper describes two mutually complementary biomechanical models for the human back. The first deals with the external forces using Newtonian mechanics. This model assumes the body to be made of an upper and lower segment separated by an imaginary transverse cutting plane at the level of interest. Using the kinematic information, the net reaction forces are calculated on the lumbar disc of choice for compression and shear. The second model deals with forces generated inside the trunk by muscular contractions, connective tissue tensions, intra-abdominal pressure, and the resistances of the spine motion segments. Using the electromyographic activity of the erector spinae muscles and the net force required by these muscles, the authors have validated their model.

C. LOCAL MUSCULAR LOAD; NECK AND UPPER EXTREMITY DISORDERS

Björkstén M, Jonsson B 1977 Endurance limit of force in long-term: intermittent static contractions. Scandinavian Journal of Work Environment and Health 3: 23–27.

The authors studied the effects of intermittent and sustained muscle contractions over long periods (60 min) and concluded that the endurance limit for intermittent contractions was 14% of the maximal force contraction, while that for sustained contractions was about 8%. This was about half the limit found by Rohmert. In addition, and in contrast to Rohmert's findings, weaker subjects appeared to have a higher endurance limit than strong subjects.

Christensen H 1986 Muscle activity and fatigue in the shoulder muscles of assembly-plant employees. Scandinavian Journal of Work Environment and Health 12: 582–587.

In responding to a questionnaire, 16% of the subjects reported pain in the neck only, 8% pain in the shoulders only and 48% pain in both areas. The muscle activity in the deltoid, infraspinatus and trapezius muscles was analysed by means of the amplitude distribution probability function. The recordings were performed on eight occasions during a full working day. Although electrical activity in muscles indicate a high degree of muscle activity, there was no decrease in mean power frequency, i.e. no sign of muscle fatigue.

Duncan J, Ferguson D 1974 Keyboard operating posture and symptoms in operating. Ergonomics 17: 651–662.

This is one of a series of papers published by this physiotherapist–doctor research team from 1971 to 1978 which reported the result of investigations into symptoms in the neck and upper extremities of process workers, telephonists and telegraphists in Australia. They were the first to detail reports of postural fatigue and pain experienced by these workers, hitherto only described in terms of clear-cut diagnosable entitites or not reported at all. In particular, this paper examines the relationship between posture and symptoms and the authors concluded that keyboard design and work height predispose to postures which in some operators gave rise to symptoms.

Hagberg M 1981 On evaluation of local muscular load and fatigue by electromyography. Arbete och Halsa: 24.
This dissertation suggests the possibility of using EMG as a determinant of estimated local muscle load and indicates that EMG amplitudes can be used to measure muscle fatigue. It also shows that EMG signs of muscle fatigue develop within a minute in the forward flexion arm position and that EMG measures on the pars descendens trapezius muscle correlate closely with the external torque in the glenohumeral joint.

Hagberg M 1981 Work-load and fatigue in repetitive arm elevations. Ergonomics 24(7): 543–555.
The aims of this experimental study were to evaluate the work-load and the shoulder muscular exertion in repetitive arm elevations. Six female subjects performed a continuous series of concentric and eccentric flexion movements in the shoulder between 0° and 90°, with 0 to 3.1 kg weights held in the hand using a power grip. The local muscular load determined by EMG on the trapezius muscle was found to be correlated closely with the external load moment about the bilateral axis of the glenohumeral joint. Symptoms and complaints 24 hours after the task were often localized to the descending part of the trapezius muscle. Thus, exertion of the descending part of the trapezius muscle may promote discomfort and complaints referred to the neck.

Harms-Ringdahl K 1986 On the assessment of shoulder exercise and load-elicited pain in the cervical spine. Biomechanical analysis of load—EMG—methodological studies of pain provoked by extreme position. Scandinavian Journal of Rehabilitation Medicine, Supplement No 14(18): 1–40.
This thesis by a physiotherapist for a doctoral degree examines how connective tissue structures counteract induced load moment and cause load-elicited pain. The time course for such pain varies with load, joint and load direction. The validity and reliability of pain induced by load in extreme position is high when assessed either on a visual analogue scale or on the Borg scale for perceived pain. In spite of good sitting ergonomics using a tilted work desk, extreme flexed neck positions were found when the thoracolumbar spine was slightly inclined backwards in combination with a flexed cervical spine. Thus, not only muscle activity but also thorough recordings of work postures should be included in ergonomic analyses to provide a basis for the avoidance of extreme joint positions.

Harms-Ringdahl K, Arborelius U P 1987 One year follow-up after introduction of arm suspension at an electronics plant. In: Proceedings of the Xth International Congress of the World Confederation for Physical Therapy, Sydney, pp 69–73.
To reduce the symptoms from extensive muscular load, approximately 60 work stations at an electronics plant were equipped with a device for arm suspension. The periods before and after the balancer was introduced were followed with assessments of perceived discomfort/pain in different body regions, using a visual analogue scale. Twice-daily assessments were made on eight occasions during the first year and three occasions the following year. In the follow-up period, 93% still used the suspension device during work. Fewer workers experienced pain from the neck and/or shoulder at the end of the work day. For those who still perceived pain, there was a decrease in intensity levels. It is suggested that if the work organization cannot be changed and long periods of assembly work avoided, arm suspension might be one way to decrease extensive neck/shoulder load.

Harms-Ringdahl K, Ekholm J 1986 Intensity and character of pain and muscular activity levels elicited by maintained extreme flexion position of the lower-cervical-upper-thoracic spine. Scandinavian Journal of Rehabilibation Medicine 18: 117–126.

The maintenance of an extreme flexion position of the neck in a sitting posture induces pain, and possibly plays a role in work-related disorders with cervicobrachial pain. In the reported study, 10 healthy subjects assessed the intensity of experimentally-induced pain on a Visual Analogue Scale. The quality and location of the pain were indicated on a drawing of the body. The pain was experienced within 15 minutes, increased with time, disappeared within 15 minutes after the provocation, but was again experienced by nine subjects the same evening or next morning and lasted up to 4 days. The activity level in some neck-and-shoulder muscles, as recorded with EMG, was low and cannot explain the perceived pain.

Herberts P, Kadefors R 1980 Arm positioning in manual tasks. An electromyographic study of localized muscle fatigue. Ergonomics 23(7): 655–665.

The concept of localized muscle fatigue is discussed within this text as being of basic ergonomic interest. The electromyographic method to quantify muscle fatigue through the myoelectric activity is used. Particular changes are shown in different arm positions. The results indicate the possibility of finding positions which reduce the total muscular load in different working positions. The study is valuable in considering the influence of various working positions on the muscles.

Jonsson B 1978 Kinesiology with special reference to electromyographic kinesiology. In: Cobb W, van Duijin H (eds) Contemporary clinical neurophysiology (suppl 34) Elsevier, Amsterdam, pp 417–428

The use of EMG as an objective measure for muscle fatigue is presented. Signs of fatigue are related to the percentage of maximum muscular force exerted and to the period for which the muscular activity is sustained. It is suggested that maintained (static) muscular force of more than 2–5% MVC during the work day is excessive. Mean muscular force should be below 10–14% MVC for avoidance of fatigue.

Kilbom Å 1988 Intervention programmes for work-related neck and upper limb disorders—strategies and evaluation. Proceedings of 10th International Ergonomics Association Congress, Sydney, pp 33–47.

Within this paper, the design and results of controlled interventions against work-related neck and upper limb disorders are discussed. The role of researchers, as active interventionists or as passive recorders of effects, is discussed and the importance of an active contribution from management and employers is stressed.

Kilbom Å, Persson I, Jonsson B G 1986 Disorders of the cervicobrachial region among female workers in the electronics industry. International Journal of Industrial Ergonomics 1:37–47.

In this study, female employees in the electronics industry were investigated. It was found that subjects' symptoms in the neck and shoulder are related to such factors as time spent in neck flexion, shoulder elevation or upper arm abduction, or total duration of arm activity. Large inter-individual differences in working technique were found. Static muscle strength of five shoulder and arm muscle groups, as well as static endurance, were not related to symptoms, nor were medical and work history, productivity, leisure, physical activity or hobbies.

Kilbom Å, Persson J 1987 Work technique and its consequences for musculoskeletal disorders. In: Musculoskeletal injuries in the workplace. Ergonomics 30(2).
This is a report of a prospective study conducted to identify factors that could contribute to the high prevalence of cervicobrachial disorders in the manufacturing industry. Women from one Ericsson factory were studied. 'At the one and the 2-year follow-up it is obvious that some of the work technique variables are important. Other risk factors include perceived stress, previous sick-leave, individual productivity, and previous work in physically heavy jobs.'

Kukkonen R, Luopajärvl T, Riihimäki V 1983 Prevention of fatigue among data entry operators. In: Kvålseth T O (ed) Ergonomics of work station design. Butterworths, London, pp 28–34.
This is one of the few intervention studies for neck and upper extremity disorders which has been reported in the literature. It is important because of the approach taken and the results. The intervention, planned and conducted by physiotherapists, consisted of an ergonomics survey of the workplace, and the implementation of changes arising out of this. In addition, employees were given a short course in the pertinent aspect of ergonomics, health education and the minimization of fatigue through breaks and exercises, and encouraged to modify their workplace where necessary. The study was different from other attempts at prcvention because it was accompanied by training on the optimum use of ergonomically- designed equipment and information on why it was important. The separate effects of ergonomics and health education, mini-breaks and exercises are likely to be considerably enhanced if combined, because the effectiveness of each depends to a large extent on the other.

Kvarnström S 1983 Occurrence of musculoskeletal disorders in manufacturing industry, with special attention to occupational shoulder disorders. Scandinavian Journal of Rehabilitation Medicine Supplement 8: 1–114.
This is a series of papers published in one supplement of this Scandinavian Journal. It examines the reporting of musculoskeletal disorders among blue collar workers in light, medium and heavy engineering jobs, and associated work, personal and social factors. Its importance lies in the range of aspects studied and the findings which support the theory that physical, psychological and social factors in combination lead to an increased reporting of musculoskeletal disorders in the workplace.

Luopajärvi T, Kuorinka I, Virolainen M, Holmberg M 1979 Prevalence of tenosynovitis and other injuries of the upper extremities in repetitive work. Scandinavian Journal of Work Environment and Health 5 (suppl 3): 48–55.
A Finnish team of researchers in the late 1970s investigated different clinical and epidemiological aspects of neck and upper extremity disorders, and a series of papers from this work were compiled into one supplement of an international journal. The devoting of one supplement of this highly regarded journal to these disorders focused attention on them, for the first time, as a legitimate and important area of study in occupational health. This paper reviewed the prevalence of disorders in a high-risk (assembly-line packers) and a low-risk (shop assistants) group. The packers were found to have a significantly higher prevalence of the disorders which were considered to be related to different aspects of their work.

Maeda K 1977 Occupational cervicobrachial disorder and its causative factors. Journal of Human Ergology 6:193–202.
Occupational cervicobrachial disorders have been noticed among workers in offices and factories since about 1955. The prevalence and the causative factors

of the disease are described in this text. There are two main factors: the ways in which the workers use their musculature and strain the nervous system; and the way in which the job is organized within the work system and how it is controlled. In the discussion, Maeda points out that an important feature in assessing the relevant work-load is that it includes both localized muscle loading and mental strain.

Maeda K, Horoguchi S, Hosokawa M 1982 History of the studies on occupational cervicobrachial disorder in Japan and remaining problems. Journal of Human Ergology 11: 17–29.

Japanese researchers, more than any other group, pioneered the study of work-related disorders of the neck and upper extremities in the 1960s, 1970s and the early 1980s. Unlike western countries at this time they did not concentrate on already recognizable and easily diagnosable disorders such as tenosynovitis and carpal tunnel syndrome, but they attempted to describe and classify a wide range of symptoms and disorders which clearly had psychological and social components as well as primary physical work-related causes. This paper summarizes the development of research in this area in Japan.

Rodgers S H (ed) 1987 Repetitive motion injuries: seminars in occupational medicine. Thieme, New York, vol 2, No 1

This journal features a well-rounded view of cause, types, evaluation and treatment of repetitive strain disorders. Several authors use ergonomic intervention as an important aspect of prevention. Other authors delineate evaluation and treatment of workers at risk of suffering this trauma. Authors from many specialties participate in the journal. Represented are the fields of ergonomics, medicine, physiology, physical therapy, occupational therapy and industry. The overall journal provides a holistic look at repetitive trauma with emphasis on the upper extremity.

Rohmert W 1973a Problems in determining rest allowances I. Applied Ergonomics 4: 91–95
and
Rohmert W 1973b Problems in determining rest allowances II. Applied Ergonomics 4:158–162.

On the assumption that fatigue is a precursor to many symptoms in the neck and upper extremities, the taking of work breaks and task variation is central to the prevention of these disorders. However, the estimation of the frequency and length of work breaks depends largely on the load on specific muscles and their capacity for work. In this set of two papers, a highly regarded work physiologist and ergonomist discusses how these may be estimated and the inherent problems in doing so.

Some researchers believe, however, that Rohmert's estimations are too high.

Sigholm G, Herberts P, Almström C, Kadefors R 1984 Electromyographic analyses of shoulder muscle load. Journal of Orthopaedic Research 1: 379–386.

In the study reported in this article, the myoelectric activity in shoulder muscles was recorded and analysed with respect to amplitude. The degree of upper-arm elevation was shown to be the most important parameter influencing shoulder muscle load. Short rotator muscles stabilizing the shoulder joint were found to be more hand-load dependent than was the deltoid muscle. The ergonomic implications of this study are that the work situation should be designed so that the arm can be kept close to the body, thus minimizing the hand load.

Silverstein B A, Fine L J, Armstrong T J 1987 Occupational factors and carpal tunnel syndrome. American Journal of Industrial Medicine 11: 343–358.
A good deal of research into neck and upper extremity disorders, particularly carpal tunnel syndrome, in industry in the USA has been carried out by researchers based at the University of Ann Arbor in Michigan. The work of various researchers from the group has been marked by the use of rigorous research methods, particularly epidemiological and ergonomic, and highly selective outcome measures of disorders. This paper is typical of many produced by the group and discusses work-related factors, particularly force and repetition and the occurrence of carpal tunnel syndrome in a range of industrial workers.

Valencia F 1986 Local muscle fatigue. Medical Journal of Australia 115: 327–330.
The difficulties of studying small and local muscle fatigue have hampered efforts to fully understand possible mechanisms which might provoke it. It is widely believed, however, that such fatigue is the precursor of many disorders of the neck, shoulders or arms and may be induced by repetitive work in fixed postures. Nonetheless, there is still considerable scepticism, particularly among the medical profession in Australia, about the causes of these disorders. This paper, written by a physiotherapist and published in a well-respected medical journal, attempts to explain the possible mechanisms of fatigue, together with their plausible clinical and workplace implicatons.

D. LOW-BACK, SPINAL FUNCTION

Ayoub M M, Dryden R, McDanial J, Knipfer R, Dixon D 1979 Predicting lifting capacity. American Industrial Hygiene Association Journal 40: 1075–1084.
The primary purpose of this paper was to determine quantitatively the appropriate operator variables to use in the prediction of the psychophysically-determined maximum acceptable work-load for lifting loads from (a) floor to knuckle height, (b) knuckle height to shoulder height, and (c) shoulder height to overhead reach height. The authors instructed their subjects to adjust the weight in a tote box to the maximum weight they could lift repetitively without excessive strain or fatigue. The subjects performed load lifting under different conditions, namely height of lift, frequency of lift, load size. Using the data obtained. the authors developed a statistical predictive model based on the operator characteristics and the task variables.

Borg G 1962 Physical performance and perceived exertion. Glerup Lund, Sweden.
It is generally accepted that individual levels of low-back pain (LBP) are impossible to judge objectively. In order to be able to measure possible changes in experienced pain in patients, an appropriate scale is required. Borg's approach is widely acclaimed as a category ratio scale for perceived exertion (C-R-10). The scale is well tested and documented and makes it possible to measure individual changes in LBP patients.

Brown J R 1972 Manual lifting and related fields. An annotated bibliography, Labour Safety Council of Ontario, Ontario Ministry of Labour, 583 pages.
At the time of its publication, this work must have been a very rich source of bibliographical material on the subject. Though out of date, it is still a good source of early works in the 1930s, 40s, 50s and 60s. References up to 1972 are included. This book categorized references in chapters on aetiology, statistical incidence, injury, spinal mobility and weight-bearing, posture, physiological problems, lifting techniques, radiography and

psychogenic low-back pain. Above all, this work, in an interesting and readable form, has synthesized a composite picture of medical, surgical, physiological and psychological aspects of the problem of back injury and low-back pain. This is a ready reference of several hundreds of papers published on the subject up to 1972. Its 28-page long preface is a particularly interesting chapter. It is here that a difference in the physiological cost of lifting with different techniques was stated.

Davis P R 1985 Industrial back pain in Europe. Special Issue Ergonomics 28(1).
 This special issue is a rich source of information on manual materials handling and low-back pain. The 405-page issue contains 44 scientific articles on different aspects of lifting and related subjects, and 671 references. The broad areas of epidemiology, spinal diseases from physical work, biology and materials handling, effects of age and sex differences, environmental considerations, methods of measurement, permissible loads and limiting factors, and training and prevention, are covered by a variable number of papers in each section.

Drury C G 1978 Safety in manual material handling. Report on International Symposium: Manual Materials Handling, State University of New York, Buffalo, July, 1976 DHEW (NIOSH). Publication Number 78–185, Department of Health and Human Services, US Government Printing Office, Washington 20402.
 This 209-page book is a report on an international symposium, including all the papers of the individual participants and authors, preceded by an introduction and followed by a chapter summary. The book has six chapters: (1) safety problems, (2) measurements and standards, (3) models of human performance, (4) factors affecting performance, (5) implementing research, and finally (6) manual material handling in the future. In each of these chapters, several authors have presented their specific work focused on a project in a given area of interest. These have then been pooled for general conclusion and summarized in the summary of the chapter. The purpose of this exercise was to determine the course of direction for manual materials-handling research, after consolidating the current state of knowledge. Each paper has its own reference list which may prove to be useful to the reader.

Eklund J 1986 Industrial seating and spinal loading. Thesis, University of Nottingham, England. ISBN 91–7870–144–9.
 A model for evaluating industrial seats is proposed, listing demands and restrictions created by the task and the workplace. A shrinkage method is developed for in-vivo assessments of spinal load using body height changes as a measure of disc creep. Discomfort ratings, body mapping, interviews, video recordings and prototype equipment suitable for the recording of head postures are also used. The work task is shown to have a major influence on the adopted work posture and must be thoroughly considered.

Kirkaldy-Willis W H 1988 Managing low-back pain. Churchill Livingstone, Edinburgh.
 This large book, which is subdivided into three major sections—'Essential principles', 'The clinical Picture' and 'Treatment', would be a very useful resource for those concerned with either prevention or management of low-back pain.

Kumar S 1984 The physiological cost of three different methods of lifting in sagittal and lateral planes. Ergonomics 27: 425–433.
 The author investigated the physiological cost of lifting and lowering activities between floor and 91 cm. A weight of 10 kg was lifted and lowered

at three-quarters reach in sagittal, 30° lateral, and 60° lateral planes using stoop, squat and free-style techniques. Comparisons of steady-state values of oxygen uptake during these activities were made. The subjects also made a subjective assessment of the relative degree of tiresomeness of these activities. The physiological costs of the three techniques were significantly different from each other, squat being the most and free-style being the least. However, the asymmetry of the tasks did not increase the metabolic cost significantly. Whereas the subjective assessment adequately reflected the physiological cost differential, the asymmetry, though identical in physiological cost requirement, caused significantly different subjective assessment ratings.

Mayer T, Gatchel R, Kishino N, Keeley J, Capra P, Mayer H, Barnett J, Mooney V 1985 Objective assessment of spine function following industrial injury. A prospective study with comparison group and one-year follow-up. Spine 10: 482–493.

This is the lead article of several related articles in the same study. It won the Volvo Award in Clinical Sciences for 1985. It chronicles a comprehensive, multidisciplinary programme designed for chronic non-working back patients. The treatment group underwent thorough evaluation by therapists, psychologists, vocational specialists and physicians. The intense physical conditioning, work hardening and counselling programme that followed is described. One-year follow-up comparisons are made with a similar group that did not participate in the programme. Results indicate that not only did the treatment group make considerable gains in strength and endurance, but they also had a high success rate in returning to gainful employment.

NIOSH (National Institute for Occupational Safety and Health) 1981 Work practices guide for manual lifting. NIOSH Technical report, publication number 81–122. US Department of Health and Human Services.

Work practices guide is an extensive work on manual materials handling. Its primary purpose was to design criteria by which guidelines could be established for sagittal plane, ground to knuckle height lifts. This 183-page book has not only achieved this, but in the process it has also addressed most of the germaine issues of lifting and manual materials handling considerably. This book is divided into eight chapters dealing with (1) the rationale of the exercise, (2) epidemiological basis for the guide, (3) biomechanical basis for the guide, (4) physiological basis for the guide, (5) psychophysical basis for the guide, (6) administrative controls, (7) engineering controls, and finally (8) recommendations. Each of these chapters is written in reasonable detail and provides a good source of references for papers published before that time. The guide has also included recommendations on the selection and training of workers who are required to perform manual materials handling.

Troup J D G, Edwards F C 1985 Manual handling and lifting. An information and literature review with special reference to the back. Her Majesty's Stationery Office, High Holborn, London.

The authors have synthesized an informative and comprehensive picture of the entire area of manual materials handling, in point form, consisting of sections on (1) statistical and epidemiological aspects, (2) biological aspects, (3) individual variation, assessment and screening, and (4) additional approaches to prevention. At the end of each section, the authors have added an interpretive commentary on the content area of the section. This 70-page book is information packed. It has tried to highlight European workers and has been less inclusive of work conducted outside Europe, though such works are contained in it. It is a useful source book for concise reading, and it also contains a good bibliography which can be followed for further reading.

Twomey L, Taylor J R (eds) 1987 Physical therapy of the low back. Churchill Livingstone, Edinburgh.

This book is principally directed at the clinical management of low-back pain and offers descriptions of various treatment techniques. Nevertheless, its coverage of basic areas such as anatomy, biomechanics and mechanisms of pain production makes it a useful resource also for those concerned with providing education in preventive back care.

E. ASSESSMENT, EVALUATION AND WORK INJURY MANAGEMENT

Coates H, King A 1982 The patient assessment. Churchill Livingstone, Edinburgh.

This book is written by two physiotherapy lecturers, primarily as a simple handbook for both physiotherapy and occupational therapy students and qualified practitioners. The book comprises six chapters covering: the gathering of information; the physical examination of the patient; the recording and evaluation of physical findings; the examination of some body systems; special tests and an assessment for a wheelchair. A list of daily living activities which may be used to form the basis of an assessment chart is included in the appendices in conjunction with anatomical outlines of the body, face and lower limbs and a sequence of diagrams representing patterns of normal developmental growth.

Cornes P 1984 The future of work for people with disabilities: a view from Great Britain. World Rehabilitation Fund, New York.

This monograph is one of a series of publications produced by the World Rehabilitation Fund through a grant from the National Institute of Handicapped Research, US Department of Education. The monograph traces historical changes that have occurred in technological production over the years and offers various perspectives on the meaning of work in industrial society. The origins of British vocational rehabilitation policy are examined, together with the scope and effectiveness of existing policy and services. Finally, contrasting scenarios on the future of work for disabled people in Great Britain are discussed.

Cornes P, Hunter J 1985 Work, disability and rehabilitation. UCIR, Michigan.

This book comprises a number of papers on vocational rehabilitation and employment of disabled people presented at the First European Conference on Research in Rehabilitation, Edinburgh, 6–8 April, 1983. The papers are grouped under four main sections (the first three being prefaced by an editorial commentary). Part I is entitled 'Work and disability' and includes papers concerned with the incidence of disability in a large public sector workforce, work accidents and absences, and work design for disabled people. Part II is called 'Vocational habilitation and rehabilitation' and includes review papers, studies which have evaluated the outcome of employment rehabilitation practices, and appropriateness of training and job experience opportunities. Part III, 'Some clinical perspectives', presents papers addressing the causes. consequences and rehabilitation of hand injuries, working capacity following myocardial infarction, and the effect of back pain on employment. Part IV, 'Work, disability and rehabilitation in perspective', provides an editorial overview of the subject.

Isernhagen S (ed) 1988 Work injury management and prevention. Aspen, Rockville, USA.
The spectrum of professional intervention in physical work injury is covered by this multidisciplinary text. Both the introductory and final chapters discuss the scope and direction of this field. The first group of chapters describe prevention of injury through education, exercise. governmental guidelines and ergonomics. A majority of the text describes programmes specifically designed to minimize the effects of work injury and maximize rehabilitation. These include early intervention, physical therapy measures, occupational medicine guidelines, functional capacity evaluation and work hardening. Chronic spinal dysfunction and pain management programmes are also described. A specialized chapter is devoted to the roles and viewpoints of professionals involved in the work injury management system. These include therapists, physicians, employers, attorneys, rehabilitation consultants and the employee/patient. Points of view stressed by the authors include the team approach, empowerment of the employee-patient, and immediate and thorough evaluation and treatment after injury.

Luopajärvi T 1987 Workers education, Ergonomics 30(2): 305–311.
The article is on health education among workers in order to prevent musculoskeletal injuries. Follow-ups have shown that health education has no lasting effect if given as lectures in a traditional way. The author, a physiotherapist, advocates new educational programmes based on the concept of 'learning by doing'.

Matheson L 1987 Work capacity evaluation. Employment Rehabilition Institute of California, Anaheim.
Utilizing a vocational, psychophysical and psychological approach, the author describes the process of evaluating and rehabilitating stabilized or chronic injured workers. Described in detail are methods of determining work capacity, reliability of effort and physical-vocational matches. The treatment programme used at ERIC is a model of how the system works. A specialized section creates and defines a new method of categorizing patients who do not put forth full effort in their programme. This syndrome of symptom magnification is divided into several categories and each is explained by definition and example. Other areas of interest covered are psychophysical testing apparatus, correlative charts to the US Dictionary of Occupational Titles and specific case studies.

National Occupational Health and Safety Commission 1987 The prevention and management of occupational overuse syndrome. Australian Government Publishing Service, Canberra.
This book is intended to be of assistance in the prevention and management of occupational overuse syndrome. The only acceptable policy must be directed towards prevention, which means addressing the occupational causes of occupational overuse syndrome at their source, by modifying the working environment to remove those causes or reduce their influence by excluding them at the design stage. Prevention and control strategies, developed by management in consultation, should be circulated in writing, acknowledging the responsibilities of all parties in implementation. These strategies should be part of an overall occupational health and safety policy. The effective implementation of a preventive strategy will generally require the allocation of appropriate personnel and financial resources.

Parry A 1980 Physiotherapy assessment. Croom Helm, London.
  It is claimed that this is the first book in Great Britian to have been written
for physiotherapists about the clinical skill of patient assessment. The first
chapter considers the principles of history taking, of objective examination and
of interpretation and presentation of findings. Subsequent chapters
discuss particular assessments in relation to the respiratory, nervous and
musculoskeletal systems. Finally, the last chapter offers a series of summaries
for types of assessment which result in statements concerning the aims and
methods of treatment.

Index